1985
YEAR BOOK OF
HAND SURGERY

.

THE 1985 YEAR BOOKS

The YEAR BOOK series provides in condensed form the essence of the best of the recent international literature in medicine and the allied health professions. The material is selected by distinguished editors who critically review more than 500,000 journal articles each year.

Anesthesia: Drs. Miller, Kirby, Ostheimer, Saidman, and Stoelting

Cancer: Drs. Hickey, Clark, and Cumley

Cardiology: Drs. Harvey, Kirkendall, Kirklin, Nadas, Resnekov, and Sonnenblick

Critical Care Medicine: Drs. Rogers, Booth, Dean, Gioia, McPherson, Michael, and Traystman

Dentistry: Drs. Cohen, Hendler, Johnson, Jordan, Moyers, Robinson, and Silverman

Dermatology: Drs. Sober and Fitzpatrick

Diagnostic Radiology: Drs. Bragg, Keats, Kieffer, Kirkpatrick, Koehler, Sorenson, and White

Digestive Diseases: Drs. Greenberger and Moody

Drug Therapy: Drs. Hollister and Lasagna

Emergency Medicine: Dr. Wagner

Endocrinology: Drs. Schwartz and Ryan

Family Practice: Dr. Rakel

Hand Surgery: Drs. Dobyns and Chase

Infectious Diseases: Drs. Wolff, Gorbach, Keusch, Klempner, and Snydman

Medicine: Drs. Rogers, Des Prez, Cline, Braunwald, Greenberger, Bondy, Epstein, and Malawista

Neurology and Neurosurgery: Drs. De Jong, Sugar, and Currier

Nuclear Medicine: Drs. Hoffer, Gore, Gottschalk, Sostman, and Zaret

Obstetrics and Gynecology: Drs. Pitkin and Zlatnik

Ophthalmology: Dr. Ernest

Orthopedics: Dr. Coventry

Otolaryngology: Drs. Paparella and Bailey

Pathology and Clinical Pathology: Dr. Brinkhous

Pediatrics: Drs. Oski and Stockman

Plastic and Reconstructive Surgery: Drs. McCoy, Brauer, Haynes, Hoehn, Miller, and Whitaker

Podiatric Medicine and Surgery: Dr. Jay

Psychiatry and Applied Mental Health: Drs. Freedman, Lourie, Meltzer, Nemiah, Talbott, and Weiner

Sports Medicine: Drs. Krakauer, Shephard, and Torg, Col. Anderson, and Mr. George

Surgery: Drs. Schwartz, Najarian, Peacock, Shires, Spencer, and Thompson

Urology: Drs. Gillenwater and Howards

1985

The Year Book of
HAND SURGERY

Editor
James H. Dobyns, M.D.
*Professor of Orthopedic Surgery, Mayo Medical School, Mayo Foundation;
Consultant in Orthopedic Surgery and Surgery of the Hand, Mayo Clinic*

Associate Editor
Robert A. Chase, M.D.
*Emile Holman Professor of Surgery and Professor of Anatomy,
Stanford University*

Year Book Medical Publishers, Inc.
Chicago

The editor for this book was Roberta A. Mendelson and the production manager was H. E. Nielsen. The Managing Editor for the Year Book series is Caroline Scoulas.

Table of Contents

The material covered in this volume represents literature reviewed up to March 1983.

Journals Represented

Acta Chirurgica Scandinavica
Acta Orthopaedica Scandinavica
Acta Radiologica (Diagnosis)
American Journal of Diseases of Children
American Journal of Neuroradiology
American Journal of Roentgenology
American Journal of Surgery
American Surgeon
Annals of Emergency Medicine
Annals of Plastic Surgery
Archives of Environmental Health
Archives of Internal Medicine
Archives of Neurology
Archives of Pathology and Laboratory Medicine
Archives of Physical Medicine and Rehabilitation
Archives of Surgery
Arthritis and Rheumatism
Brain
British Journal of Plastic Surgery
British Journal of Radiology
British Medical Journal
Cancer
Chirurg
Clinical and Experimental Dermatology
Diagnostic Imaging
International Journal of Dermatology
International Journal of Leprosy
International Orthopaedics
International Surgery
Israel Journal of Medical Sciences
Journal of Adolescent Health Care
Journal of the American Academy of Dermatology
Journal of the American Medical Association
Journal of Applied Physiology: Respiratory, Environmental and Exercise
    Physiology
Journal of Bone and Joint Surgery (American volume)
Journal of Bone and Joint Surgery (British volume)
Journal of the Canadian Association of Radiologists
Journal of Cardiovascular Surgery
Journal de Chirurgie
Journal of Dermatologic Surgery and Oncology
Journal of Hand Surgery
Journal of Investigative Dermatology
Journal of the Japanese Orthopaedic Association
Journal of the Neurological Sciences
Journal of Neurology, Neurosurgery and Psychiatry

Journal of Occupational Medicine
Journal of the Royal College of Surgeons of Edinburgh
Journal of Trauma
Journal of the Western Pacific Orthopedic Association
Lyon Chirurgical
Nervenarzt
Neurology
Neurosurgery
New England Journal of Medicine
New York State Journal of Medicine
Orthopedics
Pain
Physical Therapy
Plastic and Reconstructive Surgery
Proceedings of the National Academy of Sciences
Radiology
Revue de Chirurgie Orthopedique et Reparatrice de l'Appareil Moteur
Scandinavian Journal of Plastic and Reconstructive Surgery
Scandinavian Journal of Rheumatology
Semaine des Hopitaux de Paris
Skeletal Radiology
South African Medical Journal
Southern Medical Journal
Transplantation
Wiener Klinische Wochenschrift

Publisher's Preface

Publication of the 1985 YEAR BOOKS marks the eighty-fifth anniversary of the original PRACTICAL MEDICINE YEAR BOOKS. To mark this milestone, the YEAR BOOKS are being issued with a more contemporary cover design, and the format for the contents has been modified to identify the article title, authors' names, and journal citations more readily. The substance of the YEAR BOOK—the abstracts of scholarly articles with substantive editorial comments—is unchanged. What is new is the isolation of the reference information as a discrete block of copy. Other, less-visible changes will continue to be made as we strive to make the YEAR BOOKS the very best they can be.

We are proud to offer this first edition of the YEAR BOOK OF HAND SURGERY as a new service for those surgeons who specialize in treating diseases of and injuries to the hand.

Acknowledgments

The development of a new YEAR BOOK in a medical specialty required an open ear, an open mind, critical expertise, and a strong commitment from Year Book Medical Publishers, Inc., of Chicago, Illinois. The first open ear was a friend from prior publishing efforts, Mr. Edward Wickland, now transferred to still other publishing arenas. However, steady support has been received from the entire organization throughout, with close guidance and warm support particularly from Mr. John Matusik and Mrs. Caroline Scoulas. Work began on a handshake, with contractural elements added later as they became available. Amiable relationships initiated the project, have persisted to date, and are now the anticipated norm.

The value of YEAR BOOKS for those of us who have been YEAR BOOK fans has been due more to the informed and trenchant comments of the reviewers than to any other single feature. Without a group of such dedicated reviewers, the excitement of learning information of immediate utility will not develop. It has been our privilege to utilize the following physicians' services in this first volume. The list may be expanded in future volumes, but all of these have proved their worth and are accorded heartfelt thanks for their contributions.

James H. Dobyns, M.D.

———

Peter C. Amadio, M.D., *Assistant Professor of Orthopedic Surgery,* Senior Associate Consultant in Orthopedic Surgery and Surgery of the Hand†

Robert D. Beckenbaugh, M.D., *Associate Professor of Orthopedic Surgery,* Consultant in Orthopedic Surgery and Surgery of the Hand†

Robert H. Cofield, M.D., *Associate Professor of Orthopedic Surgery,* Consultant in Orthopedic Surgery and Adult Reconstruction†

William P. Cooney, M.D., *Associate Professor of Orthopedic Surgery,* Consultant in Orthopedic Surgery and Surgery of the Hand†

Jasper R. Daube, M.D., *Professor of Neurology,* Director of Clinical Electromyographic Laboratory†

George B. Irons, Jr., M.D., *Associate Professor of Plastic Surgery,* Consultant in Plastic Surgery and Surgery of the Hand†

Ronald L. Linscheid, M.D., *Professor of Orthopedic Surgery,* Consultant in Orthopedic Surgery and Surgery of the Hand†

Bernard F. Morrey, M.D., *Associate Professor of Orthopedic Surgery,* Consultant in Orthopedic Surgery†

Burton M. Onofrio, M.D., *Professor of Neurosurgery,* Consultant in Neurosurgery†

Ann H. Schutt, M.D., *Associate Professor of Physical Medicine and Rehabilitation,* Consultant in Physical Medicine and Rehabilitation†

Franklin H. Sim, M.D., *Professor of Orthopedic Surgery,* Consultant

*Mayo Med. School.
†Mayo Clinic.

13

in Orthopedic Surgery, Adult Reconstruction, Orthopedic Oncology and Sports Medicine†

Nicki R. Viggiano, M.D., *Instructor in Anesthesiology,* * *Consultant in Anesthesiology*†

Peter R. Wilson, M.B.B.S., Ph.D., *Associate Professor of Anesthesiology,* * *Consultant in Anesthesiology*†

Michael B. Wood, M.D., *Associate Professor of Orthopedic Surgery,* * *Consultant in Orthopedic Surgery and Surgery of the Hand*†

*Mayo Med. School.
†Mayo Clinic.

Introduction

This first year of a new enterprise, the "YEAR BOOK OF HAND SURGERY," is probably overdue. The development of a discipline whose adherents come from three surgical specialties and with no separate Board or Certificate to signal their competence is difficult to trace. While many of the pioneers of hand surgery are still alive and the half dozen or so who first restricted their practice to hand surgery are still active, it is easy to overlook the fact that hand surgery has become a major subspecialty involving the interest and practice of many physicians. Yet the signs are there. As longtime laborer for the YEAR BOOK OF ORTHOPEDIC SURGERY, it became more and more noticeable to me that an increasing number of articles were devoted to the upper limb. Although the professional activities included in hand surgery are still the part-time interests of many surgeons, they are the full-time interest of an increasing number, and practices restricted to hand surgery are becoming the rule rather than the exception. Two major national societies now represent this specific interest—each one of them nearing the 1,000 mark in membership. More and more national and international meetings are devoted to the special interest of this group and more and more countries have developed their own national hand surgery societies, a number now in excess of 30. Another signal is that followers of this discipline have arrived at positions of leadership in research, in education, and in medical administration. There are now so many involved in the practice of hand surgery that the usual division into subareas of special interest is beginning. Only the fact that articles relevant to these interests were split up among many different specialties and their vast array of publications held back development of hand surgery's own special literature. However, the *Journal of Hand Surgery* has made a very successful appearance in the past decade, along with many textbooks. Even the *Journal of Reconstructive Microsurgery* has preceded the YEAR BOOK OF HAND SURGERY. It is, therefore, with some apology at being so dilatory that this first YEAR BOOK OF HAND SURGERY is offered. It is new, it is immature, and it, too, will grow and change. We would like it to grow into what its readers desire. Comments, suggestions, and criticisms are therefore most welcome and will be taken into account.

James H. Dobyns, M.D.

1 Skeletal Trauma and Reconstruction

Mallet Thumb
K. M. Din and B. F. Meggitt (Cambridge, England)
J. Bone Joint Surg. [Br.] 65-B:606–607, November 1983   1–1

Four patients with mallet thumb were encountered in a 4-year period. Forty-eight cases of mallet finger were treated during the 4 years.

Man, 33, a right-handed computer programmer, was seen with a left mallet thumb 4 days after having been kicked on the tip of the digit while playing rugby. Swelling and tenderness were present in the distal part of the dorsum of the thumb and there was a 40-degree flexion deformity at the interphalangeal joint. There was a full range of passive extension. Radiographs showed no bone injury. Exploration showed complete avulsion of the extensor pollicis longus tendon from its insertion with a gap of 1 cm between the end of the tendon and site of insertion. The tendon was reattached to the base of the distal phalanx by passing 00 silk mattress sutures through holes drilled in the bone. The thumb was splinted in extension for 3 weeks in a forearm plaster cast. Flexion-extension motion of 0 to 45 degrees was present at the interphalangeal joint 8 weeks postoperatively. The patient was able to resume his normal activities.

The term "mallet" finger is appropriate for a flexion deformity at the interphalangeal joint of the thumb or distal interphalangeal joint of a finger when there is loss of continuity of the extensor mechanism at or close to its insertion. The term "dropped" is used for loss of continuity of the extensor mechanism proximal to the metacarpophalangeal joint of the thumb or finger. Injury distal to the metacarpophalangeal joint, tenderness at or close to the insertion of the extensor pollicis longus tendon, and injury to the base of the distal phalanx favor a diagnosis of mallet thumb. Operative treatment is recommended because successful conservative treatment has not been reported, and the tendon is thick enough to hold sutures well.

▶ The authors have pointed out the necessity for making an accurate diagnosis when failure of extension of the distal phalanx of the thumb is noted. One must differentiate among a distal extensor mechanism rupture, a proximal disruption, and a paralysis. Although the authors advocate operative treatment of this injury, they point out that conservative treatment has not been reported, and I believe this should be tried, as I would anticipate that secondary reconstruction is quite possible.—R.D.B.

Sesamoid Fracture of the Thumb

Peter Clarke, Ethan M. Braunstein, Barbara N. Weissman, and J. Leland Sosman (Harvard Med. School)
Br. J. Radiol. 56:485, July 1983   1–2

Only three previous reports of fracture of a first metacarpophalangeal sesamoid bone have appeared in the English literature. The fracture fragment must not be confused with bipartite sesamoids or two normal sesamoids of the thumb. A case of fracture of the thumb sesamoid is reported.

Man, 42, fell on his outstretched hand while playing basketball and presented with tenderness over the first metacarpal and first metacarpophalangeal joint. The ulnar collateral ligament complex did not seem to be disrupted. Radiography showed a fracture of the thumb sesamoid (Fig 1–1). Splint immobilization led to prompt relief of pain. The patient was doing well when the splint was removed 3 weeks later.

The sesamoid bone can behave as an extension of the articular surface and can be avulsed by trauma. The diagnosis of fracture is more difficult when the sesamoid is incompletely ossified. The thumb sesamoid that is embedded in the adductor pollicis tendon can be avulsed when the thumb is forcefully abducted from a position of flexion and opposition, as in skiers. Sesamoid fracture must be distinguished from ulnar collateral ligament disruption, or "gamekeeper's thumb." The absence of joint instability virtually rules out a ligamentous tear.

▶ The mechanism of injury in these cases is apparently similar to that which also causes ulnar collateral ligament disruption. Mere presence of a sesamoid

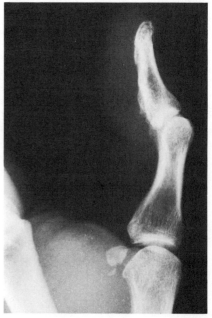

Fig 1–1.—Fracture of sesamoid bone near first metacarpophalangeal joint. Notice the cortical discontinuity establishing the diagnosis of fracture. (Courtesy of Clarke, P., et al.: Br. J. Radiol. 56:485, July 1983.)

fracture does not rule out associated ulnar collateral ligament injury, and stress testing under suitable anesthesia and arthrography may be necessary in order to rule out the more serious joint injury.—P.C.A.

Standardized Roentgenologic Examination in New and Old Capsular Ligament Injuries of the Thumb Metacarpophalangeal Joint
A. Rubach and O. Paar (Univ. of Munich)
Chirurg 54:423–424, June 1983   1–3

The diagnosis of a new ligament injury is not easily established, but because of the therapeutic consequences the differentiation between the partial and total rupture is of great importance. Besides the clinical examination, determination of the hinging function of the thumb metacarpophalangeal joint is recommended. The function of the joint is diminished when the guiding ligament of the joint is lifted and the active muscular stabilization is not enough to hold the thumb. Until now, the x-ray films were taken by the examiner placing the injured thumb on the roentgenograph cassette and holding the joint open during the filming. The result of this method depends on the strength used by the examiner.

The authors developed a simple holding device for radiologic examination of ligament and metacarpophalangeal joint injuries. The apparatus consists of a pulling device with a supporting pedestal. By means of a spring scale, a pull power of 100N is possible. Experimental postmortem studies showed that the thumb metacarpophalangeal joint can tolerate a considerable pull power. When the x-ray film is taken, the spring scale is set for 50N. Only half of the film is exposed; the other half is used for the opposite side, which allows comparison of both pictures.

The roentgenologic examination with the holding device has several advantages: standardization of the hinging power, objectivity and reproductivity of the joint instability, objective documentation, and no radiation exposure for the examiner. With the use of the holding device, pull power of 30N to 50N is needed and further traumatization is prevented. With the holding film technique, comparison with the opposite side is possible and, depending on the opening of the hinge, partial and total rupture of the collateral ligament can be differentiated.

▶ Both standardization of the force applied to the thumb for stress testing achieved by this model and comparison films of the opposite thumb are desirable. The clinical testing of resistance in flexion as well as in extension and also palpation of the ligament itself remain as important as the roentgenogram.—R.L.L.

The Looping Procedure: An Alternative Method of Thumb Restoration
Oddvar Eiken and Lars Ekerot (Malmö, Sweden)
Scand. J. Plast. Reconstr. Surg. 17:73–75, 1983   1–4

The thumb contributes about 40% of total hand function, warranting

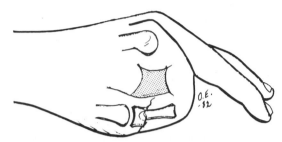

Fig 1–2.—The looping procedure. The idea is to reverse a seriously injured finger as a composite pedicle. The proximal and digital phalangeal bones are removed, whereas the midphalangeal bone is used for restoration of the thumb. (Courtesy of Eiken, O., and Ekerot, L.: Scand. J. Plast. Reconstr. Surg. 17:73–75, 1983.)

great efforts at restoring an amputated thumb. The authors describe a repair method for thumb amputations that uses a damaged finger of inferior functional value as a composite pedicle. After the proximal and distal phalangeal bones and the nail region are removed, the finger, carrying the midphalangeal bone only, is reversed and attached to the thumb remnant, forming a loop. The distal end of the phalangeal bone is fixed to the remnant of the thumb. After 3 weeks, the base of the finger is divided and the tip of the new thumb trimmed and fashioned (Fig 1–2).

This procedure is useful after severe mutilating injuries when phalangization of the first metacarpal is of little or no value and when more sophisticated procedures are not feasible. The method basically is a pollicization of a finger that is applicable when the blood supply is seriously impaired. It is a reliable and easy means of restoring a stable thumb post. In many instances, the procedure meets most functional requirements. Subsequent restoration of sensibility should be considered in young and otherwise suitable patients.

▶ This method would appear to leave an insensate thumb tip with marginal vascularity, but under some circumstances probably provides a reasonable use of a nonfunctioning finger and a satisfactory thumb post. Some might opt for a direct microsurgical transfer of the injured digit to provide vascular and neurologic continuity.—R.L.L.

Hyperextension Mallet Finger
R. H. Lange and W. D. Engber (Univ. of Wisconsin, Madison)
Orthopedics 6:1426–1431, November 1983   1–5

Mallet finger injury involves the loss of functional continuity of the extensor mechanism to the distal joint. A classification is presented in the table. Type I injuries can be managed adequately by closed reduction and immobilization in mild hyperextension. Suture repair of lacerations is generally recommended. Similar results are obtained in type II cases with splinting in mild hyperextension. Internal fixation is not necessary in these

	MALLET FINGER CLASSIFICATION
TYPE I	Extensor Tendon Injury A. Rupture or attenuation B. Laceration
TYPE II	Extensor Mechanism Avulsion (Fracture fragment less than 20% of articular surface)
TYPE III	Mallet Fractures A. Transepiphyseal plate fractures of children B. Hyperflexion bony mallet (20% to 50% articular surface fracture without subluxation) C. Hyperextension bony mallet (Generally ≥ 50% articular surface fracture with volar subluxation)

(Courtesy of Lange, R.H., and Engber, W.D.: Orthopedics 6:1426–1431, November 1983.)

cases. Type IIIA and IIIB injuries are treated by reduction through extension of the distal phalanx. Most physeal injuries are managed closed. It has been claimed that type IIIC injuries require accurate reduction to minimize posttraumatic arthritis, and the authors agree with this recommendation. Unsatisfactory results have been obtained where persistent volar subluxation is accepted.

Initial management failed to restore joint congruity in 4 of 6 cases of hyperextension mallet fracture, and persistent volar subluxation resulted. Three of these cases had been managed by open reduction with a pull-out wire technique. One patient has subsequently required distal interphalangeal joint arthrodesis for chronic pain and deformity. Two other patients underwent operative joint and fracture reduction, reduction being delayed for 2 months in both instances. The base of the distal phalanx was stabilized in mild flexion with a longitudinal Kirschner wire, and the dorsal fracture fragment was advanced and reduced with a pull-out wire (Fig 1–3). The early results have been much more satisfactory. Pain was relieved, and distal interphalangeal joint motion was much better than in any of the cases in which the joint was not reduced.

The principle of congruous reduction of intra-articular fractures is applicable to hyperextension mallet fractures. Closed reduction should always be tried in cases of acute type IIIC injury, but open reduction usually will be necessary. Both the joint and the fracture fragment should be reduced.

▶ The authors have pointed out the very subtle but very important difference between hyperextension and hyperflexion injuries, each with dorsal fracture fragments, in injuries of the distal interphalangeal joint. They hypothesize that treatment of the joints in flexion may produce reduction of the hyperextension injury fragment in the type IIIC mallet deformity. However, they are careful to

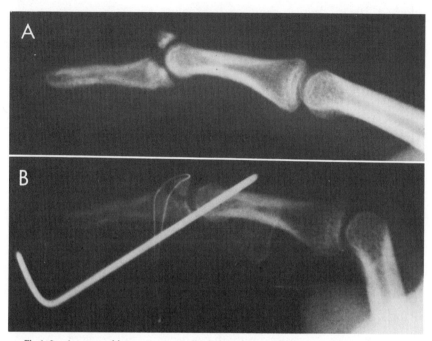

Fig 1–3.—A, untreated hyperextension mallet fracture with persistent pain 2 months after injury. B, operative management with joint reduced by mild flexion and stabilized with a buttress pin. Dorsal fragment reduced with a pull-out wire. (Courtesy of Lange, R.H., and Engber, W.D.: Orthopedics 6:1426–1431, November 1983.)

point out that open reduction may not be necessary in these cases. The addition of flexion to the position of the joint to maintain the reduction is certainly an appropriate and useful concept.—R.D.B.

Proximal Interphalangeal Joint Fracture-Dislocation Associated With Mallet Finger

R. H. Lange and W. D. Engber (Univ. of Wisconsin, Madison)
Orthopedics 6:571–575, May 1983   1–6

Proximal interphalangeal (PIP) joint fracture-dislocations and distal interphalangeal (DIP) joint mallet finger injuries are common as isolated injuries, but their association in the same digit is unusual. Three patients were seen who had combined injuries that were managed in a closed manner using a modified form of extension-block splinting described by Strong. The splint is made from two pieces of Alumafoam and tape, each ½ in. in width. Closed reduction is achieved by longitudinal traction followed by PIP joint flexion and DIP joint extension. The DIP joint is secured in mild, not forced, hyperextension. The degree of PIP joint extension block depends on the position of instability; extension of the joint is blocked 10–15 degrees short of this point. The PIP joint extension-block splint is reduced by 25% each week and generally is discontinued after 4 weeks, whereas DIP joint splinting is maintained for 6–8 weeks, with protection provided during sports activity for another month.

Man, 21, injured the right index finger while playing softball. He noted moderate swelling and tenderness at both the DIP and PIP joints 48 hours later. Radiography showed a dorsal fracture-dislocation of the PIP joint and a large area of articular surface comminution on the volar base of the middle phalanx. A type III mallet finger was present distally. Closed reduction was achieved with digital block anesthesia, and extension-block splinting was begun a week later. Examination at 8 months showed active PIP joint motion of 0–100 degrees and no DIP joint extensor lag. The final x-ray films showed satisfactory healing.

All of the fractures in this series healed uneventfully. Only 1 patient lacked full PIP joint extension at the time that splinting was discontinued, and all patients had at least 90 degrees of flexion. Mild weather-related discomfort was noted by all, but was not a significant problem, and use of the finger did not produce pain.

Modified extension-block splinting is a useful means of managing patients with combined PIP joint fracture-dislocation and DIP joint mallet finger injury in the same digit. The approach generally is limited to fractures involving not more than half of the articular surface of the PIP joint. In the presence of 30% to 50% involvement, one should ensure that motion occurs through the joint and not through the fracture line.

▶ This is a remarkably simple and clever technique for management of this difficult problem. It is important to remember in treating patients with fracture-dislocations of the proximal interphalangeal joint that constant radiographic control with lateral x-ray films in flexion is necessary to be sure that subluxation is reduced in flexion and, therefore, that late degenerative arthrosis is prevented.—R.D.B.

Palmar Dislocation of the Proximal Interphalangeal Joint
Clayton A. Peimer, Donna J. Sullivan, and Daniel R. Wild (SUNY at Buffalo)
J. Hand Surg. 9A:39–48, January 1984   1–7

Palmar proximal interphalangeal (PIP) joint dislocation is produced by combined varus or valgus stress that ruptures one collateral ligament and the palmar plate and by an anteriorly directed force displacing the middle phalanx anteriorly and disrupting the central slip.

The outcome in 11 male and 4 female patients with closed palmar dislocation of the PIP joint was reviewed 6 to 49 months after treatment. Average follow-up was 18 months. Average age of the patients was 24 years. Eight injuries occurred during athletic activity and 3 in fights. All patients had disruption of the extensor mechanism, palmar plate, and one collateral ligament. The loss of joint support resulted in palmar subluxation, malrotation, and a boutonnière deformity (Fig 1–4).

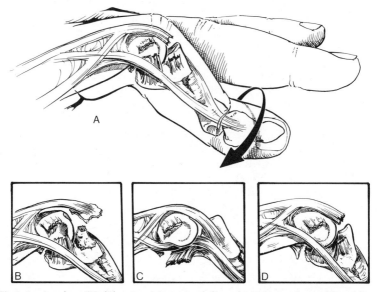

Fig 1–4.—A, palmar PIP dislocations injure central slip, palmar plate, and one collateral ligament. Loss of both static and dynamic joint support causes palmar subluxation and malrotation about intact collateral ligament. **B**, with fractures, central slip remains attached to avulsed, dorsal fragment from middle phalanx. **C**, irreducible dislocations may be due to interposition of lateral band in joint, and in these, central slip is not torn. **D**, irreducibility can also be caused by entrapment of torn collateral ligament. (Courtesy of Peimer, C.A., et al.: J. Hand Surg. 9A:39–48, January 1984.)

Twelve patients required operation for joint reduction and tendon and ligament repair; the other 3, seen earlier, had closed reduction and percutaneous pinning. The average interval from injury to referral exceeded 11 weeks. Two of the patients who were operated on had irreducible dislocations. Three had an associated dorsal avulsion fracture of the middle phalanx. A Kirschner wire was used to maintain joint reduction. All injured collateral ligaments were reattached at the site of repair. No tendon grafts were necessary. Joint alignment, comfort, and stability were restored, and all patients returned to full activities. The range of active PIP joint motion improved in all patients except a child with fibrous ankylosis, but no patient regained a full range of motion. Motion was better after closed treatment than in the patients requiring open reduction and extensor reconstruction. No patient had pain on active joint motion after treatment.

Joint stability is restored in cases of palmar dislocation of the PIP joint by closed reduction and pinning early in the course or by surgical repair at any stage. Stability and comfort are consistently restored, but some loss of PIP joint motion must be expected.

▶ The complexity of the problem and the need for accurate recognition and early repair are well emphasized in this article.—R.L.L.

Intra-articular Metacarpal Head Fractures

Edward C. McElfresh (St. Paul, Minn.) and James H. Dobyns (Mayo Med. School)

J. Hand Surg. 8:383–393, July 1983   1–8

Data was reviewed on 100 patients having 103 intra-articular metacarpal head fractures. The peak incidence was in the second and third decades. The second metacarpal most often was injured; the least injured metacarpal was the thumb. The most common types of injury were comminuted fracture, oblique (sagittal) fracture, and collateral ligament avulsion. Athletic injuries caused the largest number of fractures, followed by striking objects and fights. Twenty-two patients had open injuries. All of these patients and 8 others had operative treatment. Fractures involving large intra-articular defects generally should be reconstructed to obtain a congruent metacarpal head, and the digit should be mobilized as soon as possible.

Epiphyseal injuries have healed after closed treatment with splinting and early motion. All the collateral ligament avulsion fractures were closed. Four of 17 were operated on early, and 3 were operated on late. The 5 patients with closed osteochondral fractures did well, but infection developed in 1 of the 3 with open injuries. Among the 22 patients with oblique fractures, 7 required open reduction and internal fixation. Any displacement associated with joint incongruity in these cases should be reduced and fixed internally, and open reduction usually is required. Vertical (coronal) fractures involving a significant area of the utilized joint surface should be fixed internally with Kirschner wires. Horizontal (transverse) fractures have a poor prognosis unless they are reduced well and stabilized.

Five of 28 patients with 31 comminuted metacarpal head fractures had open reduction and internal fixation with Kirschner wires, and another had percutaneous Kirschner wire fixation. Fourteen patients had a substantial decrease in range of motion. Three had rotatory deformities. The treatment of these injuries depends on the integrity of the articular surfaces and the amount of displacement. The treatment of boxer's fractures and injuries with loss of bony substance is individualized. Avascular necrosis without an obvious fracture is rare.

▶ This article serves as a documentation of the surprisingly frequent occurrence of intra-articular metacarpal head fractures. Excellent classification is provided. Unfortunately, the article does not provide recommendations or indications for operative treatment with respect to large osteochondral defects. Osteochondral defects should be drilled for the stimulation of fibrocartilage or possibly should be covered by perichondrial grafts. I certainly agree that operative treatment of intra-articular fractures of the metacarpal head is essential. Good anatomic restoration of the articular anatomy can be obtained. If there is greater than 1 mm of displacement or greater than 2 mm of osteochondral defect, an operative intervention in the form of open reduction and internal fixation with the use of small Kirschner wires is needed.—W.P.C.

Isolated Dislocation of the Pisiform: A Case Report and Review of the Literature
Michio Minami, Jun Yamazaki, and Seiichi Ishii (Hokkaido Univ., Sapporo, Japan)
J. Hand Surg. 9A:125–127, January 1984   1–9

Isolated dislocation of a carpal bone other than the lunate and perilunate bones is rare.

The authors report the case of a patient with isolated dislocation of the pisiform who had the bone removed after attempted repositioning failed.

Man, 27, had the left wrist joint forced into dorsiflexion by a blow to its ulnar aspect as he grasped a jack handle. He reported pain in the palm when seen 8 days after injury. Hypothenar swelling and a tender bony prominence were noted; wrist motion was limited by pain. The pisiform bone lay over the hamate in the posteroanterior view, and dislocation distal to the triquetrum was evident in the lateral view. The bone was rotated 180 degrees. Exploration 10 days after injury showed the pisiform to be dislocated distally and toward the ulna. The pisohamate and pisometacarpal ligaments were torn. The bone was returned to its normal position and fixed to the triquetrum with two Kirschner wires, and the torn ligaments were repaired. A short-arm plaster was applied. After 8 weeks, the wires and cast were removed. Symptoms persisted at 3 months, and x-ray studies showed redislocation of the pisiform toward the palm. The bone was resected 3½ months after injury. Normal wrist motion was present without pain 6 years after surgery. Grasp was measured at 42 kg. The patient had returned to his original work.

Isolated dislocation of the pisiform bone probably is due to strong traction by the flexor carpi ulnaris tendon on acute dorsiflexion of the wrist with the wrist in palmar flexion. Direct external force also is a possible mechanism. Redislocation is liable to occur even if surgical repositioning of the bone is accompanied by ligament repair. Removal of the pisiform bone has given favorable results with no apparent disability, and it prevents the development of arthritis in the pisiform-triquetral joint.

▶ The authors imply that the primary treatment of a dislocated pisiform should be excision. The article presents the end-stage of a poorly recognized condition of pisotriquetral instability and pisotriquetral arthrosis after trauma. Hand physicians need to pay more attention to this area in examination and diagnostic evaluation following wrist injury.—R.D.B.

Idiopathic Avascular Necrosis of the Scaphoid: Report of Two Cases
Paul R. Allen (St Thomas' Hosp., London)
J. Bone Joint Surg. [Br.] 65-B:333–335, May 1983   1–10

The author describes two cases of idiopathic avascular necrosis of the proximal pole of the carpal scaphoid, a condition not previously reported in the English literature.

CASE 1.—Woman, 24, with wrist pain for 2 months and no history of injury, had normal x-ray findings. The symptoms became worse over the next 18 months,

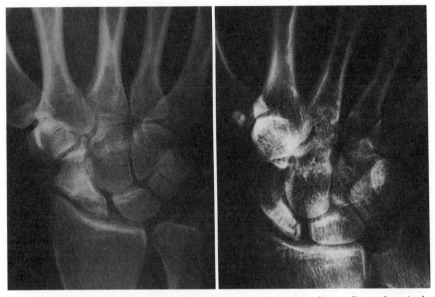

Fig 1–5 (left).—Radiograph taken 20 months after onset of symptoms shows collapse of proximal pole of scaphoid and secondary degenerative changes.

Fig 1–6 (right).—Radiograph taken 6 months after onset of symptoms shows definite increase in density of proximal pole and early fragmentation.

(Courtesy of Allen, P.R.: J. Bone Joint Surg. [Br.] 65-B:333–335, May 1983.)

and a repeat study showed increased density and some collapse of the proximal pole of the scaphoid and degenerative changes in the radioscaphoid joint (Fig 1–5). The initial symptoms appeared when the patient began knitting a sweater. A technetium bone scan showed increased uptake in the bone. Arthrodesis was carried out; histologic study confirmed the diagnosis of avascular necrosis.

CASE 2.—Woman, 38, seen after 3 months of wrist pain, was found to have a small cyst in the distal pole of the scaphoid. Increased density of the proximal pole was more evident a month later, and was definite 6 months after the onset (Fig 1–6). The patient was managed conservatively with a removable splint.

Two lateral volar vessels enter the waist of the scaphoid and supply the main body of the bone; a dorsal branch supplies the proximal pole, while a distal branch supplies the tuberosity. In the first patient, knitting could have produced a stress fracture through repetitive trauma; in the second, use of a new lawn mower could have caused the initial symptoms. Such stress fractures could well go unnoticed, but if the blood supply is disrupted, avascularity of the proximal pole could produce symptoms and lead to collapse. The rarity of the disorder might be related to an anomalous blood supply that places a person at risk from very minor trauma to the structures in the region.

▶ The authors present two interesting cases that appear to be unrecognized fractures of the proximal pole of the scaphoid, rather than a typical spontaneous avascular necrosis. Certainly, the films show in Figures 1–10 and 1–11 that fracture has occurred. I would anticipate that high-resolution tomography might have demonstrated these fractures prior to the onset of the collapse and the obvious fragmentation. It is still possible that these cases may have been a result of a primary vascular injury, a concept difficult to rule out.—R.D.B.

Bone Scintigraphy in the Evaluation of Fracture of the Carpal Scaphoid Bone
Poul T. Nielsen, Jess Hedeboe, and Per Thommesen (Randers, Denmark)
Acta Orthop. Scand. 54:303–306, April 1983   1–11

The authors evaluated wrist scintigraphy with ^{99m}Tc-methylene diphosphate for excluding or detecting carpal scaphoid fractures when performed 10 days after injury. Sixty-one male and 39 female patients with a mean age of 33 years were seen prospectively during 1 year. They had 101 injured wrists. Scintigraphy of both wrists 10 days after injury was performed while a cast remained in place, and clinical evaluation was repeated 2 days later. Scintigraphy was done 3 hours after administration of 10 to 15 mCi of ^{99m}technetium-methylene diphosphate.

Tenderness in the anatomical snuff box persisted 12 days after injury in 51 wrists. Radiographs showed 19 fractures of the carpal or surrounding bones, including 7 scaphoid fractures. None of the 50 wrists without tenderness had fractures. Fifty-four scintigrams were designated positive, and 13 were inconclusive. Twenty-five fractures were detected in this group. All 11 patients with scaphoid fractures had positive scintigrams. Three other patients had scapholunary dissociations, and there was 1 case each of Kienböck's disease of the lunate, osteoarthrosis of the first carpometacarpal joint, and de Quervain's tendovaginitis. Four patients with scaphoid fractures had normal radiographs but positive scintigraphic findings.

A normal wrist scintigram done 10 days after injury rules out fracture of the scaphoid or surrounding wrist bones. Routine scintigraphy, however, is of limited value in detecting or predicting scaphoid bone fractures. If wrist scintigraphy is done in doubtful cases after secondary clinical and radiographic evaluation, the number of such examinations can be minimized and the time of unnecessary casting shortened.

▶ The authors have demonstrated that fractures of the scaphoid will produce a positive bone scan in all cases at 2 weeks after injury. The recommended program is utilization of bone scintigraphy in the patient with persistent snuff box tenderness following a 2-week period of immobilization after wrist injury. If the scan is normal, one can rule out a fracture; if it is abnormal, the index of suspicion of fracture must be raised and tomography should be performed to detect subtle or oblique fractures not seen on routine x-ray films.—R.D.B.

Regional Scintimetry in Scaphoid Fractures

Niels Olsen, Peer Schousen, Hans Dirksen, and Jens Krogh Christoffersen (Univ. of Copenhagen)
Acta Orthop. Scand. 54:380–382, June 1983   1–12

Suspected fractures of the carpal scaphoid must be diagnosed and treated early in order to prevent complications and avoid overtreatment. The authors used a quantitative scintigraphic method to examine the regional distribution of activity in the scaphoid bone in 4 male and 2 female patients, aged 17–59 years, clinically suspected of having a fresh scaphoid bone fracture. All 6 patients were seen within 24 hours of injury. Initial radiographs showed a scaphoid fracture in 4 patients; the other 2 had negative radiographs at all intervals and no symptoms when last seen. Scintigraphy with ^{99m}Tc-Sn-pyrophosphate and a gamma camera having a pinhole collimator was done 3–4 days after trauma in patients with fractures. Small ^{51}Co sources were placed on the contour of the scaphoid drawn on the skin and visualized on the same oscilloscope.

In all 4 fractured scaphoid bones, increased activity was present in all regions of the bone, but not in scaphoid bones without symptoms. The region of injury in fractured bones had higher activity than the others when the proximal, middle, and distal thirds of the bone were assessed separately. The smallest gradient of activity between the region of fracture and the adjacent areas was significantly greater than the largest gradient between regions in control bones.

Quantitative scintigraphy of the scaphoid bone can provide a precise diagnosis of scaphoid bone fractures. This is especially useful in cases of fracture of the proximal third of the scaphoid, where lengthier immobilization is required for union and where avascular necrosis can develop. The method appears to be a useful supplement to positive survey scans in the early diagnosis of clinically suspected scaphoid bone fractures where initial radiographs are nondiagnostic. Scintimetry also may be helpful in diagnosing nonunion and avascular necrosis and in assessing the healing of scaphoid fractures.

▶ This technique also may have value for studying avascular necrosis of the proximal fragment of scaphoid fractures. It seems doubtful at present that this method has definite value in the diagnosis of scaphoid fractures that is not already obtainable with tomography and simpler scanning techniques.—R.L.L.

Management of the Fractured Scaphoid Using a New Bone Screw

Timothy J. Herbert and William E. Fisher (Univ. of New South Wales, Sydney)
J. Bone Joint Surg. [Br.] 66-B:114–123, January 1984   1–13

Symptomatic nonunion of the scaphoid is a common and disabling disorder, but internal fixation has never been popular, partly because firm fixation has been difficult to achieve. The authors have used a new double-

threaded bone screw to provide rigid internal fixation of all types of scaphoid fracture. The length of thread on the leading end of the screw is
short enough to allow firm fixation of small proximal-pole fractures of
the scaphoid. Absence of a protrusive screw head permits the screw to be
inserted through articular cartilage where necessary. The screws, of tita-
nium alloy, are 4 mm in diameter and 16–30 mm in length. Drilling and
tapping are done by hand. The method of positioning the jig on the scaphoid for proper screw insertion is illustrated in Figure 1–7.

A total of 158 operations using the new bone screw were done in 1977–
1981. Symptomatic sclerotic nonunions predominated. There were 15 fracture-dislocations in the series. Fifty-four proximal pole fractures were
treated. Relative ischemia of the proximal fragment is not a contraindication, but long-standing pseudarthrosis with severe arthritis usually con-
traindicates reconstruction. Excellent fixation was obtained in 83% of
cases. Plaster immobilization is necessary only in cases of unstable fracture
with significant associated ligament damage. Patients not entitled to compensation were away from work an average of 5½ weeks after the operation. All but 4% of the 138 patients followed up were highly satisfied
with the outcome, and 91% of patients had satisfactory clinical results.
No failures of union followed operations for acute unstable fractures. No
serious complications occurred. Six patients required revision, 2 after further marked wrist trauma.

These results justify continued use of this technique in the open man-

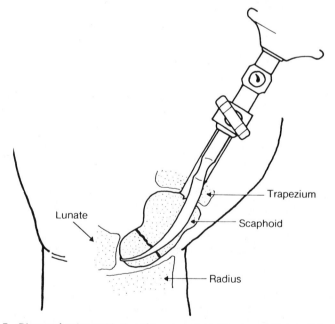

Fig 1–7.—Diagram showing positioning of jig on scaphoid. (Courtesy of Herbert, T.J., and Fisher,
W.E.: J. Bone Joint Surg. [Br.] 66-B:114–121, January 1984.)

agement of scaphoid fractures, particularly acute unstable injuries. Primary bone grafting may be indicated in cases of unstable comminuted fracture, especially if associated with midcarpal joint dislocation.

▶ This is a timely article with a unique solution to the problem of scaphoid fracture. I agree with most of the authors' statements that nonunited scaphoids lead to progressive degenerative change, that an expedient method of internal fixation is desirable, and that prolonged immobilization is undesirable. I would also agree that union itself is only one parameter of establishing the final result, as functional use is also important. While the authors have classified the latter, they have not provided us with an objective range of motion or grip strength with which to assess the postoperative state. I would certainly agree with the authors that this technique of opening the collapsed volar portion of the bone is important. The authors do not state how they maintain midcarpal alignment, which particularly in nonunions is so often disrupted by dorsiflexion of the lunate. The authors also state that this is a simple method, and in one figure in the original article suggest that this screw is much easier to insert than the standard corticocancellous screw; however, in their audiovisual presentations they have indicated that sometimes it is desirable to nibble away a portion of the trapezium in order to apply the jig and insert the screw. Compression of the jig across an unstable bone seems likely to result in distortion unless this is carefully controlled either by inserting the bone graft first or fixing the fragments during jig application. Lastly, although the authors indicate that firm compression persists, previous series have shown backing out of the screw to be fairly common. A temporary adjacent Kirschner wire to prevent rotation of the fragments about the longitudinal axis of the screw would appear to be a reasonable precaution.

Leyshon, Ireland, and Trickey (*J. Bone Joint Surg.* [*Br.*] 66-B:124–127, 1984) recently described a somewhat related technique in which, however, in situ fixation always is used regardless of the position of the scaphoid. No immobilization is used postoperatively. They report an 87% union rate with an average healing time of 6–7 months and return to work an average of 8 weeks postoperatively.

The authors suggest that a relatively simple technique of inserting a cancellous compression screw in the scaphoid results in quite satisfactory results, and they have found little indication of mechanical instability at the midcarpal area secondary to their nonunions. There apparently were no significant instances of screws backing out, and the rate of unions was remarkably high. If there were erosion of the palmar cortex of the scaphoid, this type of approach obviously would fix that deformity in the scaphoid resulting in a malunited scaphoid. The authors show no lateral roentgenogram, and their method of taking a single anteroposterior roentgenogram at the time of the operation obviously would not indicate the condition of the midcarpal alignment. Carpal union was assessed by means of standard roentgenograms, always somewhat difficult. No tomography was used for assessment. This obviously has worked in the authors' hands, but there is a considerable body of evidence to suggest that biomechanics of carpal scaphoid nonunion are considerably more complicated than the authors have addressed in this article.—R.L.L.

On a different track, Kim, Shaffer, and Idzikowski (*J. Bone Joint Surg.* [Am.] 65-A:985–991, 1983) in a review of scaphoid nonunions that failed additional treatment, suggest that underlying psychiatric problems were the primary cause. The authors have separated their series into two groups of patients: those in whom the scaphoid fracture united and those in whom it did not. Six of the 13 patients with persistent nonunion were found to have definite psychiatric abnormalities. The patients in whom union occurred were not studied as carefully, however, and follow-up in this group was not complete. The type of treatment used and anatomical features relating to the individual fractures were not discussed, nor was the way in which the psychiatric diagnosis arrived at explained. Thus, the authors' conclusion that psychiatric factors may take priority over anatomical and surgical ones in dealing with the patient with scaphoid nonunion are not truly supported by the study. Although it is certainly important to keep psychiatric background information in mind when selecting patients for reconstructive surgery of any sort, particularly after the failure of initial treatment modalities, the overwhelming majority of clinical evidence would indicate that factors such as fracture stability and treatment modality are more important in determining whether ununited fractures of the scaphoid will heal after treatment–W.P.C.

Arthrography of the Traumatized Wrist: Correlation With Radiography and the Carpal Instability Series
E. Mark Levinsohn and Andrew K. Palmer (SUNY, Upstate Med. Center)
Radiology 146:647–651, March 1983   1–14

Arthrography was used with fluoroscopic monitoring to assess the soft tissues of the wrist in 100 patients who had chronic traumatic pain but did not have rheumatoid arthritis. The 52 male and 48 female patients had an average age of 27.8 years. Routine radiographs were followed by a carpal instability series in 93 cases. Single-contrast arthrography then was done for all patients, under fluoroscopic control, using a mixture of methylglucamine diatrizoate, lidocaine, and epinephrine 1:1000. Six patients had bilateral arthrography, and 3 had repeat unilateral studies. No significant complications occurred.

Twenty-six arthrograms were considered normal. The most common abnormalities were capsular tears or localized ganglia, radiocarpal and midcarpal communication, and perforation of the triangular fibrocartilage. Lymphatic opacification and tendon sheath filling were less frequent findings. Communication between the radiocarpal and pisiform-triquetral joints was present in 69% of the cases. Perforation of the triangular fibrocartilage was significantly associated with both ulna-plus variance and carpal instability. No other significant correlation was evident between preexisting wrist instability and any combination of arthrographic abnormalities.

Carpal instability was associated with perforation of the triangular fibrocartilage in this series of patients with chronic post-traumatic wrist pain. Identification of the site of radiocarpal or midcarpal leakage may be useful in repairing the intracarpal ligament. Capsular tears or ganglia were present in 31% of the cases.

▶ The correlation of ulnar length with arthrographic communication through the lunotriquetral area is an important finding that suggests the force relationship between the functioning components of the wrist joint. The correlation between positive arthrographic findings and carpal instability is to be anticipated, but is important to document. Arthrography combined with differential lidocaine injections into the wrist joints has diagnostic value, especially when the joints are intact and leakage is not seen through either the triangular fibrocartilage or through the interosseous membranes.—R.L.L.

Dynamic Radiography of the Wrist
F. Schernberg and Y. Gerard (Reims, France)
Rev. Chir. Orthop. 69:521–531, 1983   1–15

The diagnosis of ligamentous lesions may be achieved by dynamic radiographs in radial or ulnar angulation and in forced torsion, traction,

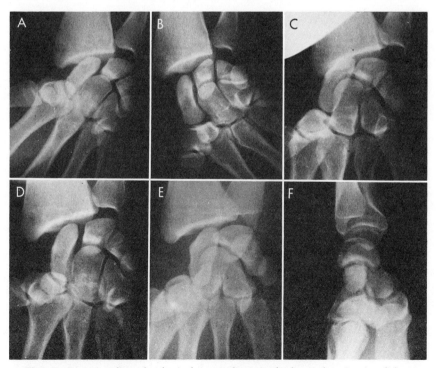

Fig 1–8.—Dynamic radiographs of wrist for use in diagnosis of radiocarpal sprains: A, radial angulation; B, cubital angulation; C, radial displacement; D, cubital displacement; E, pronation; and F, posterior slide or displacement. (Courtesy of Schernberg, F., and Gerard, Y.: Rev. Chir. Orthop. 69:521–531, 1983.)

and radial, ulnar, anterior, and posterior displacement. The authors used a strictly defined initial position in frontal and sagittal planes for comparable films in the study of the shape of the bones, their relationship to each other in different positions, and radiocarpal and intracarpal joint lines. A thorough study of the normal wrist is followed by illustrations of pathologic conditions, including dislocations, disjunction between the scaphoid and lunate, and midcarpal and radiocarpal sprains. In one example, a patient aged 22 incurred a wrist injury in a motorcycle accident, and considerable swelling of the wrist was noted on clinical examination. Although standard frontal and profile films showed no evident lesion, dynamic radiographic examination in translation, pronation, and posterior displacement showed possible displacement of the carpal bone in relation to the inferior extremity of the radius, allowing the diagnosis of pulled ligaments (Fig 1–8), which was confirmed by surgical intervention. Certain bone injuries also may appear on these dynamic films, for instance, the notoriously difficult to diagnose fractures of the carpal scaphoid bone, which may well go undetected on standard radiographs. It consequently is considered indispensable that a traumatized wrist be observed in five views: four in the frontal plane (radial and ulnar angulation and radial and ulnar displacement) and one in the sagittal plane.

▶ The authors have expanded admirably on a concept touched on by others that force displacements in the three planes of the wrist may show ligamentous injuries and occasionally fractures that are not apparent on standard radiographs. They have correlated these well with clinical and operative findings. Similar conclusions were drawn by Nielsen and Hedeboe (*J. Hand Surg.* 9A:135–138, 1984), who found cineradiography useful in identifying scapholunate dissociation in patients in whom routine wrist x-ray studies were normal. They emphasize the importance of obtaining comparison views of the symptomatic and asymptomatic wrists.

Both dynamic and cineradiography should improve our diagnostic accuracy in patients with symptoms compatible with intercarpal instability. Earlier treatment should lead to better long-term results.—R.L.L.

Posttraumatic Palmar Carpal Subluxation: Report of Two Cases
Hans-Wolfgang Bellinghausen, Louis A. Gilula, Leroy V. Young, and Paul M. Weeks (Washington Univ.)
J. Bone Joint Surg. [Am.] 65-A:998–1006, September 1983   1–16

Traumatic carpal instability can present both diagnostic and management problems. Posttraumatic palmar carpal subluxation has been mentioned only as a theoretic type of instability. A satisfactory functional outcome after closed reduction and nonoperative management was achieved in two patients followed up for 3 years after such an injury. The patients were a man aged 73 who had tried to catch a heavy falling object and a man aged 27 who was holding the handles of a motorcycle during a collision as the wrists were hyperextended. Immobilization was continued for 4–6 weeks after reduction of the injuries. The older patient reported frequent recurrences of radiocarpal subluxation when he moved his wheelchair, and x-ray studies showed degenerative changes and remodeling deformities of the radiocarpal joint. The younger patient had occasional wrist pain after heavy work. Roentgenography showed persistent palmar carpal subluxation associated with ulnar translocation.

A hyperextending distraction injury at the level of the radiocarpal joint can tear the palmar radiocarpal ligaments, if taut, while leaving the bone structure intact. Ulnar translocation can result from rupture of the ventral radiocarpal and ulnocarpal ligaments. The presence of an avulsion fracture of the base of the ulnar styloid process in one case suggested that the ulnar collateral ligament was intact. Both injuries are thought to have been due to distraction, causing rupture or severe stretching of the volar and dorsal radiocarpal and ulnocarpal ligaments, because no carpal fracture was present. Delayed adequate management of carpal ligament instabilities can lead to scar formation in and about the carpus and early degenerative arthritis.

The surgical management of carpal ligament instabilities is still evolving. Anatomical repositioning of the carpus appears necessary to avoid longstanding disability causing degenerative joint disease. An argument can be made for reduction and immediate stabilization of a palmar carpal subluxation, with possible ligament reconstruction.

▶ This article documents two case reports of palmar carpal subluxation of the wrist and provides an excellent review of the anatomy and kinematics involved in posttraumatic carpal instability. The authors' concept of the pathology—tearing of the volar and dorsal radiocarpal ligaments—as a result of distraction and shear forces across the wrist is probably correct, particularly if ulnar translation of the carpus is also a result of these ligament tears. We agree with the subtle and overt x-ray findings of the authors and believe that this report helps clarify the natural history of palmar carpal subluxation. The authors correctly point out that conservative treatment of such injuries has not given satisfactory results and that surgical repair or reconstruction of the volar and dorsal radiocarpal ligaments with complete reduction of the carpus is necessary to diminish the long-term problems of carpal instability and degenerative arthritis. It is unfortunate that the authors were unable to confirm the suspected pathology anatomically by surgical exploration. Tearing of the scapholunate ligaments, for example, may have been only partial, because in one case the arthrogram did not show a dye leak between the radiocarpal and intercarpal joints despite a slightly increased scapholunate gap. Similarly, there is uncertainty about the degree of disruption of the lunotriquetral ligaments and perhaps some of the other ligament restraints; however, it is likely that the pattern of ligament disruption varies from case to case. Increasing recognition of palmar carpal subluxation will result in further delineation of the pathomechanics, and the effort has been advanced by the authors' analysis of these cases. —W.P.C.

External Fixation of Complex Hand and Wrist Fractures

Stanley A. Riggs, Jr., and William P. Cooney, III (Mayo Clinic and Found.)
J. Trauma 23:332–336, April 1983   1–17

Indications for external fixation have increased because of the problems associated with internal fixation of comminuted or open fractures of the hand, wrist, and forearm. The authors reviewed the results obtained in 33 patients with upper extremity injuries in whom external fixation with the Jaquet minifixateur was used. Twenty-two patients had unstable Colles' fractures, 10 had fractures of the hand, and 1 had an osteotomy for Madelung's deformity. The patients' average age was 47 years. The external fixateur was used primarily in 19 cases; in 14, it was used after cast or Kirschner wire fixation had failed to hold the reduction. The procedure was done with the use of an axillary block, Bier's intravenous anesthesia, or general anesthesia.

All the hand fractures united within 12 weeks, the average time being 6 weeks, and no secondary procedures were necessary. The distal radial fractures united in an average of 6.8 weeks. Grip strength averaged 60% of that on the uninjured side a median of 10 months after treatment.

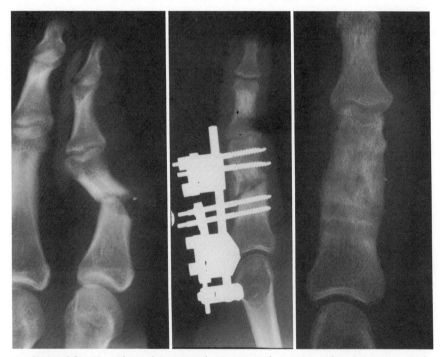

Fig 1–9 (left).—No evidence of union 5 weeks postoperatively in patient with comminuted proximal phalangeal fracture.

Fig 1–10 (center).—Stabilization with mini-external fixateur.

Fig 1–11 (right).—Healed fracture 13 weeks after application of external fixation.

(Courtesy of Riggs, S.A., Jr., and Cooney, W.P., III.: J. Trauma 23:332–336, April 1983.)

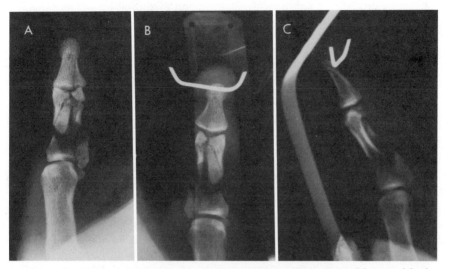

Fig 1–12.—**A,** comminuted fracture of proximal phalanx and minimally displaced fracture of distal phalanx. **B,** skeletal traction. **C,** gauntlet cast. (Courtesy of Riggs, S.A., Jr., and Cooney, W.P., III: J. Trauma 23:332–336, April 1983.)

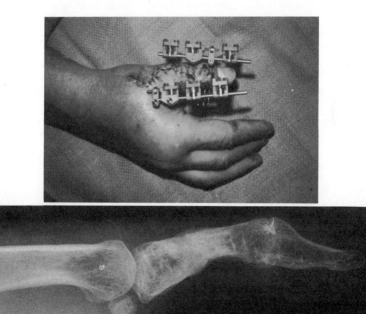

Fig 1–13 (top).—Mini-Hoffmann external fixateur applied after bone grafting.
Fig 1–14 (bottom).—Healed fracture after 10 weeks of immobilization with external fixateur.
(Courtesy of Riggs, S.A., Jr., and Cooney, W.P., III: J. Trauma 23:332–336, April 1983.)

Complications occurred in 22% of cases, and included two pin-site infections but no cases of osteomyelitis. Two patients had transient radial neuritis. The outcome in a patient with a comminuted proximal phalangeal fracture is shown in Figures 1–9 to 1–11 and that in a patient with a comminuted fracture of the proximal phalanx and a distal phalangeal fracture, in Figures 1–12 to 1–14.

Exoskeletal fixation is a useful approach to compound, segmental, and very comminuted fractures of the hand, unstable distal radial fractures, and septic nonunions. It is an excellent salvage method where more traditional methods of closed or open fracture treatment have failed. The external minifixateur provides rigid stability and has wide adaptability, allowing pin placement in a wide range of angles and positions without interfering with soft tissue care or overall hand function.

▶ This potpourri of cases clearly demonstrates the usefulness of external skeletal fixation in the management of complicated hand fractures and the necessity for facility with the instrumentation in the armamentarium of all hand surgeons.—P.C.A.

Hoffmann Pelvic Stabilization for Injuries to the Hand and Wrist
C. Craig Crouch and James B. Bennett (Baylor College of Medicine)
J. Hand Surg. 8:211–212, March 1983   1–18

Immobilization is a problem after pedicle flap coverage of upper extremity injuries with extensive soft tissue loss. The authors successfully used a modification of the Hoffmann apparatus in two patients requiring flap coverage.

Man, 47, was shot at close range in the right hand with a 12-gauge shotgun. The entrance wound was on the palmar-radial aspect of the wrist and the exit wound at the dorsal wrist area. Decreased sensibility was noted in the area of the

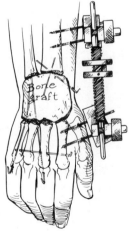

Fig 1–15.—Hoffmann external fixation device in place, with large soft tissue and bony defects. (Courtesy of Crouch, C.C., and Bennett, J.B.: J. Hand Surg. 8:211–212, March 1983.)

dorsal thumb web. The extensor mechanism and soft tissue coverage were absent. The distal radius and ulna were comminuted, and the carpal and metacarpal bones were injured. A Hoffmann device with percutaneous pins and connecting rods was used for stabilization after debridement. The dorsal skin defect later was covered by a tensor fascia lata pedicle flap and stabilized by a pelvic Hoffmann device (Fig 1–15). The device was kept in place for 3 weeks. The base of the flap then was detached, and iliac bone was grafted 6 weeks later. Bony union ensued, with excellent soft tissue coverage. Tendon transfers to the thumb and fingers are planned.

Use of the pelvic Hoffmann device to stabilize pedicle flap coverage facilitated wound care and flap inspection and stabilized the flap while it was revascularized. No complications resulted, but pin tract infection and pin loosening are possibilities. Upper arm stiffness can be minimized by having the patient exercise. This type of fixation has significant advantages in the management of avulsion injuries of the hand and forearm where flap coverage is indicated for extensive soft tissue loss.

► The authors describe a unique technique for combining external skeletal fixation of a distal forearm fracture with soft tissue coverage using a tensor fascia lata flap. As described, with an additional outrigger the hand can be fixed to the flap site, insuring "cooperation" in patients who present more difficult management problems.—W.P.C.

Delayed Primary Bone Grafting in the Hand and Wrist After Traumatic Bone Loss
Alan E. Freeland, Michael E. Jabaley, William E. Burkhalter, and Andre M. V. Chaves
J. Hand Surg. 9A:22–28, January 1984   1–19

The results of 21 bone graft procedures, done as part of the overall delayed primary management of hand and wrist wounds in 17 patients, were reviewed. The average follow-up was 22 months. The 13 male and 4 female patients had an average age of 26 years. Most patients had low-velocity gunshot wounds or close-range shotgun wounds. Metacarpals and proximal phalanges usually were damaged. Bone grafting was done within 10 days after injury in all cases, and usually after 3–7 days. A unicortical cancellous iliac bone graft was used in 10 defects and a pure cancellous graft from the ilium or distal radius in 5. Several fixation methods were utilized. Flaps were used in 7 cases, and skin grafts in 3 cases.

All but 1 of the 21 bone grafts united clinically and radiographically. One patient had delayed union of a graft that was not rigidly fixed. No infections occurred, and no grafts were lost. Patients with only segmental metacarpal bone loss had early recovery, usually within 2–3 months. Total recovery took longer when tendon loss also was present. Grafting of the phalanges usually was followed by some residual loss of motion from adhesion formation. Two patients required surgery to release adhesions. In 2 other cases, the proximal interphalangeal joint ankylosed in an acceptable position.

Bone grafting can be done safely within a context of delayed primary repair in patients with traumatic bone loss in the hand and wrist. Grafting is carried out within 10 days after injury. The overall time of repair and reconstruction is significantly shortened, and conditions for early functional return are optimized. A surgically clean wound and a good blood supply are important, as is stable fixation. Autogenous bone should be used. Deep structures and fixation devices must be covered with viable tissue.

▶ The authors have pointed out the excellent utilization of delayed primary treatment of wounds. We have known for some time that internal fixation may be used safely on a delayed basis after primary wound cleansing has occurred. The authors have added the utilization of late primary cortical-cancellous bone grafting. Recent experience at our institution indicates that bone from a bone bank may be a satisfactory substitute in many situations where previous bone grafting materials were removed from the iliac crest, and it is likely that this material will be useful in the authors' setting also, eliminating the need for morbidity from the removal of iliac grafts.—R.D.B.

Long-Term Results of Ulnar Lengthening for Kienböck's Disease
J. Roullet, G. Walch, and G. Spay
Lyon Chir. 79:255–260, July–Aug. 1983   1–20

Eleven of 21 patients treated prior to 1970 for Kienböck's disease were reexamined. Eight had undergone ulnar lengthening by the same technique. Patients' ages ranged from 17 to 34 years. Radiologically, according to Decoulx's classification of necrosis, 1 patient represented stage I; 2, stage II; and 5, stage III. All patients had a short ulna with a radioulnar index of from 1 to 5 mm. The internal covering defect of the lunate bone described by Razemon was found to be in excess of 40% in 5 of the 8 patients, and in 7 the lunate bone was of Antuna Zapico type I with an oblique upper edge and an upper internal projection, as if the bone were drawn in by the digital fossa of the ulna. On profile films the faulty posture of the mediocarpal is the rule, causing instability of the wrist in palmar flexion. Dorsal radiolunar angle was found to be more than 20% in all patients.

Functional results were evaluated on the basis of Michon's criteria. Results were best in terms of freedom from pain and restoration of strength but were less satisfactory with regard to mobility. Conservation of the shape of the lunate bone could be demonstrated roentgenographically in 6 of the 8 patients, but arthrosis invariably developed. However, the arthrosis is well tolerated after 15 years, and patients are completely free of pain. Arthrosis does not appear to be associated exclusively with lengthening of the ulna, because it has been reported by almost every author regardless of technique used. In the authors' opinion, ulnar lengthening is the treatment of choice in all stages of Kienböck's disease.

▶ The authors have reported late degenerative changes, despite clinical comfort and reconstitution of the lunate, following ulnar lengthening for Kienböck's disease. Despite this, I still believe that the lengthening procedure or the radial shortening procedure is worthwhile as a clinical, non-bridge-burning, procedure that will provide for pain relief and at least clinically delay incapacity.— R.D.B.

Plate Fixation of Unstable, Displaced Fractures of the Anterior Margin of the Radius

B. Augereau, D. Lance, and M. Kerboul (Paris)

Int. Orthop. 7:55–59, 1983   1–21

The authors successfully managed these unstable fractures by using a preformed epiphyseal plate that, by its adaptation to the epiphyseal profile, maintains the reduction and assures sufficiently solid fixation for early mobilization (Fig 1–16). Five Smith fractures and 23 fractures of the anterior margin of the lower end of the radius were treated in this manner. The essential points of the technique were (1) a large enough incision to allow opening of the carpal tunnel and good exposure of the fragments, (2) precise reduction of the fragments with endoarticular control and temporary wire fixation, and (3) screwing of the plate into an appropriate position to stabilize the obtained reduction.

The results obtained by this method confirm its superiority: 78% very

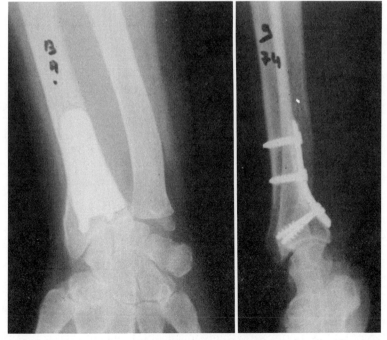

Fig 1–16.—Surgical treatment. Osteosynthesis by plate fixation was performed, with a very good result. (Courtesy of Augereau, B., et al.: Int. Orthop. 7:55–59, 1983.)

good results compared with 32% by orthopedic means. When correctly carried out, osteosynthesis persistently allows very satisfactory anatomical reconstitution and excellent function regardless of the complexity of the fracture, and this technique is suggested for all unstable fractures of the radius with anterior displacement.

▶ The authors present their experience with 28 Smith-type fractures of the distal radius, including 23 fractures of the anterior margin and 5 intra-articular Smith fractures. The Smith fractures have been subdivided into three types. We would agree that the authors' method of internal fixation with an anterior buttress plate is superior to techniques in which an AO plate is just used for buttress purposes only. We have seen displacement of the anterior lip margin when internal fixation of intra-articular fractures has not been obtained. Unfortunately, the manufacturer of the plate is not mentioned in this report, but this information may be obtained by writing the authors.

A related article by Freising and Walter (*Chirurgie* 54:742–748, 1983) also reflects the increased concern for more aggressive surgical management of intra-articular fractures of the distal radius. As in other joints, precise fracture reduction is necessary. We support the principle espoused in these two articles of open reduction and internal fixation (or combined internal and external fixation) of intra-articular fractures of the distal radius to achieve a satisfactory wrist joint.—W.P.C.

Fracture of the Radius With Instability of the Wrist
Daniel I. Rosenthal, Matthew Schwartz, Warren C. Phillips, and Jesse Jupiter (Harvard Med. School)
AJR 141:113–116, July 1983   1–22

Because the pathomechanics of distal radial fracture and carpal dissociation overlap, the two injuries can occur simultaneously. The findings in 190 consecutive distal radial fractures in skeletally mature patients were reviewed to determine the frequency of coexisting carpal instability. Fracture displacement was measured in 91 consecutive patients. Rotatory subluxation of the navicular was diagnosed in the anteroposterior view when there was a 3-mm or larger space between the scaphoid and lunate and when the scapholunate articular space was significantly larger than the other joint spaces. Dorsiflexion instability was diagnosed in the lateral film when the lunate was dorsiflexed with respect to the axes of the radius and capitate and the scapholunate angle exceeded 60 degrees.

Ligamentous intercarpal instability was observed in 14 patients (7.4%). Nine of these had a Colles' fracture, 4 a radial styloid fracture, and 1 a Smith fracture. None of the patients had scaphoid fracture. Ligamentous instability was more likely to occur in older patients and in those with a lower combined cortical thickness. The severity of fracture-displacement, shortening, angulation, and presence of an ulnar styloid fracture could not be related to the risk of ligament damage occurring. Carpal instability was apparent on the initial x-ray films in all but 1 patient, but it was not diagnosed correctly at this time in any.

The pathomechanics of the radial styloid fracture involve forced extension, ulnar deviation, and supination. An intra-articular vertical fracture component was seen between the scaphoid and lunate in several patients with Colles' fracture, presumably reflecting the same mechanism. Effective treatment requires recognition of posttraumatic carpal instability within a few weeks of its occurrence. Otherwise, severe, disabling radiocarpal joint degeneration may develop. Fluoroscopically positioned spot films may help confirm the diagnosis in doubtful cases. Comparison films of the opposite wrist also may be helpful.

▶ The authors are calling attention to a problem that is much more common than generally is recognized, a concomitant sprain of the wrist leading to instability through the carpus. It is particularly important in younger patients with distal radial fractures and should actively be considered and treated, particularly when the radial styloidal break mentioned is present. By causing a secondary realignment dorsiflexion of the proximal carpal row, a dorsal angulation of the radial fragment may simulate a scapholunate dissociation because of the apparent widening of the scapholunate space. As the authors point out, the lack of an increased scapholunate angle and the relative silhouettes of the scaphoid and lunate should help to resolve this differentiation. If there still is doubt, arthrography is indicated.—R.L.L.

Impending Rupture of the Extensor Pollicis Longus Tendon After a Minimally Displaced Colles' Fracture: Case Report
R. E. Bunata
J. Bone Joint Surg. [Am.] 65-A:401–402, March 1983   1–23

Rupture of the tendon of the extensor pollicis longus at the wrist is an uncommon complication occurring several weeks or months after Colles' fracture, often after a fracture not requiring reduction. Possible causes include laceration of the tendon at the time of injury, attrition as the tendon rides over a bone spicule, and devascularization of the tendon at the time of injury. The author reports a case of impending rupture of the extensor pollicis longus tendon after a minimally displaced distal radial fracture.

Woman, 48, had a long cast applied for an undisplaced radial fracture. Pain occurred with all movements of the thumb and was felt on the dorsum of the wrist near Lister's tubercle. During a decompression procedure, abrasion of the extensor pollicis longus tendon was seen just beneath the retinaculum over a length of 3 cm, with loss of about one third of its diameter. The tendon was placed subcutaneously. The sheath was sutured after failure to find a sharp edge of bone, and a short cast was applied. The fracture healed satisfactorily, and the pain subsided gradually. Complete motion and good strength were re-established in 6 months.

Attrition was probably the mechanism of tendon injury in this case. Kinking of the tendon sheath or inapparent fibrosis in the sheath could have been the cause. Pain in the dorsal part of the wrist with thumb motion or crepitus with thumb motion lasting more than 7–10 days suggests the possibility of extensor pollicis longus tendinitis in a patient with minimally displaced Colles' fracture. Removal of the tendon from its compartment can prevent rupture and preclude the need for reconstructive therapy.

▶ Historically, extensor pollicis longus injuries after Colles' fracture have been detected only at the time of rupture. This article points out the importance of careful observation of extensor pollicis longus function after Colles' fracture. In the case described, impending rupture was detected, precluding the need for tendon reconstruction. Although reconstruction in the form of tendon repair or, more usually, tendon transfer has a high likelihood of success, diagnosis and treatment before rupture clearly provide the patient with the shortest period of disability and should be more reliable in terms of restoration of function.— P.C.A.

Role of Radiography and Computerized Tomography in Diagnosis of Subluxation and Dislocation of the Distal Radioulnar Joint

David E. Mino, Andrew K. Palmer, and E. Mark Levinsohn (SUNY, Uptown Med. Center)
J. Hand Surg. 8:23–31, January 1983   1–24

Subluxation or dislocation of the distal radioulnar joint (DRUJ) may initially go undiagnosed because of inability to obtain x-ray confirmation. The authors evaluated routine roentgenography and computed tomography (CT) for diagnosing distal DRUJ subluxation and dislocation in 3 cadaver upper extremities transected at the midhumerus level. Reproducible forearm positioning was possible with a Steinmann pin inserted through the metacarpals. Studies were repeated after excision of all soft tissue structures supporting the DRUJ in different positions of rotation, with 50% palmar and dorsal subluxation and with dorsal dislocation.

Both subluxation and dislocation were diagnosed accurately from a true lateral roentgenographic projection of the wrist with the forearm in neutral rotation. Minimal supination or pronation of the forearm, however, compromised diagnostic accuracy. A single CT scan through the DRUJ was diagnostic of both subluxation and dislocation in all positions of forearm rotation. The DRUJ was best visualized by a section projecting the ulnar styloid process, sigmoid notch, and Lister's tubercle. The ulna in the reduced DRUJ translocated dorsally with pronation and palmarly with supination, but it remained reduced at all times within the confines of the sigmoid notch of the radius.

An accurate diagnosis of DRUJ subluxation and dislocation can be made from a true lateral wrist roentgenogram. Such a study may be impossible because of wrist pain or plaster immobilization; in these circumstances, a single CT scan can be used to diagnose subluxation or dislocation of the DRUJ in any position of forearm rotation.

▶ The interpretation of positioning of the distal radioulnar joint is taking on increased importance with the realization of its significance as a determinate of the final functional status after trauma or disease. Although cost considerations must be kept in mind, the CT scan has clear utility for evaluating the distal radioulnar joint when there is clinical indication of disease in this area. An additional benefit is that it is easy to obtain studies of both wrists simultaneously for comparative purposes.

A related paper by Cone et al. (*Invest. Radiol.* 18:541–545, 1983) demonstrates similar utility of these techniques at the proximal radioulnar joint.— R.L.L.

Clinical and Roentgenographic Evaluation of Nonunion of the Forearm in Relation to Treatment with dc Electric Stimulation
R. Bruce Heppenstall, Carl T. Brighton, John L. Esterhai, Jr., and Douglas Becker (Univ. of Pennsylvania)
J. Trauma 23:740–744, August 1983   1–25

Closed reduction and functional bracing now are recommended for managing many single forearm bone fractures, but nonunion continues to be a problem with both operative and brace methods. Data on 50 nonunions of forearm fractures in 42 patients who were referred for electric treatment between 1970 and 1982 were reviewed by the authors. There were 22 nonunions of the radius and 28 of the ulna. Seven patients had associated medical problems. Three radial nerves and 1 median nerve were injured. Vascular status was normal in each patient. Sixteen open fractures resulted in nonunion; all were debrided initially. Nine infections occurred.

Initial management of nonunion was by casts in 11 cases, compression plates in 20, intramedullary rods in 11, pins and plaster in 5, and external fixation in 3. Nearly two thirds of all the nonunions were in the middle part of the bones. There were 30 comminuted fractures, 3 transverse injuries, and 17 oblique fractures. All but 2 fractures were displaced. The average time since injury was 2 years. Success was achieved with electric treatment in 71% of 45 complete treatment courses. The success rates were 74% if 2 patients with large osseous defects were excluded and 80% if 3 patients with recurrent osteomyelitis also were excluded.

Electric therapy appears to be a promising alternative to bone grafting for nonunions of forearm bone fractures. Minimal complications have occurred with use of this semiinvasive approach, compared with open treatment methods. Electric treatment is not indicated if a gap is present at the site of nonunion; a live microvascular pedicle bone graft is preferred in such a case.

▶ The authors have demonstrated success with dc electric stimulation in established nonunions of the forearm bones. In our experience, similar success has been achieved with the noninvasive pulsed electric magnetic stimulation method. In either case, it is my opinion that electric stimulation, rather than surgery, should be considered as the first line of treatment for established nonunions of the forearm bones that can be demonstrated as not having a synovial nonunion.—R.D.B.

The Disparate Diameter: Sign of Rotational Deformity in Fractures

Allan Naimark, Judith Kossoff, and Robert E. Leach (Boston Univ.)
J. Can. Assoc. Radiol. 34:8–11, March 1983   1–26

Although clinical assessment usually is better than radiography in detecting rotational deformity at fracture sites, the forearm is an exception. It appears that in the absence of comminution, a significant rotational deformity must be considered when the diameter of a long bone changes abruptly across a fracture line. The findings in a woman, aged 40, who sustained a distal radial shaft fracture and had local pain 5 weeks later are shown in Figures 1–17 and 1–18 and compared with the normal

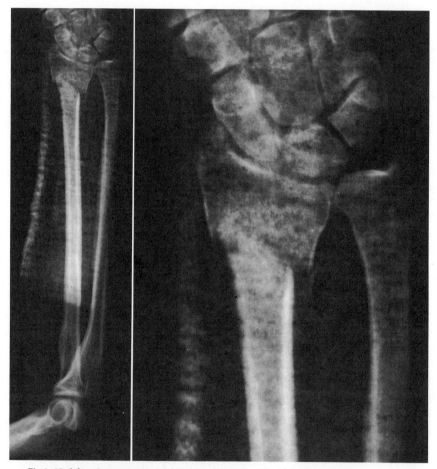

Fig 1–17 (left).—Posteroanterior radiograph of forearm through plaster of Paris splint, obtained 5 weeks after injury. Measurements of diameter of shaft immediately proximal and distal to fracture of distal radius are remarkably disparate (1.5 and 2.6 cm, respectively). Note lack of radial bow and abnormal position of bicipital tuberosity.

Fig 1–18 (right).—Close-up of fracture region.

(Courtesy of Naimark, A., et al.: J. Can. Assoc. Radiol. 34:8–11, March 1983.)

appearance in Figure 1–19. Marked rotational deformity was confirmed at surgery and corrected; after healing, full range of rotation was restored. The findings in a boy, aged 12, who injured his ring finger are shown in Figures 1–20 and 1–21. Rotational deformity was clinically apparent in this case.

Severe rotational deformity can sometimes be observed radiographically from a marked disparity in diameter between the bone just proximal and that just distal to the fracture line. If the cross section of a long bone at the site of fracture is ovoid and the diameter changes abruptly in the absence of comminution, significant rotational deformity is a good possibility. If displacement is severe, differential magnification has to be taken

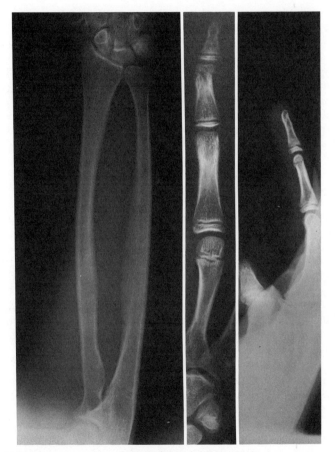

Fig 1–19 (left).—Posteroanterior radiograph of forearm of normal subject.

Fig 1–20 (center).—Posteroanterior radiograph of ring finger shows mild angulation and disparity between bone diameters immediately proximal and distal to fracture of neck of middle phalanx, indicating severe rotational deformity.

Fig 1–21 (right).—Postreduction lateral radiograph of ring finger shows that anatomical position has been restored.

(Courtesy of Naimark, A., et al.: J. Can. Assoc. Radiol. 34:8–11, March 1983.)

into account. Negative findings do not exclude rotational deformity. The disparate diameter sign is most important in assessing forearm trauma. The joints proximal and distal to the fracture site should be included in the study, preferably on the same film.

▶ There is nothing new in this short article, but almost every point that it makes concerning the identification of rotational deformities at fracture sites is commonly ignored, forgotten, misunderstood, or misapplied. Committing these few facts to memory will save many patients and many clinicians much grief, particularly in the management of forearm fractures.—J.H.D.

Traumatic Radioulnar Synostosis Treated by Excision and a Free Fat Transplant: Report of Two Cases
Ken Yong-Hing and Stanley P. K. Tchang (Univ. Hosp., Saskatoon, Sask.)
J. Bone Joint Surg. [Br.] 65-B:433–435, August 1983   1–27

Traumatic radioulnar synostosis was managed in two patients by excising the cross-union and interposing a free fat transplant, with excellent functional results. A man aged 19 had a distal ulnar fracture, incurred in a motorcycle accident and fixed with a plate and screws, but developed a radioulnar synostosis in 30 degrees of pronation. The synostosis was excised after removing the plate and screws. A free nonvascularized subcutaneous fat transplant measuring 7.5 × 3 × 1 cm was taken from the anterior abdominal wall and placed at the site of the synostosis, where it covered all the raw bone surfaces and completely filled the dead space. Movement was encouraged immediately postoperatively and the patient regained full pronation; supination remained 15 degrees less than on the uninjured side. The other patient was a man aged 19 with a synostosis in neutral rotation after fractures of both bones. In this case, the ulna was stripped circumferentially of its soft tissues for the length of the bony bridge. The final range of motion was nearly normal. The radial plate was not removed. In these cases, the treatment of radioulnar synostosis by excision and free fat transplantation has produced impressive functional results at 2–3 years. Further trial of this approach is warranted.

▶ The authors have described a new and relatively simple technique that has been successful in their two cases of distal radioulnar synostosis after trauma. It could be suggested that treatment with simple excision may have been successful in their cases, but if an interposition material were to be considered, the free fat transfer is simple and less hazardous than utilization of silicone. It appears to warrant further clinical consideration.—R.D.B.

Effects of Angular and Rotational Deformities of Both Bones of the Forearm: An In Vitro Study

Richard R. Tarr, Arthur I. Garfinkel, and Augusto Sarmiento (Univ. of Southern California)
J. Bone Joint Surg. [Am.] 66-A:65–70, January 1984   1–28

Most dual-bone fractures of the forearm are difficult treatment problems regardless of the approach used. The effects of combined deformity on forearm motion were examined in 6 intact, fresh cadaver specimens. The remaining pronation and supination were measured after the production of angular and rotatory deformities at the distal and middle levels of the forearm. The study method is illustrated in Figure 1–22.

When both forearm bones were angulated with a combined radioulnar and dorsovolar deformity of 10 degrees, a loss of 12.5% of pronation-supination was found in forearms with a distal third fracture, and a loss of 16% was found in those with a middle-third fracture. Pronation losses were similar for the distal and middle-third deformities, but supination loss was much less in forearms with distal-third deformities. Drastic losses of supination were present in forearms with middle-third angular deformities of greater than 10 degrees. Rotatory deformities produced pronation-supination losses equal to the degree of deformity, but in the opposite direction. A 10-degree pronation deformity, for instance, produced a 10-degree loss of supination motion.

This study showed greater loss of forearm motion with middle-third than with distal deformities. Pure rotatory deformities of the radius pro-

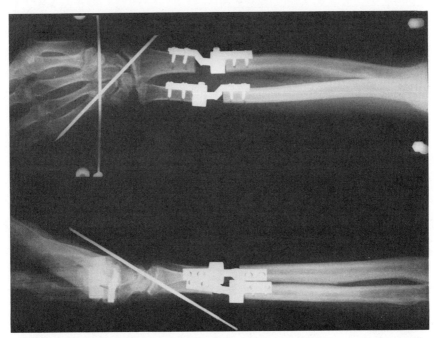

Fig 1–22.—Anteroposterior and lateral radiographs of forearm suspended in measuring frame, with specially fabricated plates positioned in distal end of radius and ulna. (Courtesy of Tarr, R.R., et al.: J. Bone Joint Surg. [Am.] 66-A:65–70, January 1984.)

duce rotational losses equal to the degree of rotatory deformity. Soft tissue tension, particularly of the interosseous membrane, limits rotation.

▶ This is an excellent early study of the effects of malalignment on rotational function of bones in a laboratory model. It is a fine beginning for what should be an ongoing study of the effects of changing various facets of the forearm rotational mechanism. One obvious case in point is the effect that variations in angulation or alignment have on the distal radioulnar and the elbow and wrist joints, as it is safe to assume there is both a change in contact area and the arc of contact during motion, particularly at the radiocapitellar joint after significant change in forearm alignment.—R.L.L.

▶ The practical implications of this work are clear. Smaller degrees of angular and rotational deformity, which when totaled sum no more than 10 degrees, are associated with minimal losses of forearm rotation. Greater degrees, particularly of angular deformity, are associated with significant losses of rotation, especially supination, and therefore must be avoided.—P.C.A.

The Os Supratrochleare Dorsale: A Normal Variant That May Cause Symptoms

Wim R. Obermann and Henry W. C. Loose (Univ. Med. Center, Leiden, The Netherlands)

AJR 141:123–127, July 1983   1–29

The os supratrochleare dorsale appears to be an accessory bone nucleus of the olecranon or a normal variant, the supratrochlear foraminal bone. Fifteen well-documented cases have been reported, all in male patients

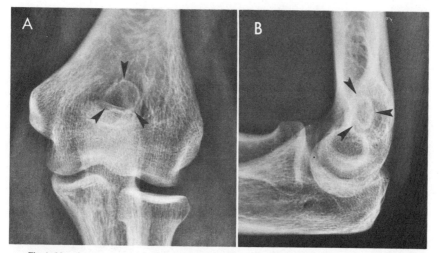

Fig 1–23.—Asymptomatic left elbow. Anteroposterior (**A**) and lateral (**B**) views. Intact "bone" in olecranon fossa (*arrowheads*) with little trabeculation is seen. Supratrochlear septum is intact. (Courtesy of Obermann, W.R., and Loose, H.W.C.: AJR 141:123–127, July 1983.)

aged 15 to 40 years. All were symptomatic. The authors report data on 4 patients (3 men and 1 woman) with an os supratrochleare dorsale (Fig 1–23). Three patients had symptoms that necessitated removal of the structure; 1 had a bilateral abnormality.

The os supratrochleare dorsale is most likely an accessory bone, but because of its location it is prone to being injured by the olecranon, leading to secondary chondrometaplasia of the bone itself. Symptomatic patients have posttraumatic bone changes, but subjects without symptoms exhibit a normal trabecular pattern. The radiographic findings after trauma may be indistinguishable from those of a posttraumatic loose body lodged in the olecranon fossa. The disorder appears unrelated to the supratrochlear septum or the bones in the coronoid fossa.

▶ This article serves as a valuable contribution not of original information but, rather, as a reminder of the unusual radiographic variation about the elbow known as the "os supertrochlea dorsale." Although there has been some controversy regarding the origin and significance of this entity, this article documents well that it should be considered a normal variant and, thus, usually can be left alone. However, because the ossicle is subject to injury, removal is the treatment of choice if symptoms persist. In our judgment, this is a valuable article with a clear discussion of the origin and significance of this radiographic curiosity.—B.F.M.

Four-Part Fractures of the Neck of the Humerus
P. G. Stableforth (Bristol Royal Infirm.)
J. Bone Joint Surg. [Br.] 66-B:104–108, January 1984   1–30

Data on 32 patients with four-part proximal humeral fractures and a prospective series of 49 cases referred in the past 12 years were reviewed. Vascular injuries occurred in 5% of cases, and brachial plexus damage in 6%. The mean patient age was 67 years. The dominant extremity was involved in 48 cases. Manipulation was used in most of the retrospective series. Three patients had primary open reduction without internal fixation. Neurologic recovery occurred in 4 of 5 patients having exploration of fracture-dislocation. Only 3 of the 32 patients had satisfactory results. Only 1 patient was free of pain, and over half the patients used analgesics regularly. The humeral head often was malrotated and the tuberosities displaced. Three patients had bony glenohumeral fusion, and 4 humeral heads exhibited avascular necrosis.

Some patients in the prospective series who had a disorganized upper humerus or displacement of the detached humeral head into the axilla underwent insertion of a Neer prosthesis. The 16 patients with severe displacement who were operated on had consistently better range of motion on follow-up than the 16 patients who were not operated on. Surgically treated patients made a more complete functional recovery. Loss of sleep and functional disability due to pain were more frequent in patients who were not operated on. Return of shoulder strength occurred more often after operative treatment. The 17 patients with minimally displaced fractures who were treated conservatively had results very similar to those obtained in cases of displaced fracture that were treated surgically.

Reconstruction of the upper humerus with insertion of a Neer prosthesis usually will restore function and relieve pain in patients with displaced four-part fractures of the humerus. Whatever treatment is used, disability is prolonged, and conscientious physiotherapy is essential. Intensive re-mobilization over 3–4 months may be necessary before these elderly patients are able to undertake activities of daily living without help. Alertness and determination are more important factors than age or physique.

▶ A particularly important aspect of this article is the analysis of those patients with four-part fractures or fracture dislocations who had nonoperative treatment. Some people have implied that patients with these fractures do well with nonoperative treatment. This study shows quite clearly that nonoperative treatment in these injuries will produce a very poor result in more than the majority of patients. It also shows that reconstruction using a prosthesis offers results that warrant surgery in this older age group. It also brings to light the importance of prolonged physical therapy and the contributions of mental alertness and determination to a successful result.—R.H.C.

Bristow-Latarjet Procedure for Recurrent Anterior Dislocation of the Shoulder: A 2- to 5-Year Follow-up Study on Results of 112 Cases
L. Körner, B. Lundberg, and T. Wredmark
Acta Orthop. Scand. 54:284–290, April 1983   1–31

The authors reviewed the results of 112 consecutive Bristow-Latarjet operations performed at four hospitals in Sweden from 1975 to 1979 for recurrent anterior shoulder dislocation. One of the patients had bilateral operations. The average follow-up was 30 months. Fifty-seven patients had operations on the dominant extremity. Most primary dislocations occurred before age 22 years. About one fifth of the dislocations were categorized as spontaneous. The goal of the procedure was to secure the tip of the coracoid process to the anterior part of the scapular neck medial to the glenoid rim. A malleolar screw was preferred.

Redislocation occurred in 6% of the cases and subluxations in another 7%. Five of the 7 redislocations occurred in the first postoperative year. Seven reoperations were necessary for reasons other than reluxation. There were 3 superficial infections but no deep postoperative infections. Operative fracture of the coracoid fragment appeared to increase the risk of recurrence or subluxation. An average of 10% of muscle strength was lost in the operated shoulder. Abduction was not significantly affected. Ten of the 12 patients who had poor results from previous operations had an excellent or good outcome. Osseous healing was seen in only about half of the cases.

The Bristow-Latarjet operation is an effective way of treating patients with chronic anterior shoulder instability. Ninety percent of the patients had excellent or good subjective results, and only 3 of the patients had a poor outcome. Most patients who had poor results after other surgery had good or excellent results after the Bristow-Latarjet procedure.

▶ This is a very good review of the Bristow type of procedure. The patient population is slightly heterogeneous. All patients had recurrent anterior dislocations of the shoulder; most dislocations were traumatic in origin, but 18% were classified as spontaneous. The 6% recurrence rate and an additional subluxation rate of 7% indicate that this procedure is certainly no more desirable than others for control of anterior shoulder instability. The loss of motion in external rotation and residual weakness also strongly suggest that this procedure is no better than others in avoidance of these postoperative limitations. Worrisome is the 10% reoperation rate to date and the knowledge that in 44% of the patients bony union did not occur between the coracoid tip and the glenoid. In fact, in 16% of these there was displacement of the coracoid tip away from the glenoid. While one may argue that this procedure is one of the acceptable alternatives for correction of anterior shoulder instability, one might also argue from this article, as well as others, that it really enjoys no advantages in terms of overall results and the complication rate may well be higher, considering the fairly frequent need for reoperation.—R.H.C.

2 Soft Tissue Trauma and Reconstruction

Gatewood and the First Thenar Pedicle
Roy A. Meals and Garry S. Brody
Plast. Reconstr. Surg. 73:315–319, February 1984   2–1

The authors discuss the career of Gatewood, a physician without a given first name who provided the first recorded description of the thenar flap in the *Journal of the American Medical Association* in 1926. Gatewood was much admired because of his honesty, modesty, and sincerity of purpose. Those who trained under him recall his consideration of their needs and aspirations. Gatewood was a general surgeon in the broadest sense, and was the author of 50 journal articles on subjects ranging from amebiasis, patellar fracture, and peptic ulcer to epiphyseal growth and esophageal stricture. His special interest was surgery of the stomach and duodenum. He was considered to be one of the best teachers on the faculty of Rush Medical School. His surgical leadership was widely recognized. Apart from Gatewood's devising the thenar flap, his advocacy of outpatient surgery was a prophetic effort.

► This simple but effective biographic essay by Meals and Brody should be read by every surgeon. It simply generates admiration for Gatewood and reviews one's own personal resolves to remain individual.—R.C.

Treatment of Nail Bed Avulsions With Split-Thickness Nail Bed Grafts
Glenn H. Shepard (Riverside Hosp., Newport News, Va.)
J. Hand. Surg. 8:49–54, January 1983   2–2

Available methods of treating nail bed avulsions are deficient. The author established the feasibility of split-thickness grafting of nail bed segments in the squirrel monkey and then applied the method to patients. The nail structure of the squirrel monkey resembles that of human nails grossly and microscopically. Thin grafts from the nail bed achieved an excellent take over avulsed areas in this model, following full-thickness excision of the nail bed distal to the proximal nail fold. Grafts 0.007- to 0.009-in. thick were used. Grafts were sutured over the defects. Most nails treated by split-thickness nail bed grafting were normal at follow-up, and microscopy showed a thinned but otherwise normal nail bed.

Thirty-one patients with avulsion of segments of the nail bed were treated in this way. The injured nail bed had enough residual tissue to serve as a donor site in 24 cases, while 7 patients received grafts from the

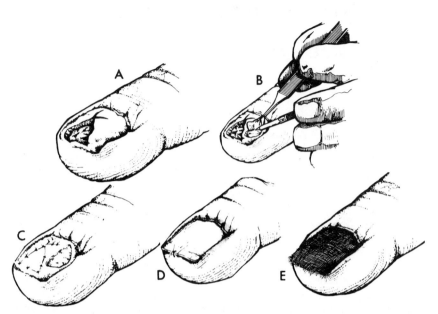

Fig 2–1.—A, full-thickness nail bed avulsion. **B,** split-thickness nail bed graft is removed using magnification. **C,** split-thickness nail bed graft is sutured over defect with 7-0 chromic catgut. **D,** the nail, when available, is replaced over the defect and a pressure dressing is applied. **E,** when the nail is not available, a single thickness of Betadine gauze is placed over the defect with the proximal portion slipped under the proximal nail fold. (Courtesy of Shepard, G.H.: J. Hand Surg. 8:49–54, January 1983.)

lateral third of the great toe. The technique of graft placement is illustrated in Figure 2–1. Five patients had either nonadherence of the nail or an irregular nail surface, while 26 had normal-appearing nails. No deformities occurred in graft donor areas. In contrast, nail deformities were present in all 4 other patients treated by rotation pedicle flaps, and nonadherence was seen in all 4 given dermal grafts.

Split-thickness nail bed grafting has the advantages of frequent availability of tissue on the injured digit and the absence of donor site deformity, whether on the injured digit or a donor great toe. Grafting is not necessary if microscopy shows that the avulsion is of partial thickness. The key to the procedure is the use of thin grafts that provide enough tissue to restore function to the lost nail bed segment without producing functional loss in the donor region.

▶ In recent years, much greater attention has been given to reconstruction of nail bed injuries. In most reports, it has been clear that acute repair provides much better results than late reconstruction. This technique has the advantage that local tissue often can be used, leaving no secondary donor deformity.— P.C.A.

Free Nail Bed Graft for Treatment of Nail Bed Injuries of the Hand
Hidehiko Saito, Yorio Suzuki, Keiji Fujino, and Tatsuya Tajima (Niigata Univ.)

J. Hand Surg. 8:171–178, March 1983

2–3

Split-skin grafting, intermediate dermal and reverse dermal grafting, and secondary healing all have failed to provide normal-appearing nails in patients with a severely crushed or avulsed nail bed but an intact matrix. The authors have achieved normal-appearing nails by free grafts of full-thickness nail bed from the lesser toes or from an amputated finger. This approach is useful in restoring fingertip length when used in conjunction with local skin flaps such as V-Y advancement or rotation flaps (Fig 2–2). The nail bed and matrix are removed in one piece, and the donor defect is covered with a small split-skin graft from the side of the foot. The graft is trimmed and placed in the finger defect. In type II and III injuries the hyponychium is reconstructed before the nail bed is grafted. In type IV injuries the eponychium may have to be reconstructed with local skin flaps.

This approach was used in 11 fingers of 10 patients. There were 4 type I injuries localized to the nail bed; 2 type II avulsion injuries of the dorsal part of the fingertip; 4 type III injuries, with amputation at the level of

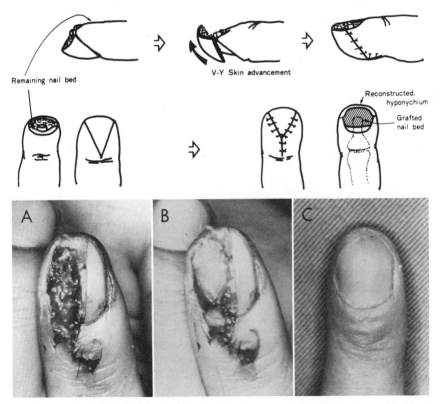

Fig 2–2 (top).—Lengthening of fingertip with V-Y advancement flap and reconstruction of nail bed with full-thickness nail bed graft.

Fig 2–3 (bottom).—Man, 28, with type I injury. A, before treatment; B, after nail bed graft has been sutured in place; and C, 15 months after operation.

(Courtesy of Saito, H., et al.: J. Hand Surg. 8:171–178, March 1983.)

the proximal part of the nail bed; and 1 type IV injury involving both the nail bed and the matrix. The outcomes in 2 cases of type I injury are shown in Figure 2–3. All 4 patients with type I injury regained normal-appearing nails. One with a type II case had a slightly rounded nail. The 3 evaluable patients with type III cases had nearly normal-appearing nails. The patient with a type IV injury regained a smooth, relatively good-looking nail. All grafts were from the lesser toes. No donor site problems have occurred.

Free full-thickness grafting of nail bed from the toe has given good cosmetic results in patients with severe injury of the nail bed but an intact matrix. The procedure can be combined with local skin flaps when length of the fingertip is being restored after amputation.

▶ Free nail bed grafts including a segment of the nail matrix from the toes, amputated segments, or discarded digits are important in reconstructing acute nail bed injuries. We have used reverse dermal grafts with fairly similar results (Clayburgh, R. H., et al.: *J. Hand Surg.* 8:594–599, September, 1983). Only one case of a chronic (late) nail bed injury is included in this series, and the result was only fair to good. Late nail bed reconstruction remains the real challenge. The importance of this article is the reminder to reconstruct nail bed fingertip injuries acutely with "like" tissues for the best result.—W.P.C.

The "Antenna" Procedure for the "Hook-Nail" Deformity

Erdogan Atasoy, Alan Godfrey, and Michael Kalisman (Univ. of Louisville)
J. Hand Surg. 8:55–58, January 1983   2–4

The hook-nail deformity often follows distal fingertip amputation with loss of part of the distal pulp, phalanx, and nail bed. The deformity may be of cosmetic importance, or it may be disabling to those with certain occupations. Four patients with the hook-nail deformity have been managed by an "antenna" procedure involving multiple Kirschner wires and were followed up for 1 to 4 years.

TECHNIQUE.—The nail plate is elevated from the nail bed along its full length, the part distal to the lunula is discarded, and the pulp skin is incised and reflected out to a normal contour. Scar tissue may have to be removed from the deep surface and margin of the pulp. The full-thickness nail bed is elevated from the distal phalanx back to where it is straight and is splinted there with two or three Kirschner pins inserted into the dorsum of the distal phalanx. The defect is covered by a cross-finger flap from the dorsum of the adjacent finger, which is divided after 2 weeks. The Kirschner pins are left in place for 3 weeks.

The antenna procedure supports the nail bed, and the cross-finger flap reconstructs the lost pulp and relieves the deforming tension. The viability of the elevated nail bed is not compromised as long as its continuity with the remaining proximal matrix and paronychial skin fold is not interrupted.

▶ Secondary nail reconstruction remains a difficult problem. In a select group of patients, this procedure may be of cosmetic value.—M.B.W.

The Extended Palmar Advancement Flap
A. Lee Dellon (Johns Hopkins Hosp.)
J. Hand Surg. 8:190–194, March 1983   2–5

Use of the palmar advancement flap in thumb reconstruction provides local tissue that is normally innervated and leaves acceptable scarring at the donor site. An extended version of this flap permits defects of up to 30 mm to be resurfaced without joint contracture resulting. The flap is extended proximally onto the thenar eminence, and the donor-site defects are closed using local rotation flaps. The procedure is illustrated in Figure 2–4. The classic midlateral incisions are extended so that both sets of neurovascular bundles are included within the flap. The incisions stop about 1 cm distal to the thenar crease. The princeps pollicis artery may have to be mobilized, as may the radial digital artery. The flap is elevated superficial to the tendon pulley system distally and the thenar muscle fascia proximally. The width of the flap over the thenar eminence is not critical. The distal tip of the flap is tailored as needed to provide a contoured profile to the thumb. The advanced palmar flap is sutured to the dorsal skin in reconstructing avulsed distal thumb segments, preserving a maximal amount of the remaining phalanx.

This approach has been used four times, with excellent functional and cosmetic results in all cases. All the patients returned to their previous work. Morbidity at the donor site was minimal, and first web space contractures did not develop. The only complication was an area of dorsal marginal necrosis on the radial side of the thumb, which healed secondarily with local wound care.

The extended palmar advancement flap is a reliable means of providing a greater supply of normally innervated tissue for resurfacing extensive distal palmar thumb defects. The use of local rotation flaps to close the donor site defects permits full extension of the thumb web space and prevents flexion contractures of the metacarpophalangeal and interphalangeal joints. No cortical relearning is necessary, but sensory reeducation does facilitate functional recovery.

▶ This flap may be useful in the reconstruction of certain thumb amputations; it does require extensive dissection, however. A cross-finger flap also may be used for the same injury, and it may avoid the extensive dissection of the flap described in this article. Sensibility may be restored by dissecting the branches of the radial nerve going to the cross-finger flap and anastomosing these to the digital nerves of the thumb.—P.C.A.

Open Treatment of Fingertip Amputations
R. P. Lamon, J. J. Cicero, R. J. Frascone, and W. F. Hass (St. Paul-Ramsey Med. Center, St. Paul, Minn.)
Ann. Emerg. Med. 12:358–360, June 1983   2–6

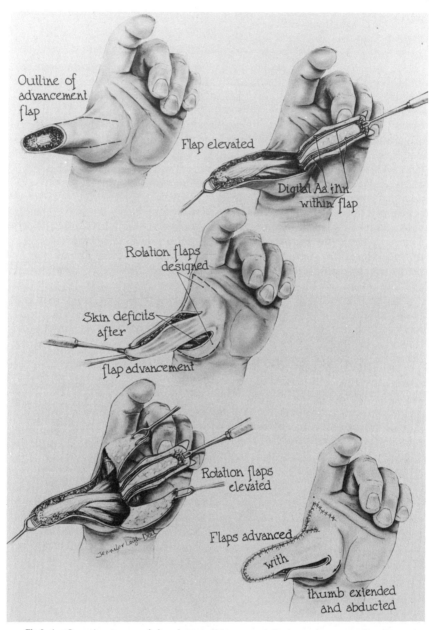

Outline of advancement flap

Flap elevated

Digital Ad. Nn. within flap

Rotation flaps designed

Skin deficits after flap advancement

Rotation flaps elevated

Flaps advanced with thumb extended and abducted

Fig 2–4.—Operative stages needed to elevate and inset extended palmar advancement flap. (Courtesy of Dellon, A.L.: J. Hand Surg. 8:190–194, March 1983.)

The results of open treatment of fingertip injuries were reviewed in 22 male and 3 female patients aged 5–77 years. Three patients were children. Eighteen injuries occurred at work and 7 at home. Crush injuries were most frequent, followed by cutting injuries. The left thumb and left index finger were the most frequently injured digits. Amputation occurred at or distal to the distal half of the fingernail in all cases. The finger was cleaned and the wound irrigated with saline under digital block anesthesia. The open wound was covered with bacitracin ointment, and a tubular gauze bandage and four-pronged plastic splint were applied. Systemic antibiotics were not given unless deep contamination was strongly suspected. Seven patients required debridement of fingernail, bone, or devitalized tissue. The wound was soaked in warm, mild soap solution and redressed 3 times a day, starting at 48 hours. Active range of motion exercises were done during the soak periods.

Patients often were able to return to work after 24 hours. Only 5 patients received systemic antibiotics. No wound infections occurred. The average time to complete reepithelialization was 29 days. All but 2 patients had normal sensation at this time. One patient had minimal partial loss of flexion at the distal interphalangeal joint. The outcome in 1 case is shown in Figure 2–5.

Open treatment of distal fingertip amputations provides for complete healing without infection, a return of normal sensation, preservation of joint mobility, and normal fingerpad contours. Systemic antibiotics need not be routinely administered if the wound is thoroughly cleansed and the devitalized tissue debrided.

▶ Healing by second intention is achieving more and more acceptance for the management of selected fingertip amputations. In appropriately selected patients, healing and return to work time are not prolonged over traditional sur-

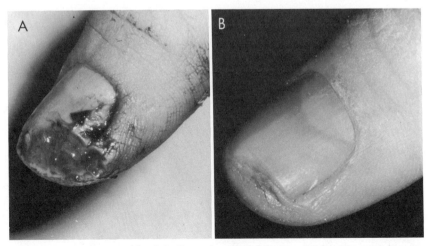

Fig 2–5.—**A**, amputation of thumb tip. **B**, complete reepithelialization at 43 days. (Courtesy of Lamon, R.P., et al.: Ann. Emerg. Med. 12:358–360, June 1983.)

gical methods that include skin grafting and local or remote flaps, and non-surgical treatment has the additional benefit of avoiding surgical complications.

It is important, however, to select patients properly. It is appropriate for any age group, but should be restricted to patients without significant pulp loss. Although volar, oblique wounds will contract and heal by second intention, frequently the resulting scar is adherent to the distal phalanx and rather tender. Procedures designed to provide additional soft tissue bulk, such as the thenar flap, may be more appropriate for these patients. Open treatment would appear ideal for patients with minimal or no bone exposed with transverse or dorsal oblique amputations of the fingertip.—P.C.A.

Local Arterialized Island Flap Coverage of Difficult Hand Defects Preserving Donor Digit Sensibility
Elliott H. Rose
Plast. Reconstr. Surg. 72:848–858, December 1983   2–7

Arterialized island pedicle flaps were used to resurface difficult hand wounds in 6 patients (average age, 30 years). The flaps were transferred from the lateral surface of a nearby digit beneath a subcutaneous bridge. The flap design (Fig 2–6) includes only the digital artery and small venules in the pedicle, preserving the digital nerve in continuity in the donor finger. This minimizes sensory loss, eliminates the need for cortical reeducation, and precludes multistage procedures for coverage. The lengthy pedicle permits a wide arc of coverage over the palm, dorsum of the hand, and adjacent digits. Defects as large as 6 × 2.5 cm can be covered. Where the flap is placed on the dorsum of the hand, the deep transverse metacarpal ligament can be partially divided to reduce traction on the pedicle. The donor site is covered with full-thickness skin from the groin. No specific systemic anticoagulants are used.

All 6 flaps survived totally. They were slightly plethoric for 2–3 days but developed normal capillary fill by the fourth postoperative day. The average flap was 4.25 cm long and 2.1 cm wide. The largest flap measured 5.5 × 2.5 cm. Two-point discrimination at the donor defect averaged 4.5 mm. Mild hypertrophic scarring occurred at the donor site in 1 case. Secondary neurolysis of the donor nerve was performed in 1 case, with full sensory return.

Use of a neurovascular island flap including only the digital artery and venae comitantes at its pedicle to cover difficult hand wounds has given favorable results. It is a single-stage procedure, and its versatility and proximity to the site of injury encourage its use for primary coverage. Either the radial or the ulnar surface of a nearby digit can be utilized. Pliable soft tissue coverage facilitates secondary reconstructive procedures. Larger defects should be covered by a more conventional distant flap or free microvascular flap.

▶ The author has presented another method of resurfacing the hand with critical soft tissue defects such as in joint coverage problems. This method ap-

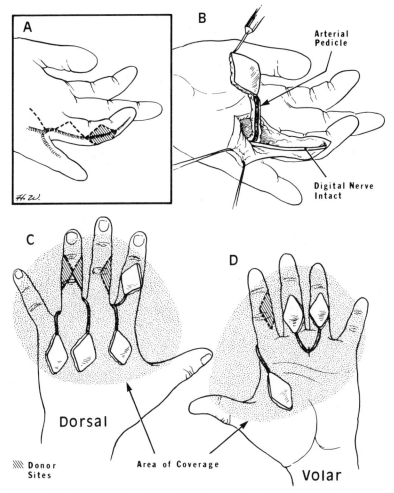

Fig 2–6.—Flap design. **A,** diamond-shaped island centered over digital artery. **B,** arterial pedicle is separated from donor digital nerves microscopically. **C** and **D,** the arc of coverage includes the adjacent digits and dorsum of the hand and palm. (Courtesy of Rose, E.H.: Plast. Reconstr. Surg. 72:848–858, December 1983.)

pears to have significant potential. Most authors would be reluctant to jeopardize the radial aspect of the index or long finger as the author's diagram suggests.—R.L.L.

One-Stage Flap Repair With Vascularized Tendon Grafts in a Dorsal Hand Injury Using the "Chinese" Forearm Flap

C. D. Reid and A. L. H. Moss (Frenchay Hosp., Bristol, England)
Br. J. Plast. Surg. 36:473–479, October 1983   2–8

Injuries of the dorsum of the hand with damage to the extensor mechanism are not infrequent and cause considerable morbidity. Skin flap transfer requires several stages over a considerable period. The authors describe a one-stage approach to repair of dorsal hand injuries with loss of both skin and tendon that does not require microvascular anastomoses. A radial forearm flap, or "Chinese" flap, is raised to provide skin cover along with the palmaris longus tendon and part of the tendinous portion of the brachioradialis for reconstructing the finger extensors. The tendons lie within condensed deep fascia or close to the intermuscular septum, and therefore remain well-vascularized when the flap is harvested. The radial nerve is preserved.

The "Chinese" flap is a local one-stage reconstruction that provides rapid healing, with a possible reduction in adhesion formation between the tendons and recipient bed. No thinning of the flap is necessary. There is no functional deficit at the donor site. Postoperative mobilization is possible with a shorter hospital stay. The flap is very versatile. Vascularized bone from the radius can be incorporated in it, as can the cutaneous nerves of the forearm. The donor site in female patients can be repaired with other skin flaps. Cold intolerance and claudication in the hand may occur after radial artery division, especially in young manual workers. The vessel could be vein-grafted if indicated. Flap edema can be minimized by reconstructing a superficial vein or by early use of a pressure garment.

The disadvantages of the "Chinese" flap repair of dorsal hand injuries are outweighed by the advantages. Early restoration of normal function is possible using this method in cases of loss of skin on the dorsum of the hand and the extensor tendon.

▶ The radial forearm flap as described is very useful for dorsal, volar, or combined dorsal and volar skin coverage of the hand. Extensor tendon reconstruction is often simultaneously necessary. We have found a conventional tendon grafting approach in combination with the described flap to be very successful. It is questionable whether a "vascularized tendon graft" in combination with this flap represents a significant advantage.—M.B.W.

Antecubital Fasciocutaneous Flap
B. G. H. Lamberty and G. C. Cormack
Br. J. Plast. Surg. 36:428–433, October 1983   2–9

Anatomical studies of the vascular territories of the forearm have suggested that a significant length-to-breadth fasciocutaneous flap can be raised on the inferior cubital artery. The authors have used this flap as a pedicle flap in one case and as a free flap in another case after doing cadaver studies. Ideally, the axial line of the flap lies along the cephalic vein, directed from the origin of the vessel below the midinterepicondylar point to the radial styloid process. In one case the flap midline was in the midforearm line because of a previous skin graft procedure, but the flap survived on a 4:1 length-to-breadth ratio. The flap has a wide arc of

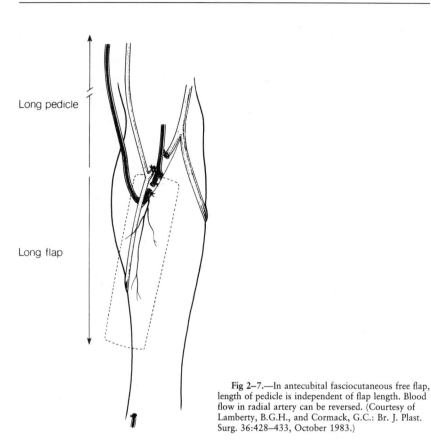

Long pedicle

Long flap

The antecubital
fasciocutaneous free flap

Fig 2–7.—In antecubital fasciocutaneous free flap, length of pedicle is independent of flap length. Blood flow in radial artery can be reversed. (Courtesy of Lamberty, B.G.H., and Cormack, G.C.: Br. J. Plast. Surg. 36:428–433, October 1983.)

rotation and can be used as cover for the elbow or as a distant flap. The flap is not used in the absence of an adequate-sized inferior cubital artery or when this vessel arises from a radial recurrent coming from the brachial artery rather than the radial.

The current design of a fasciocutaneous skin flap raised on the radial artery depends on septal perforators for its blood supply. In the distal forearm these perforators are small and their axiality is directed transversely. Use of a flap based on the inferior cubital artery permits a large skin flap to be raised along with a long vascular pedicle (Fig 2–7), overcoming a constraint of the present design and permitting more versatile flap orientation at the recipient site. Circulatory complications are likely to be significantly less frequent with use of this flap. Venous drainage is best achieved via the cephalic vein, rather than via a reverse flow in the radial venae comitantes.

▶ This article presents two clinical cases using a fasciocutaneous flap based on the inferior cubital artery. A pedicle flap was used in one case and a free flap in the other; both represent clinical applications of previous work done by Lamberty and Cormack in defining a blood supply to the skin of the forearm. These studies were published in the *British Journal of Plastic Surgery* in October, 1983. This work should be referred to for a better understanding of the blood supply on which this flap is based.

The authors compare this flap to the "Chinese" or radial arm flap. They state that the antecubital flap has a longer pedicle and is not related to the length of the flap, whereas in the Chinese flap, the length of the pedicle is inversely proportional to the length of the flap. However, it should be noted that when they speak of "pedicle," they are only referring to the vein, which can be quite long. The arterial pedicle is limited, as it can only be taken up to the bifurcation of the brachial artery. It would be nice if this flap could be harvested based entirely on the inferior cubital artery, with the radial artery left intact, but apparently this vessel is too small (0.5 to 1 mm in the authors' studies) for routine use, so the authors included a segment of the radial artery. Despite this, it would still have some advantage over the radial arm flap in that only a small segment of radial artery need be taken and, thus, could be reconstituted with a shorter vein graft.

I think this represents a nice piece of laboratory investigation followed up with clinical application in two cases.—G.B.I.

Simultaneous Bilateral Staged Groin Flaps for Coverage of Mutilating Injuries of the Hand

Paul M. Heath, Ian T. Jackson, William P. Cooney III (Mayo Clinic), and R. G. Morgan (Norwood, Australia)
Ann. Plast. Surg. 11:462–468, December 1983   2–10

The groin flap is useful in early wound closure of massive hand injuries because it is less hirsute than the hypogastric flap and is in a better site for comfort and for donor site scarring. It is the only axial flap that can be comfortably paired with an adjacent axial pattern flap to cover both aspects of the hand completely. The flap is based on the superficial circumflex iliac artery. Collateral vessels are present that may allow extension of the flap to the lateral border of the erector spinae. Immediate or early coverage of relatively uncontaminated degloving injuries is preferred. Bilateral groin flaps are designed slightly larger than the defects to be covered. The flap width can be as great as 20 cm, but usually averages 10 cm. The safe flap length has been reported as being 30 cm, extending to the posterior axillary line, or to the lateral border of the erector spinae muscles. The flaps are tubed when possible, and the donor defects are closed directly. Whether or not to delay the flap depends partly on its appearance and on the inset size. Division usually is carried out at 3 weeks, with insetting 2 to 3 days afterward.

The groin flap procedure is a safe and reliable means of covering extensive mutilating hand injuries. A flap has survived after accidental division of the artery. Thumb reconstruction can be undertaken simultaneously with coverage by bilateral groin flaps. The second flap may allow bone graft transfer with at least some intact periosteal blood supply. Extension of the groin flap to its limits provides coverage that is adequate for reconstructing defects that extend proximal to the wrist.

► The particular suitability of bilateral groin flaps for resurfacing circumferential injuries to the hand is pointed out by this article. I would think that a single free groin flap also could be wrapped around the hand and the 3 weeks of immobilization necessary for flap vascularization from the recipient site could be avoided, at least in some cases.—P.C.A.

Flaps of the Latissimus Dorsi Muscle in Difficult Wounds of the Trunk and Arm
William D. Morain (Dartmouth-Hitchcock Med. Center, Hanover, N.H.)
Am. J. Surg. 145:520–525, April 1983   2–11

The latissimus dorsi muscle has the largest surface area of any extremity-related muscle unit of the human body. This fact, along with the muscle's dual blood supply, gives it special value for use in reconstructive surgery. Its location makes it of potential value in reconstructing the abdomen, thorax, vertebral area, and arm. The chief vascular supply to the latissimus dorsi is the thoracodorsal artery and vein. The entire muscle with overlying skin can be rotated around the thoracodorsal vessel pivot point to reach the anterior or posterior trunk or arm. A series of large, paraspinous, perforating vessels is used as a secondary blood supply and can carry a sizeable part of the muscle with overlying skin as a distally based flap.

Variations in flap design have been used successfully to reconstruct large wounds in the scapular region, the sternocostal region, the anterior thoracicoabdominal area, the axilla and breast, the vertebral and paravertebral areas, the intrathoracic cavities in pleurocutaneous fistula, and the arm. The flap can be transferred as a single unit or split longitudinally. The origin and insertion of the muscle should be divided in complex reconstructive settings. Transfer without skin is advocated when a flap is placed intrathoracically for pleurocutaneous fistula closure. The latissimus dorsi has excellent two-dimensional tensile strength, and alloplastic mesh or bone graft support usually will not be necessary after abdominal or moderate-sized chest wall reconstructions. The risk of infection is greater in an area of ulceration of an irradiated or malignant lesion if nonvascular materials are present.

► Doctor Morain has elaborated on additional applications of the versatile and highly adaptable latissimus dorsi flaps in split modes, with or without overlying skin, and based either laterally or medially. In a more fundamental sense, he has shown in the case presentations the important contribution of blood supply of the sort brought by muscle flaps to difficult, contaminated, postirradiation wounds. Either the pectoralis muscle flap that I have used or the latissimus dorsi flap may be very effective in intrathoracic plumbage to fill empyema spaces with vascularized autogenous tissue.

Flaps of the sort described by Doctor Morain make curative, albeit destructive, irradiation more acceptable and legitimate in treatment of advanced malignancies, as demonstrated in 5 of his 7 cases. This principle also applies to curative surgery that requires removal of important muscles in the upper extremity. Such ablation is done less reluctantly when replacement with trunk muscle, as an innervated and vascularized flap, is possible. The choice of donor muscles multiplies tremendously when free, microneural, and microvascular transfers are considered when dealing with difficult wounds that demand coverage or muscle function, or both.—R.A.C.

3 Thermal, Chemical, and Radiation Burns

Prospective Study of Burn Wound Excision of the Hands
Cleon W. Goodwin, Molly S. Maguire, William F. McManus, and Basil A. Pruitt, Jr. (Brooke Army Med. Center)
J. Trauma 23:510–517, June 1983   3–1

The exact role of early excisional therapy of burns of the dorsa of the hands is undefined. Ninety-eight consecutive patients with 164 burned hands involving the entire dorsum and all digits. The patients had second-degree, deep second-degree, or third-degree injuries above the level of the tendons and joint capsules. Mean age was 29 years, and the mean burn was 37% of the body surface area. Sixty-seven patients had early excision and grafting of their hand burns; the other 31 were managed nonoperatively at the outset. Early excision was done in the first or second week after injury. Unexpanded 1.5:1 mesh grafts were used in most cases. The control patients had eschar débridement as indicated and received continuous topical antimicrobial therapy.

Early operation did not affect survival adversely. Excision and grafting of deep dermal burns offered no apparent advantage over primary healing with physical therapy with regard to maintenance of hand function. Hands with more superficial injuries also responded as well to nonoperative as to early operative management. Early excision and grafting of third-degree injuries tended to worsen the outcome, but the differences were not statistically significant.

The findings fail to support the widespread belief that early excision and grafting preserve hand function better than a conservative approach after thermal injury of the dorsum of the hand. Early excision and grafting of selected full-thickness injuries of the hands may be indicated in patients with small total body surface burns to reduce the hospital stay. Patients with massive injuries, however, should have early operation for area coverage, not for excision of hand burns.

▶ This is an excellent article that addresses an area of controversy about the treatment of burns of the hands. The very basic question is whether to treat such burns conservatively with topical antibiotics, hydrotherapy, and physical therapy and then later skin graft the ones that don't heal or to treat them more aggressively by early surgical excision and grafting; the bottom line is the functional end result.

There has been a trend in recent years toward early surgical excision and grafting, and the claim has been that this provided a superior functional result. This article would tend to contradict that thinking. The study comes from the

Brooke Army Medical Center, which has one of the largest burn units in the United States. This is a large series involving 164 burned hands. It's a prospective study, although not randomized, because most of these patients had burn injuries involving other parts of the body, which limited the authors' ability to randomize the hands completely.

The most controversial hand burn is the deep dermal burn because such burns are often difficult to assess accurately as far as the depth of injury, and the best form of treatment to select has been a problem. The very superficial dermal burns are no problem because they heal spontaneously. The obviously full-thickness burns are no problem as far as determining what to do because they will all need to be skin grafted. These two latter groups were eliminated from this article, and only the problem of the deep dermal burn was addressed. The authors concluded that there was no significant difference in the end result whether this group of patients was treated aggressively by surgical excision and grafting or conservatively, allowing the wound to heal or allowing the eschar to slough and then grafting the wound.—G.B.I.

The Trapezoid Flap for the Correction of Burn Scar Contractures
A. D. Scotland and A. M. Morris
Br. J. Plast. Surg. 36:291–294, July 1983   3–2

Correction of flexion contracture due to scarring is particularly difficult after burn injury of the hand, where posttraumatic syndactyly may be marked. The authors describe a method of scar contracture release that appears to circumvent many of the difficulties associated with Z-plasty, V-Y advancement, and incision of the contracture with split-skin grafting of the defect. A sliding trapezoid flap that is wider distally and includes scar tissue or old skin graft in its substance is used (Figs 3–1 and 3–2). The flap shrinks and slides proximally as it is elevated on a deep subcutaneous base, permitting distorted structures adjacent to the contracture to resume normal position. Small back cuts can be made to allow the end of the flap to be inset in its new position. The secondary defect is covered with a split-skin graft. Active and passive exercises are begun as soon as the graft is stable.

Thirteen trapezoid flaps were used in 5 patients without any flap necrosis occurring. Full release of all contractures was obtained except in a boy with dense contracture of the elbow joint capsule due to electric burn injury. The preoperative deformities have not recurred on follow-up for 6–18 months.

The trapezoid flap technique is a means of providing a considerable two-dimensional release of scar contractures. At the same time, it allows the free release of adjacent normal tissues previously distorted by scarring and returns them to their natural position.

▶ This looks like a reasonable approach to this problem. The main advantage is that it leaves skin with subcutaneous tissue at the flexion crease where

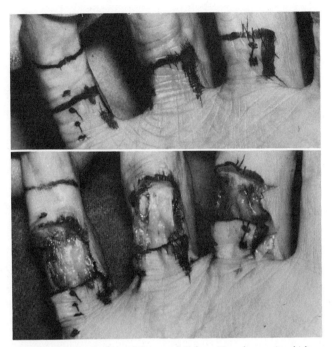

Fig 3–1 (top).—Preoperative marking of the trapezoid flaps. Note the way in which normal skin at the base of the digits has been distorted and drawn distally.

Fig 3–2 (bottom):—After release of all the trapezoid flaps, note how the flaps have retracted proximally and allowed the distorted normal tissue in the web spaces to return to their natural position.

(Courtesy of Scotland, A.D., and Morris, A.M.: Br. J. Plast. Surg. 36:291–294, July 1983.)

there is movement, resulting in a defect for skin grafting over a stationary area. This maneuver is basically the same in principle as a V-Y procedure, the difference being that the release incision is rectangular rather than triangular and the resultant defect is grafted rather than closed. Unless the skin is normal on both sides of this flap and very pliable, one would likely have to add back cuts at the base of the flap that would leave small, triangular defects that would have to be skin grafted (see Figure 3). The authors do not mention how long these flaps could be relative to their base. They do mention that 1 of the 13 flaps necrosed.

An alternative way to release contracture in a flexion crease is with a double apposed Y incision. This would create an effect similar to that described by Scotland and Morris, but with combined proximal and distal releases, again leaving a central rectangular area to be grafted.—G.B.I.

▶ For smaller degrees of contracture, Nathan (*J. Hand Surg.* 9A:43–53, 1984) has recommended double V-Y flaps at the interphalangeal joints. In essence, a diamond-shaped incision is made over the contracted joint, and length is obtained proximally and distally as one would for a Kleinert-Atasoy type flap at the fingertip with perpendicular dissection without undermining, followed by V-Y closure.—P.C.A.

Clinodactyly Following Electric Burn: Observations on Two Cases

A. Fingerhut, M. Brocard, and R. Ronat (Poissy, France)
Sem. Hop. Paris 59:2131–2134, September 1983   3–3

Rare as they are, most clinodactylies after burns are essentially due to cutaneous or ligamentous lesions, osseous involvement being rather the exception. Two patients with unilateral epiphyseal lesions at the level of the distal interphalangeal articulation recently were encountered and treated. In the first case, an angular deformity at the distal interphalangeal joint was discovered several months after a seemingly minor electric burn of the hand in a patient aged 16. A similar case of minor electric burn to the hand of a child aged 7 was subsequently discovered to have produced incipient deformity and was treated successfully with percutaneous pinning.

Voltage and duration of contact are the two major factors in determination of possible sequelae; the bloodstream acts as a conductor for the current, which explains the occurrence of ischemic lesions at a distance from the burn site. Recent anatomical studies (e.g., Braun, 1977) have revealed the existence, in certain persons, of an asymmetric digital vascularization with a prominent collateral artery, which is internal for the thumb and index finger and external for the fourth finger. It is known that ischemia may be responsible for cartilaginous articular lesions of the phalanges without involvement of the diaphysis. The latest arteriographic studies suggest that the vascularization of the epiphyses is assured by an arteriole other than the one that supplies the diaphyses. These epiphyseal arteries arise either perpendicularly from the distal phalangeal arc or, mainly in the young, from the predominant collateral artery itself at the level of the phalangeal head. One hypothesis merits attention: a thrombosis related to selective unilateral involvement by electric diffusion along one of these epiphyseal arteries could explain the progressive necrosis of a condyle or flange at the base of a phalange. It would then be a matter of an epiphysiolysis by ischemia.

In light of these observations, regular and prolonged surveillance appears to be necessary in cases of even seemingly insignificant electric burns of the extremities. If a deformity appears, a splint or temporary pinning can prevent a significant clinodactyly.

▶ This article brings to our attention a particular complication of electric burns, namely, late osteonecrosis of a phalangeal condyle. The authors present two cases in children and postulate that this complication may be more prominent in children because of the increased blood supply to the condylar or epiphyseal area in persons in this age group.

Their first case was discovered retrospectively after the development of angular deformity at the distal interphalangeal joint several months after an apparently minor electric burn to the hand.

A second similar case of minor electric burn to the hand in a child subsequently was treated, and early deformity was detected and managed successfully by percutaneous pinning.

The authors' recommendations are sound: patients, particularly children, with electric burns of the hand need to be observed for late complications of osteonecrosis. These complications may develop several months after the initial burn has healed. Early diagnosis may provide for successful treatment by splinting either internally or externally. Even if splinting is unsuccessful in preventing a collapse of the osteonecrotic segment, secondary soft tissue contractures can be avoided. I also agree with the authors that arthrodesis is appropriate for cases with existing collapse or those in whom splinting is unsuccessful.

It should be noted also that similar deformities can occur after cold injury, although frostbite growth deformities usually are symmetrical. Brown, Spiegel, and Boyle have recently reviewed this topic (Pediatrics 71:955–959, 1983).—P.C.A.

Assessment of Tissue Viability in Frostbite by ^{99m}Tc Pertechnetate Scintigraphy
Zarrindokht Salimi, Wenzel Vas, Premsri Tang-Barton, Rama G. Eachempati, Lucy Morris, and Michael Carron (St. Louis City Hosp.)
AJR 142:415–419, February 1984   3–4

Pertechnetate scintigraphy for assessment of tissue viability was used in 6 cases of severe frostbite injury of the extremity. A total of 14 extremities were involved, including the feet in 1 patient. A flow study was carried out using 15 mCi of ^{99m}Tc-pertechnetate and a large-field-of-view gamma camera having a low-energy collimator. Static images then were obtained. Normally finger activity appears in the same frame as the palmar arch or the next frame when sequential images are recorded for 16 frames at a rate of 2 seconds per frame. When flow in the radial and ulnar arteries is equal, all the fingers fill at the same time and with the same intensity.

All 5 patients with perfusion defects in the fingers required surgical excision of the involved areas. A patient with hyperemia of the hands but no perfusion defects and another patient with hyperemic changes in the feet required only conservative management. One of the patients followed up showed reperfusion of 2 distal phalanges with initially reduced perfusion. They did not require surgery, but the other 3 distal phalanges, with persistent defects, eventually required amputation. The other patient followed up also had surgery for digits with persistent defects.

Pertechnetate imaging can distinguish viable from nonviable tissue in patients with severe frostbite injury of the hands and feet. The test is simple and noninvasive, and the findings are easy to interpret. Nonviable tissue appears as a perfusion defect that persists on follow-up imaging. Viable but hyperemic tissue exhibits increased soft tissue uptake and indistinct vascular structures. Initial imaging should be done within 24–48 hours after injury, and a repeat study should be done 7–10 days later.

▶ We have used technetium scanning, early phase, for the evaluation of peripheral vascular disease over the past 5 years. We feel this offers quantitative data as to the degree of peripheral blood flow and, correspondingly, tissue viability. The authors have extended this technique to the assessment of frostbite injuries. The series is small (only 6 patients) and the results are qualitatively interpreted by the examining physician as to the amount or degree of radiographic uptake, i.e., blood flow. Improved counting techniques should provide a more quantitative number for future references. The study, even as it stands, presents an excellent technique for evaluation and selection of treatment modalities for frostbite injuries. It is important that early counts, within the first 10 to 60 seconds, be performed and that these be standardized for each patient in order to have clinical significance. I would recommend this technique not only for frostbite injuries and burns, but also for other forms of vascular ischemia.–N.P.C.

Treatment of Frostbite With Intra-arterial Prostaglandin E₁

Richard A. Yeager, Thomas W. Campion, John C. Kerr, Robert W. Hobson, II, and Thomas G. Lynch
Am. Surg. 49:665–667, December 1983   3–5

In frostbite, tissue destruction is minimized by rapid rewarming of frozen parts. Frostbite victims often are seen after slow rewarming has taken place, however, and no effective treatment is known in these circumstances. Prostaglandin E_1 (PGE_1) could be useful because it encourages vasodilation and inhibition of platelet aggregation. The authors examined the efficacy of intra-arterial PGE_1 infusion in a rabbit hindlimb model of frostbite. Anesthetized animals had the hindlimb immersed in 50% ethylene glycol solution at -15 C. The subcutaneous temperature was maintained at this level for 15 minutes after the submerged limb reached -15 C. Either slow rewarming over 1 hour at room temperature or rapid rewarming at 42 C was carried out, followed by no treatment or intra-arterial bolus injections of physiologic saline, reserpine, or PGE_1. Prostaglandin E^1 was given in a dose of 10^{-1} $\mu g/kg^{-1}/minute^{-1}$ for 3 hours or in intra-arterial bolus injections of 10^{-1} $\mu g/kg^{-1}$. Tissue loss was estimated after 30 days.

Animals that received a 3-hour infusion of PGE_1 after slow rewarming had less tissue loss than those rewarmed slowly but not treated and those given saline only. The findings in the former animals were similar to those in rapidly rewarmed rabbits. Animals that were rewarmed slowly and given bolus injections of reserpine or bolus injections of PGE_1 had more tissue loss than those given a 3-hour infusion of PGE_1 and not significantly less loss than those animals having slow rewarming and no adjunctive treatment. Rapidly rewarmed animals that received a 3-hour infusion of PGE_1 did not differ significantly from those rapidly rewarmed animals that did not.

Intra-arterial PGE_1 may prove clinically useful in the treatment of frostbite patients. An infusion after slow rewarming led to significant tissue salvage in the present study of rabbits with cold injury to a hindlimb. Rapid rewarming alone remains the most effective treatment of frostbite. Where it is not feasible, using intra-arterial PGE_1 may be worthwhile.

▶ This is an interesting experiment. The clinical applicability will require further assessment.—R.L.L.

Hydrofluoric Acid Burns of the Hand
Ronald R. Straub (Mesa, Ariz.)
Orthopedics 6:978–980, August 1983   3–6

Hydrofluoric acid is a commonly used industrial substance, especially in the semiconductor industry. It is an extremely strong inorganic acid that readily penetrates the skin and deep tissues, causing liquefaction necrosis and erosion of underlying bone. The acid also can be absorbed through the respiratory tract, causing acute respiratory failure and pulmonary edema. The severity of tissue damage is related directly to both the concentration of the acid and the duration of exposure. Hand burns usually produce intense pain, and skin blistering and surrounding erythema often are seen. The author encountered two cases of hydrofluoric acid burn of the hand, incurred in etching circuits. One patient had a thumb injury that resolved after débridement and local calcium gluconate injections. The other was similarly treated for a burn of the thumb at the pulp and nail region, but developed reflex sympathetic dystrophy and required complete removal of the thumb nail when stellate ganglion blocks failed to produce persistent relief. Significant improvement did not occur until ulnar nerve transposition was done and a second series of stellate ganglion blocks carried out.

Initial treatment of any caustic burn of the skin involves copious irrigation with water and sodium bicarbonate solution, if available. Application of magnesium oxide paste (hydrofluoric acid burn ointment) may be helpful. Repeated injections of 10% calcium gluconate solution into the skin and subcutaneous tissues are indicated in a dose of about 0.5 ml/ sq cm of burn area. Pain may respond to digital blocks with 1% plain Xylocaine. If the subungual area is involved, partial or complete removal of the nail may be necessary so that calcium gluconate can be instilled into the underlying tissues. Any blisters or eschar should be debrided. Appropriate antibiotic coverage should be given. Cooling with iced Zephiran or hyamine soaks may restrict blood flow and reduce edema formation. Studies have suggested that magnesium acetate and magnesium sulfate may be preferable to calcium salts, but this has not been confirmed.

▶ Hydrofluoric acid burns are uncommon but cause severe injury, and immediate appropriate treatment is necessary to minimize this.

The treatment is copious irrigation, topical magnesium oxide paste, injections of 10% calcium gluconate into the involved tissues, and pain relief, in addition to standard treatment for the burn. Little is said about the mechanism of action of the magnesium oxide paste and calcium gluconate. When the hydrofluoric acid comes into contact with the skin, hydrogen gas is released and the fluoride ions penetrate the skin and combine with various salts in the skin, remaining active for some time and producing soft tissue injury. The idea of the topical and injected solutions mentioned above is to bind the fluoride ions, to either keep them from penetrating the skin or to inactivate them. The sooner this treatment is started, the less tissue damage there will be.

In the second patient, the thumb nail bed area was involved and the nail ultimately was removed. This is a particularly troublesome area, and I would recommend immediate removal of the nail if it is involved with a hydrofluoric acid burn.

A point that is not raised in this article may dictate hospitalization. The injection of calcium gluconate is usually quite painful, and consideration should be given to preceding this with an intravenously administered narcotic or regional anesthesia.—G.B.I.

Management of Extensive Doxorubicin Hydrochloride Extravasation Injuries
Ronald M. Linder, Joseph Upton, and Robert Osteen (Harvard Med. School)
J. Hand Surg. 8:32–38, January 1983   3–7

Indolent chemical burns from subcutaneous extravasation of doxorubicin is one of the major side effects of the use of this drug for treating leukemia, lymphoma, and many cancers. Forty patients seen in 1978–1981 with extensive doxorubicin extravasation injuries were followed for at least 6 months. All patients had a loss of at least 300 sq cm of tissue in the upper arm or forearm or significant soft tissue loss over the hand or palmar part of the wrist with exposure of important structures. All were managed surgically. Eighteen patients were children. The most common primary diagnosis was leukemia. The dose of extravasated drug was estimated at 3 to 10 mg in all instances.

Most injuries were in the upper extremity. Treatment consisted of initial débridement and subsequent wound closure. The operating microscope often was used to insure clearance of involved neurovascular structures. The open wounds were covered by dressings moistened in half-strength sodium hypochlorite. Most of the 34 surviving patients had wound closure by split-thickness skin grafting. Local flaps were used in 2 cases, and a distant abdominal flap in 3 cases, to protect extensor tendons without vascularized paratenon. A wide range of nosocomial organisms was present in the wounds, with very little inflammation. Ten patients presented with sepsis and positive blood cultures. Seven developed nerve compression syndromes. Eleven patients had a residual sympathetic dystrophy syndrome. Nearly all patients whose wounds were not closed within 3–4 weeks developed permanent joint stiffness. Late partial skin graft loss occurred in 11 cases.

Extensive doxorubicin paravenous extravasation injuries have a chronic, indolent course characterized by marked pain and ulceration. The best initial management remains unclear; it is hoped that agents will be found that will inactivate the drug when placed in the area of extravasation. Very few lesions heal spontaneously. Immediate excision of all red crystalline deposits will yield the most predictable results. The simplest, most expeditious means of wound coverage should be used; usually this is skin grafting. Doxorubicin should be administered only by those familiar with the risks. Peripheral infusions should be given through small, flexible polyethylene catheters, and critical anatomical sites should be avoided.

▶ The Bell curve of toxic substances introduced into the body for therapeutic purposes and most often obtaining access via the upper extremity is still on the rise. This well-documented article surveys the tragic experiences with one typical and popular agent. It tells how to cope with the resulting problems but, more importantly, it discusses how the majority of them may be avoided.— J.H.D.

Chronic Radiation Dermatitis From Radioactive Gold Jewelry
L. William Luria, H. Berman, and S. Satchidanand (Buffalo Genl. Hosp.)
N. Y. State J. Med. 83:741–743, April 1983   3–8

Three patients were seen recently with chronic radiation dermatitis of areas of the hands which were in contact with gold jewelry. None reported repeated exposure to ionizing radiation. It was learned that radioactive gold (^{198}Au) had contaminated the local gold supply, and the two pieces of jewelry tested were radioactive. At present, the problem appears to be mainly in the state of New York. The jewelry had been worn for 15 months to 18 years. Skin dryness, cracking, and bleeding were symptoms that were noticed. All 3 biopsy specimens showed chronic radiation dermatitis.

Chronic radiation dermatitis appears as thin, dry skin that is smooth, shiny, and hairless in its early stages. Telangiectasia and a wartlike keratosis may develop, followed by ulceration and development of carcinoma. The early stages can be mistaken for senile changes, secondary to actinic damage. Pain and itching may be present in acute and chronic cases. Chronic dermatitis results from repeated "suberythermal" doses of ionizing radiation. Excision biopsy should be strongly considered for lesions associated with gold jewelry if the piece of jewelry is not available for testing. The preferred treatment when the diagnosis is confirmed has been wide excision and full-thickness skin graft reconstruction. A 2-mm margin is maintained around the lesions. No complications of healing occurred in any of the patients.

▶ Hopefully, better control mechanisms for radioactive waste have eliminated potential future problems of this sort. It would appear for the present that radiation dermatitis should be included in the differential diagnosis of skin lesions in association with gold jewelry.—P.C.A.

Microwave Radiation Injury
Judith E. Tintinalli, Gary Krause (Wayne State Univ.), and E. Gursel (Detroit Receiving Hosp.)
Ann. Emerg. Med. 12:645–647, October 1983   3–9

Several uses of microwave radiation have been found in medicine and several more can be expected in the future, so the opportunities for accidental exposure are increasing. The authors report what is believed to be the third case of extremity injury in the English language literature.

Man, 35, had momentary exposure of the right hand to microwave radiation while heating a sandwich in a microwave oven at work because the appliance did not shut off when the door was opened. The hand was white and cold when it was withdrawn from the oven. Paresthesias were present in all fingers 30 minutes later and the hand was pale and cold. Capillary pulsations were reduced, and there was a 60-second delay in return of color after compression and release of the radial and ulnar pulses. Motor strength and sensation were intact. The hand was entirely normal an hour after exposure and on follow-up a week later.

The interactions of microwaves with the human body is virtually impossible to predict. Cataracts have developed in exposed laboratory animals, and irradiation also has been reported to lead to hypotension and bradycardia. Ischemic necrosis and incapacitating paresthesias in the hand have resulted from brief exposures to microwave radiation. Coagulation necrosis that cannot be reversed apparently can result from this form of irradiation. Public education in the potential adverse effects of microwave radiation exposure is necessary. Persons with total body exposure but no obvious specific injury should be followed up for possible ocular or testicular complications.

▶ This presentation is highly informative, and the reader should be referred to the original article itself for a detailed discussion of the potential hazards of microwave radiation.—R.D.B.

4 Nerve Trauma and Reconstruction

Peripheral Nerve Repairs With Clotting Substances: Experimental and Clinical
T. Futami, M. Yamamoto, A. Kobayashi, and M. Nishida (Kitasato Univ., Kanagawa, Japan)
J. West. Pacific Orthop. Assoc. 20:35–39, June 1983   4–1

Clotting substances were used by the authors for nerve anastomosis in the hope of avoiding the nerve damage that occurs even with microsurgical techniques. Human fibrinogen solutions and thrombin with calcium chloride and trasylol have been employed. Biomechanical studies using flexor carpi radialis tendons from fresh cadavers indicated that the fibrin suture is of adequate adhering strength within 30 seconds (Fig 4–1). Studies of rat sciatic nerves that were severed and repaired with the fibrin suture method showed some regeneration of nerve fibers after about 4 months and significant axonal regeneration at 5 months.

Over 20 clinical cases now have been treated and followed for less than 2 years. Significant recovery of nerve function was obtained in most cases

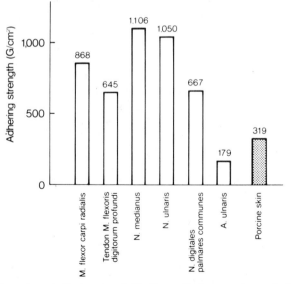

Fig 4–1.—Comparison of adhering strength. Significant adhering strength was obtained with mean value of about 800 gm/cu cm for the peripheral nerve and about 1,000 gm/cu cm for the flexor tendon. (Courtesy of Futami, T., et al.: J. West. Pacific Orthop. Assoc. 20:35–39, June 1983.)

by glueing the nerve ends with fibrin paste. The nerve ends can be approximated without producing further tissue damage, and microsurgical equipment is not needed. There is no foreign body reaction. The fibrin paste is resorbed within 3 weeks after its application.

▶ This very preliminary report again brings up the possibility of using clotting substances as a form of "biologic suture." The procedure is recommended based on its speed, simplicity, and low cost. Comparative data regarding extent of neuroma formation and quality of reinnervation are lacking. This remains an experimental procedure.—P.C.A.

Sensory Electroneurographic Parameters and Clinical Recovery of Sensibility in Sutured Human Nerves
W. Tackmann, J. Brennwald, and H. Nigst (Univ. of Basel)
J. Neurol. 229:195–206, May 1983   4–2

Thirty-seven patients with traumatic transection of 41 median and ulnar nerves at the wrist were evaluated 5 to 59 months after primary or secondary suture repair or grafting. Median age at evaluation was 34 years. Eight injured median nerves and 5 ulnar nerves were grafted. Three nerves in each group were sutured secondarily. Follow-up studies were carried out 8 to 27 months after treatment.

A significant increase in cumulative amplitude was observed over time after nerve suture, but no such change was seen in maximum sensory nerve conduction velocity or maximum nerve action potential amplitude. The recovery of two-point discrimination, vibration threshold, and sensibility could not be related to the passage of time after operation. Cumulative amplitude correlated with both two-point discrimination and recovery of sensibility, but electrophysiologic variables were not adequate predictors of overall clinical recovery. Neither maximum amplitude nor cumulative amplitude correlated with the vibration threshold.

Clinical recovery of nerve function after nerve suture or grafting could not be related to the electrophysiologic test results in this series of cases. Changes in the cortical representation of cutaneous receptive fields after nerve severance and suture have been described in animal studies and might reflect the misdirection of regenerating peripheral nerve fibers. These changes may also account for both incomplete recovery of sensibility and the poor correlation found between the clinical and the electrophysiologic findings after nerve repair in patients.

▶ This useful article points out the current limitations of electroneurographic data in charting the recovery of sensory function. Although a statistically significant correlation in trend between amplitude of the sensory nerve action potential and various parameters of sensibility was found, the scatter was extremely wide. Amplitude or other electric data would not be very useful clinically, for example, in determining whether nerve regeneration were proceeding satisfactorily, at least for the patient mix presented in this article.

Clinically, it is evident that factors such as patient age and patient motivation play a large role in determining the quality of sensibility recovery after nerve suture. Because there was a very wide variation (ages 7–72) in age and there are no details as to the type, if any, of sensory reeducation used in these patients, it is not possible to know whether these factors were important. It would be helpful to repeat this study in a more uniform patient population in which a specific program of sensory reeducation is followed.—P.C.A.

Correlation of Histology and Sensibility After Nerve Repair
A. Lee Dellon (John Hopkins Univ.) and Bryce L. Munger (Pennsylvania State Univ.)
J. Hand Surg. 8:871–875, November 1983   4–3

The partially denerated human fingertip was used as a model with which to correlate the results of a detailed assessment of sensibility with the presence of reinnervated sensory corpuscles, identified by light and electron microscopy. Specimens were obtained from 3 patients early in the recovery stage after median nerve division and repair. The moving-touch, constant-touch, tuning fork, Semmes-Weinstein monofilaments, vibrometer, and static and moving two-point discrimination tests were carried out before and after an elliptical biopsy of the tip of the long finger.

Excellent correlation was found between the results of sensibility testing and the reinnervated sensory end-organs present within the fingertip. Each

AGE 30

27 MONTHS
S/P
MEDIAN
NERVE
REPAIR

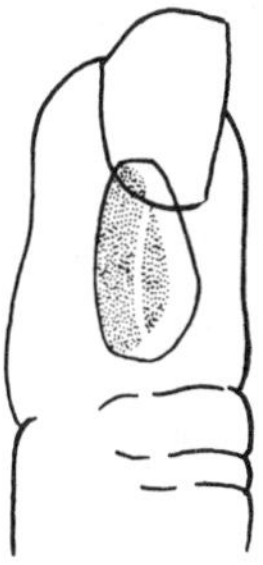

MOVING TOUCH	CONSTANT TOUCH	256 CPS	30 CPS
YES	YES (HEAVY)	YES	YES

VFH	t_{120}	M2PD	s2PD
5.46	.36	4mm	NONE

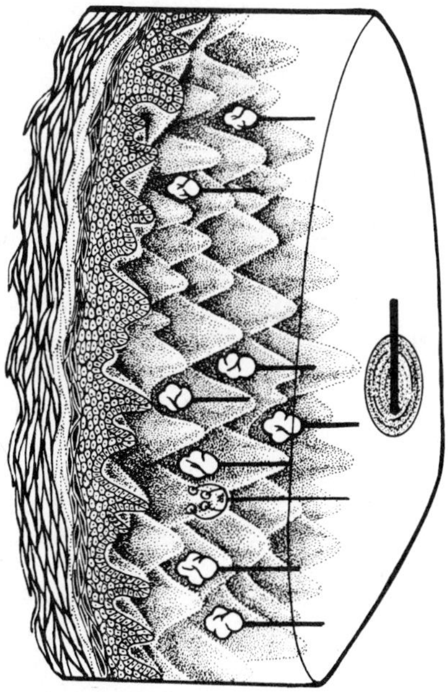

Fig 4–2.—Correlation of histology and sensibility in one female patient. (Courtesy of Dellon, A.L., and Munger, B.L.: J. Hand Surg. 8:871–875, November 1983.)

patient had sensory reeducation before the final assessment. An example is a woman aged 30, who was evaluated 27 months after median nerve repair at the wrist. The histologic and functional findings are correlated in Figure 4–2. Recovery of constant-touch in these cases was associated with a reinnervated Merkel cell-neurite complex, the receptor for the slowly adapting fiber-receptor system that mediates perception of constant-touch and pressure. Numerous reinnervated Meissner corpuscles were present when there were moving-touch and perception of vibratory stimuli at 30 cycles per second. All patients perceived vibratory stimuli at 256 cycles per second and had a reinnervated pacinian corpuscle present. These are the receptors of the quickly adapting fiber receptor system, which mediates the perception of moving-touch.

The reinnervated mechanoreceptors identified in fingertip biopsy specimens in these patients were appropriate to provide the neurophysiologic basis for the observed results of clinical sensibility testing.

▶ This report continues the pioneering work of Doctor Dellon in the field of peripheral nerve receptors. In this study, by using techniques of both light and electron microscopy, he was able to correlate the actual sensibility recovery with that which would be predicted based on the types of nerve receptors actually reinnervated in the biopsy specimen. Information of this sort increases our understanding of what happens after repair of peripheral nerves in man.— P.C.A.

Carbonic Anhydrase Activity of Human Peripheral Nerves: Possible Histochemical Aid to Nerve Repair

Danny A. Riley and David H. Lang (Med. College of Wisconsin, Milwaukee)
J. Hand Surg. 9A:112–120, January 1984   4–4

Inability to match appropriate fascicles in the nerve stumps is a major limiting factor in peripheral nerve repair. Riley et al. (1981, 1982) found that the presence of carbonic anhydrase (CA) activity in sensory neurons distinguishes them from the ventral motor root axons. Riley and Lang developed a fixation method for use in fresh human nerve biopsy specimens in order to discriminate the fascicles through their axon staining patterns. Immersion fixation in 2.5% glutaraldehyde satisfactorily and specifically demonstrated CA activity in both rat and human nerve specimens. Peripheral nerve samples from 3 male patients were obtained as diagnostic specimens. Histochemical studies were completed within 3–4 hours of receiving the tissue.

Nerve fascicles were readily discriminated from one another by the individual staining patterns of the constituent axons. Axoplasmic staining was predominantly a feature of sensory fibers, whereas myelin staining characterized skeletal motor axons. The distinction was made in rat dorsal and ventral roots and in the human peripheral nerve specimens. The findings in a patient with ulnar nerve injury are shown in Figure 4–3.

Histochemical studies for CA activity may provide a means of accurately

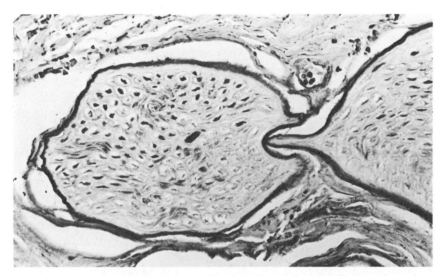

Fig 4–3.—Carbonic anhydrase staining of a fascicle in a human ulnar nerve biopsy specimen taken proximal to the site of the nerve injury. There is intrafascicular segregation of the axoplasmic reactive and nonreactive axons. Segregation of like axons is a commonly observed feature in mixed fascicles; original magnification × 335. (Courtesy of Riley, D.A., and Lang, D.H.: J. Hand Surg. 9A:112–120, January 1984.)

matching the fascicles in severed nerve ends in patients with injury to peripheral nerves in situ or in amputated parts. The heterogeneity of nerve fiber staining potentially can be used to aid nerve repair and promote enhanced regrowth of axons to the appropriate end organs. Further study is needed to determine the function of CA in axons and Schwann's cells.

▶ Techniques such as this point the way to a future in which much more accurate intraoperative nerve mapping will be available to the hand surgeon. By providing a more correct alignment of the proximal and distal stumps, presumably a better quality result will be obtained, although this remains to be proved.—P.C.A.

Peripheral Projections of Fascicles in the Human Median Nerve
W. Schady, J. L. Ochoa, H. E. Torebjörk, and L. S. Chen (Dartmouth Med. School)
Brain 106:745–760, September 1983   4–5

The localizing ability of the brain can be used to map the cutaneous projection of individual sensory fibers or groups of fibers at any point along the course of a nerve. The authors used this approach to assess both the degree of segregation of cutaneous and muscle fascicles in mixed nerves and the distribution of peripheral projections of the fiber complement of nerve fascicles within the total cutaneous nerve territory. Sixty-six studies were done on the median nerves of 4 healthy adults aged 20–44 years, 16 studies at the wrist and 50 at various levels in the upper arm. Tungsten semimicroelectrodes were used to deliver square-wave pulses at 0.1–4 V, corresponding to currents up to 130 μamp. Double electrode studies also were carried out.

Intraneural microstimulation at liminal intensities for conscious detection gave rise to an elementary sensation projected to a small, well-defined field. An increased amplitude of stimulation did not alter the intensity of the sensation, but led to the sequential recruitment of new, qualitatively different sensations. About half the fascicles at the upper arm level appeared to supply skin or muscle exclusively, while the rest substantially were committed to skin or muscle. The projection areas of skin nerve fascicles tended to be discrete at both the wrist and the arm (Fig 4–4). Confluent areas covered no more than 20% of the total median nerve territory. At the wrist, fascicular territories usually resembled the inner-

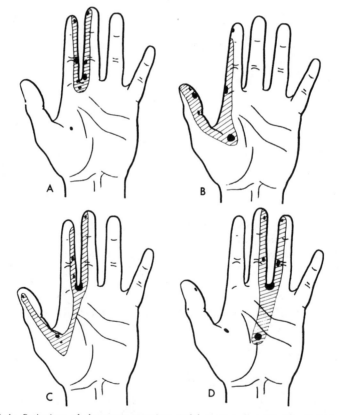

Fig 4–4.—Projections of elementary sensations *(solid areas)* and maximal projection territories *(hatched areas)* mapped during four representative experiments when the upper arm was stimulated. Evoked sensations were typically projected to a digital interspace plus a wedge of palm, although sometimes additional areas were involved. (Courtesy of Schady, W., et al.: Brain 106:745–760, September 1983.)

vation areas of single palmar digital nerves, whereas in the upper arm they tended to cover digital interspaces.

Most of the rearrangements of spinal root fibers into terminal nerve branch groupings appear to occur at the brachial plexus level. The intraneural fascicular plexus may act as a safety mechanism, permitting nondermatomal overlap at proximal levels. The findings emphasize the need accurately to match fascicular ends at all levels where this is possible, because proximal nerve fascicles retain some identity in terms of a predominant commitment to either muscle or a circumscribed area of skin.

▶ Using highly sophisticated techniques of intraneural stimulation and recording in awake human subjects, these authors provide an elegant demonstration of the distribution of single nerve fascicles at different levels of the median nerve. Most rearrangements of spinal root fibers into terminal nerve branch groupings occur at the plexus level, with only minimal additional regrouping occurring in the peripheral nerve.—J.D.

Variations in Digital Sensory Patterns: Study of the Ulnar Nerve-Median Nerve Palmar Communicating Branch
Roy A. Meals and Martin Shaner
J. Hand Surg. 8:411–414, July 1983   4–6

A connection between the ulnar and the median nerves is shown in some anatomy texts, and injury to a communicating nerve branch during carpal tunnel release has been described. The authors dissected 50 cadaver palms to delineate the surgical anatomy of the communicating branch. A communication was present in 80% of specimens. It generally was immediately deep to the superficial arterial arch and took an angular course across the palm on exiting from Guyon's canal. In some specimens it ran almost parallel to the ring finger flexor tendons. Most of the branches were single bundles, but some formed a network. Most communicating branches arose proximally from the fourth common digital nerve (ulnar) and proceeded distally to enter the third common digital nerve (median). In only 1 instance did median fibers enter the classic ulnar nerve distribution. The diameter of the communicating branch averaged one fourth of that of a proper digital nerve at the finger base. Wide variation in the number of sympathetic fibers passing from nerve trunks to the superficial arterial arch was found in all palms, regardless of whether sensory communications were present.

Aberrant sensory findings can be explained by the presence of a communicating branch between the ulnar and the median nerves in the palm. The branch may account for persistent sensibility in the long finger after complete median nerve laceration at the wrist. If a lacerated communicating branch is overlooked, a permanent sensory deficit will be present even with good recovery of adjacent lacerated and repaired nerves. The median-ulnar sensory connection is most at risk during carpal tunnel release, ring finger flexor tendon operations, Dupuytren's fasciectomy, and mobilization of neurovascular island flaps. Unrecognized lacerations of the communicating branch may explain some cases of palmar pain with perhaps only subjective distal sensory loss. These findings may otherwise be attributed to nerve traction, scarring, or another nonspecific cause.

▶ Doctors Meals and Shaner have done hand surgeons everywhere a considerable service by calling to our attention the potential clinical importance of this commonly visualized communicating nerve branch. The branch would appear to be in particular jeopardy if dissection is carried out from distal to proximal without careful visualization of the terminal branches of the median nerve. Of course, it is also at jeopardy with the blind sectioning of the transverse carpal ligaments still performed by some nonhand surgeons. As in all hand surgery, adequate visualization is the key to avoidance of injury to this particular structure.—P.C.A.

Lateral Antebrachial Cutaneous Nerve as a Highly Suitable Autograft Donor for the Digital Nerve
M. Sue Tank, Royce C. Lewis, Jr., and Penelope W. Coates (Texas Tech Univ.)
J. Hand Surg. 8:942–945, November 1983 4–7

The lateral antebrachial cutaneous nerve and the digital nerve were compared histomorphometrically in 10 patients who received digital nerve grafts with the lateral antebrachial cutaneous nerve as donor in a 14-month period. Small segments of both the lateral antebrachial cutaneous and digital nerves were obtained at operation. There were no significant differences between the lateral antebrachial cutaneous and digital nerves with respect to fascicular area, area of the entire nerve bundle, or percentage of the nerve bundle occupied by nerve fascicles. In 5 of 9 cases the fascicular area of the lateral antebrachial cutaneous nerve was the same as or greater than that of the paired digital nerve. In 6 of 9 cases the fascicular percent of the entire nerve bundle was greater in the lateral antebrachial cutaneous nerve or the same as in the paired digital nerve.

The lateral antebrachial cutaneous nerve closely resembles the digital nerve in its fascicular pattern and is highly suitable as a donor for use in digital nerve grafting. The lateral antebrachial cutaneous nerve innervates skin on the lateral aspect of the forearm, and loss of sensation in this region is not considered to be clinically significant. Overlapping innervation is usually provided. No patient has complained of dysfunction from a sensory deficit in the forearm.

▶ This article goes to some length to demonstrate that the fascicular anatomy of the lateral antebrachial cutaneous nerve is similar to that of the digital nerve; therefore, the lateral antebrachial cutaneous nerve should be considered a particularly suitable donor for digital nerve grafting. To my knowledge, the fascicular anatomy of a donor nerve, which is basically supplying Schwann tubes, has yet to be shown to have a significant effect on the results of nerve grafting. The lateral antebrachial cutaneous nerve certainly may be used as a digital nerve graft donor. It should be considered, however, that there will be a loss of sensibility on the upper extremity in an area that may be more likely to come in contact with the outside environment than the lateral border of the foot and is certainly more likely to be probed and palpated by the patient. As such, although not "clinically significant," the loss of sensation may be more noticeable to the patient and this also should be a consideration when nerve graft donor sites are chosen. One final consideration is the relative length of nerve available, which, of course, is much greater with the sural nerve. Therefore, the sural nerve probably would be a more appropriate donor if a long segment of multiple grafts are anticipated.—P.C.A.

Neuroma Formation Following Digital Amputations
Gregory T. Fisher and John A. Boswick, Jr. (Univ. of Colorado)
J. Trauma 23:136–142, February 1983   4–8

Neuromas long have been associated with amputations. Information on 100 consecutive patients, who had 144 digital amputations between 1978 and 1980, was reviewed by the authors for the occurrence of painful neuromas. There were 87 male and 13 female patients in the series. Forty-three percent of amputations were at or distal to the distal interphalangeal joint, 31% were at or distal to the proximal interphalangeal joint, and 26% were at or distal to the metacarpophalangeal joint. Nineteen patients had multiple amputations. The index finger was most often involved. Male patients had an average age of 30 years and female patients, an average age of 19 years. The neurovascular bundle was isolated, placed at slight tension, and transected at the time of amputation. Local flaps were used for wound closure in most instances.

Four of the 100 patients developed painful amputation stumps that lasted for 6 months or more after injury. Phantom phenomena were universal in the first month, but subsequently resolved in most cases; they were not painful. Only 1 of the 8 patients reporting phantom phenomena at 4 months or longer after injury had a painful amputation stump for 6 months or more.

Neuromas can form at sites of nerve transection, but whether they will transmit painful perceptions can be influenced by patient care. Reassurance regarding the relative severity of an injury and the potential for rehabilitation will help reverse the tendency for the patient to have regressive responses to injury. Little support should be given to any secondary gain desire that perpetuates disability. Patients are encouraged to use the injured part. As the patient sees that he or she can perform despite the injury, efforts at rehabilitation will increase, and loss of the part will become relatively insignificant, as will any associated symptoms.

▶ Only a small number of neuromas followed digital amputations in this series of over 100 patients. I believe the authors are correct in stating that their postoperative mental rehabilitation program is important in decreasing the phantom and neuroma-type pains. It is noted that the authors were meticulous in dissecting the neurovascular bundles and cutting back the nerves at the time of definitive amputation closure. This is a key and sometimes overlooked point of technique in these "simple" traumatic amputations of digits.—R.D.B.

Implantation of Sensory Nerve Into Muscle: Preliminary Clinical and Experimental Observations on Neuroma Formation
A. Lee Dellon, Susan E. Mackinnon, and Alan Pestronk
Ann. Plast. Surg. 12:30–40, January 1984   4–9

The authors describe two patients and the findings in a baboon model suggesting that a classic neuroma does not develop in a transected sensory nerve implanted into muscle tissue.

CASE 1.—Woman, 40, with multiple, self-inflicted lacerations of the wrist, had had a number of attempts at repair and then grafting of the median nerve. A painful distal wrist mass was found to represent a large neuroma of the palmar cutaneous branch of the median nerve. The proximal end of the median nerve was embedded in the flexor sublimis muscle and was only slightly enlarged.

CASE 2.—Man, 34, with avulsion of the right arm at the proximal humeral level, was explored for neuroma pain 9 months after injury. The nerve stumps were covered with a brachialis muscle flap. Massive, painful plexus neuromas were present proximally 6 months later. The most distal nerve stump that had been covered with muscle was asymptomatic and not swollen.

Branches of the median and ulnar nerves of baboons were transected and either left in place or implanted into an adjacent muscle flap. Reexploration 4 weeks later showed an early disorganized pattern of fibers in the transected ends of control nerves (Fig 4–5), whereas the implanted nerves exhibited parallel fibers and no disorganization (Fig 4–6).

A transected nerve will form a classic neuroma if left in the subcutaneous tissue, but a neuroma will not form if the nerve is implanted into adjacent muscle. The findings should be considered to be preliminary until a larger, prospective series of clinical cases is available and further primate studies are carried out. If the findings are confirmed, the surgical effort needed to transpose a sensory nerve into muscle and postoperative immobilization may be warranted in patients with painful cutaneous neuromas.

▶ Treatment of painful neuromas remains a controversial subject. This article provides some clinical and experimental support for implantation of nerve into muscle. Although the data are suggestive, they are certainly not conclusive. To put weight on the opposite side of the scale, I have seen a case of traction neuroma of a nerve produced by this type of procedure, with severe lancinating pain caused with contraction of the muscle into which the nerve end had been embedded.

I do agree with the authors' suggestion that the neuroma be transposed to an area where it can be protected and hopefully can be situated in a bed with good blood supply. A subdermal location is clearly inappropriate, but intramuscular implantation is not the only alternative. Transposition into deeper submus-

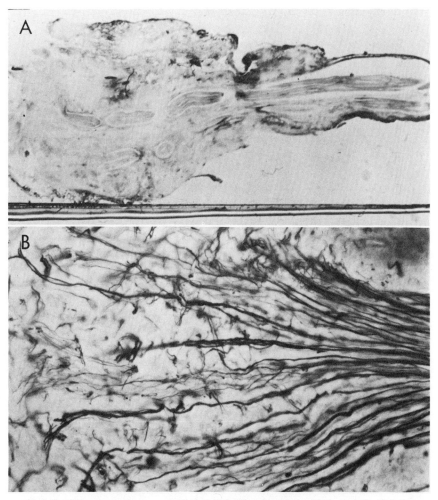

Fig 4–5.—Baboon control nerve, transected and left subcutaneously at wrist for 4 weeks. **A,** large cap of connective tissue surrounding nerve trunk; original magnification ×5. **B,** axon sprouts arborizing randomly; original magnification ×100; silver stain. (Courtesy of Dellon, A.L., et al.: Ann. Plast. Surg. 12:30–40, January 1984.)

cular layers is often possible, as is transposition away from areas of high contact such as the radial side of the forearm.

I disagree with the authors that resection of the neuroma bulb is usually necessary. It has been my practice to transpose the intact neuroma to a new location, using the criteria described above to select the location. There are a number of reports in the literature supporting this method of treatment as frequently successful. In my opinion, intramuscular implantation is an interesting but as yet unproved method of treatment for this common condition.

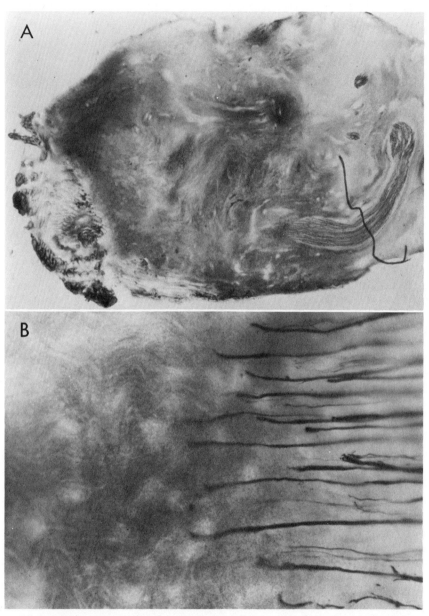

Fig 4–6.—Baboon nerve implanted into muscle. **A,** small group of muscle fibers separated by hyaline-like matrix from nerve end; original magnification ×5. **B,** terminal axon sprouts are parallel in orientation; original magnification ×100; silver stain. (Courtesy of Dellon, A.L., et al.: Ann. Plast. Surg. 12:30–40, January 1984.)

Perhaps more interesting is the solution proposed by Gorkisch et al. (*Plast. Reconstr. Surg.* 73:293–299, 1984), when paired cut nerve ends or neuromas are present. They suggest suturing the two ends together, then severing and repairing one of the two limbs in situ, creating, in effect, a segmental nerve graft between proximal segments. Preliminary clinical and experimental results seem encouraging. The authors postulate that this method inhibits axoplasmic flow by creating equal but oppositely directed axoplasmic flow gradients.

An alternative explanation, in a review of the article by Brooke Seckel, suggests that the interpolated graft acts to shield the axonal buds from neurotrophic factors secreted by denervated end organs, perhaps by secreting neurotrophic factors of its own.—P.C.A.

Investigation of Traumatic Lesions of the Brachial Plexus by Electromyography and Short Latency Somatosensory Potentials Evoked by Stimulation of Multiple Peripheral Nerves
C. Yiannikas, B. T. Shahani, and R. R. Young
J. Neurol. Neurosurg. Psychiatry 46:1014–1022, November 1983   4–10

Accurate localization of brachial plexus and cervical root injuries is necessary for the proper prognostic assessment of affected patients. Ten patients with brachial plexus trauma were studied in an attempt to improve the diagnostic accuracy of sensory evoked potential (SEP) recording by stimulating multiple peripheral nerves. The median, ulnar, and superficial radial nerves and, in 2 cases, the musculocutaneous nerve were stimulated with 0.1-msec pulses of 2 Hz adjusted to produce a small muscle twitch or be 3 times the sensory threshold. The three most prominent negative potentials were analyzed.

Four patients had major involvement of the C-5 to C-6 segments, 3 had involvement of the C-8 to T-1 segments, 2 had involvement of the C-5 to C-6 segments only, and 1 had C-5 to T-1 involvement. The SEP patterns associated with the most common brachial plexus lesions were predictable. Injury of the upper trunk predominantly altered the musculocutaneous and radial SEPs, whereas lower trunk or medial cord lesions primarily affected the ulnar SEPs. Diffuse plexus lesions altered SEPs from all stimulation sites. The SEP recording was most useful in evaluating lesions involving only the upper segments. In most cases, the requisite data were obtained by conventional electromyography.

Both conventional electromyography and SEP recording can be quite helpful in precisely diagnosing traumatic lesions of the brachial plexus. The studies are particularly useful in making a prognosis and clarifying the possible benefits of reconstructive surgery. Sensory evoked potential recording and electromyography also can help assess the progress of nerve regeneration after surgical treatment.

▶ The authors have confirmed the electrophysiologic changes occurring with brachial plexus trauma and the value of standard electromyography and nerve conduction studies. They also demonstrate that sensory evoked potentials show the expected changes after plexus trauma and in a few patients can add to the accuracy of defining the severity and location of the damage. They correctly note that recording sensory evoked potentials with multiple peripheral nerve stimulation is a time-consuming procedure that need not be applied in all patients with plexus damage. They would be most likely to be of help in patients with sensory loss, normal electromyography and normal peripheral sensory nerve action potentials.—J.D.

Dorsal Root Entry Zone Lesions (Nashold's Procedure) for Pain Relief Following Brachial Plexus Avulsion

D. G. T. Thomas and J. P. R. Sheehy (London)
J. Neurol. Neurosurg. Psychiatry 46:924–928, October 1983   4–11

Brachial plexus avulsion is an important cause of intractable pain, especially in young motorcycle accident victims. The minority of patients with severe chronic pain have proved to be especially resistant to treatment with several methods, including cordotomy, rhizotomy, and narcotics. Thomas and Sheehy evaluated Nashold's procedure of intraspinal coagulation of the dorsal root entry zones of the avulsed roots in 19 patients with partial or complete brachial plexus avulsion. Fifteen lesions resulted from motorcycle accidents. There typically was crushing or burning pain in the deafferentated limb, which tended to be felt globally throughout the arm, either proximally or distally. The pain was often constant. A completely flail extremity was most frequent. Sensory loss usually involved the entire extremity to the shoulder. Most patients had had transcutaneous stimulation, and 1 had undergone cordotomy. Root avulsion was often more extensive than was apparent myelographically.

The procedure was performed, with the operating microscope, at a laminectomy extending from C5 to T1. Thermocoagulation lesions were produced at 2-mm intervals with 40 mamp over 15 seconds. Typically 20 to 24 lesions were made over the brachial plexus outflow region. Eleven patients had 75% or more relief from pain that persisted, and 5 others had 25% to 75% pain relief. Commonly relief became slightly less in the early postoperative months before it stabilized. Six patients have been followed for over 1½ years. Ten patients had some initial deterioration in motor or sensory function in the ipsilateral leg, but in most the signs remitted. All the patients are ambulatory. The most common sensory change was a proprioceptive deficit.

All but 3 of 19 patients with severe chronic pain from brachial plexus avulsion, refractory to other measures, have improved to some degree after the production of dorsal root entry zone lesions. Only 2 patients have had significant persistent disability. This approach seems to be indicated for patients with severe, disabling pain refractory to other treatments.

▶ Doctor Nashold has been a forerunner in the pain management field for decades, and this work is added testimony to the fact that the difficult pain problem associated with brachial plexus avulsions may, in some instances, be helped with dorsal root entry zone radiofrequency lesions. It is to be noted that of the 19 patients presented in this article, 7 experienced postoperative motor weakness in addition to the neurologic deficit present preoperatively. This underscores the absoluteness of attempting all other forms of nondestructive pain management prior to resorting to the dorsal root entry zone operation.— B.M.O.

Studies on Conversion of Motor Function in Intercostal Nerves Crossing for Complete Brachial Plexus Injuries of Root Avulsion Type

Masataru Takahashi (Univ. of Tokyo)
J. Jpn. Orthop. 57:1799–1807, November 1983   4–12

The course of conversion of motor function was assessed in 25 patients in whom the third and fourth intercostal nerves were crossed to the musculocutaneous nerve to produce elbow flexion after the total avulsion type of brachial plexus injury. The patients, with an average age of 18 years, were assessed 1–9 years after operation. All voluntarily were able to flex the elbow joint after operation. Spontaneous activity that synchronized with respiration was present in the biceps brachii in the early stage of reinnervation, but then disappeared gradually as volitional control and endurance improved. Quite satisfactory function developed within a period of several years. Involuntary action potentials were not provoked by coughing or sneezing after some time had elapsed since the operation.

An electric mechanographic test was carried out in order to assess proprioceptive sense after this operation. Cutaneous sensation was found to have an important role in judgments of joint position in this setting. Patients were able to control flexion and extension of the elbow better than expected even with their eyes closed. Sensation is likely to persist over the area supplied by the second thoracic nerve root even after total brachial plexus paralysis. Pericubital sensation is likely to be preserved after intercostal nerve crossing. This sensation probably is helpful in perceiving the position of the elbow joint, because little proprioceptive feedback stimulation arises from the muscles themselves, and the joint has lost its sensibility.

▶ The author reports remarkable results from intercostal neurotization of the musculocutaneous nerve. These results, confirmed by electromyographic studies, vividly illustrate the potential for neurologic plasticity in this group of patients. It should be borne in mind, however, that an early aggresive surgical approach also can be rewarding in selected patients (Stevens, et al.: *Surg. Neurol.* 19:334–345, 1983). Additional options also may include local muscle transfer in cases of incomplete but irrepairable plexus damage. Tsai et al. (*J. Hand Surg.* 186–190, 1984) recently reviewed the indications for and surgical technique of pectoralis major and minor transfer to restore elbow flexion in selected patients with brachial plexus injury.—M.B.W.

5 Infection

Septic Arthritis of the Wrist

Evan S. Rashkoff (Columbia-Presbyterian Med. Center, New York), William E. Burkhalter (Univ. of Miami), and Ronald J. Mann (Univ. of Utah Med. Center)
J. Bone Joint Surg. [Am.] 65-A:824–828, July 1983   5–1

The findings of septic arthritis of the wrist were reviewed in 28 patients who underwent early surgical drainage, parenteral antibiotic therapy, and early motion after surgical decompression. Two patients were children, and most of the rest were young adults. Four patients were on conservative management for osteoarthritis with wrist involvement, and 3 had rheumatoid arthritis. Trauma was documented in 17 of the 29 wrists involved, most commonly from the attempted intravenous injection of a narcotic. Preexisting infection or inflammation may have predisposed the patient to carpal infection in 3 cases.

All patients reported progressive pain and a decreasing range of wrist motion. Tenderness was present, with severe pain with any wrist movement. No patient had fluctuant swelling. Symptoms and signs were more acute in patients with sepsis secondary to trauma. Radiographs showed soft tissue swelling in most cases. Aspiration of synovial fluid revealed leukocytosis on direct smear or culture, or both. Thirty-four arthrotomies were done on the 29 involved wrists, usually by a dorsal approach. Most patients were operated on within 24 hours of diagnosis. Pyarthrosis was present in most cases. Cartilage necrosis was seen in 1 patient. The usual etiologic organism was *Staphylococcus aureus*. All the arthrotomy wounds healed by secondary intention. Parenteral antibiotics were given for an average of 10 days after operation. Passive and active assisted motion was initiated 24 hours after surgery. Oral antibotics were continued on an empirical basis for up to 2 weeks after discharge. There were no recurrences in the 22 patients followed up. No patient had an unstable wrist. Good or excellent results were seen in 10 patients who were operated on within 10 hours of diagnosis. Surgery was delayed for over 16 hours in 10 of 13 wrists with a fair or poor outcome.

Trauma was the cause of septic arthritis in most of these cases. Aspiration of the wrist is an invaluable diagnostic aid. Parenteral antibiotics should not be given until a diagnosis is made. Septic arthritis of the wrist is considered a surgical emergency requiring immediate arthrotomy and early postoperative rehabilitation. Early, aggressive treatment yields the best functional results.

▶ Such a large series of cases of septic arthritis of the wrist is unusual. The authors point out correctly the necessity for early, aggressive treatment.— R.L.L.

Herpetic Whitlow: Epidemiology, Clinical Characteristics, Diagnosis, and Treatment

Henry M. Feder, Jr., and Sarah S. Long
Am. J. Dis. Child. 137:861–863, September 1983   5–2

Herpetic whitlow is a herpes simplex virus infection of the distal phalanx, occurring mainly in medical personnel and in persons with herpes infection. It is reportedly infrequent in infants and children.

Girl, aged 6 months, was seen after tenderness and erythema of the distal part of the third finger had been present for 24 hours. Temperature was 39.4 C. The pulp region of the distal phalanx was swollen, erythematous, and tender, and an enlarged epitrochlear node was present. Fever resolved with dicloxacillin therapy, but vesicles developed over the fingertip (Fig 5–1). The Tzanck test on a vesicular base revealed multinucleated giant cells. Bacterial culture of the vesicular fluid was negative; viral cultures were not obtained. The swelling and erythema resolved over the next week after antibiotic therapy was stopped, and no new vesicles appeared. The finger was normal 2 weeks later. There was a less severe recurrence 2 months thereafter.

The herpetic whitlow usually does not contain pus. The patient initially has pain and tingling or burning of a distal phalanx, followed by digital swelling and erythema, sometimes associated with fever, adenopathy, adenitis, and constitutional symptoms. Vesicles then appear and usually co-

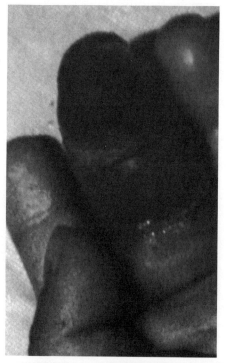

Fig 5–1.—Resolving herpetic whitlow. Finger is swollen and erythematous, and secondary vesicles are present. Distal phalanx that was site of primary vesicular eruption is crusted. (Courtesy of Feder, H.M., Jr., and Long, S.S.: Am. J. Dis. Child. 137:861–863, September 1983; copyright 1983, American Medical Association.)

alesce, remaining for about 10 days. Peeling occurs within a week, leaving normal skin. About one fifth of patients have recurrences, which are usually less severe than the initial infection. Secondary bacterial infection is not uncommon.

The initial episode of herpetic whitlow usually occurs during a primary herpes simplex virus infection. The diagnosis is rapidly confirmed by the Tzanck test or culture. Treatment is symptomatic; surgical incision is avoided. Dry dressings are useful. Aspiration of tense vesicles may relieve pain. The usefulness of topical acyclovir therapy is unclear, but local treatment with idoxuridine in dimethyl sulfoxide has been reported to shorten the course of herpetic whitlow.

▶ Even in the pediatric age group, herpetic whitlow must remain in the differential diagnosis of painful, swollen, inflamed lesions of the fingertip. Diagnosis is not as easy as in the adult because there usually is no history of exposure or an identifiable environmental risk of exposure as there is for the health professional who typically presents with this problem. A high degree of suspicion therefore is necessary, and confirmation of the diagnosis must await the development of characteristic vesicles, which then can be unroofed, for either smear or culture. As in the adult, prognosis is good in pediatric cases and antibiotics or débridement is unnecessary.—P.C.A.

Eikenella corrodens in Human Bite Infections of the Hand

David R. Schmidt and James D. Heckman (Univ. of Texas, San Antonio)
J. Trauma 23:478–482, June 1983   5–3

Eikenella corrodens increasingly has been implicated as a pathogen in human bite injuries. The authors reviewed the findings in 30 patients seen in a 5½-year period with closed fist injuries of the hand infected by *E. corrodens*. All were male patients, with an average age of 30 years. Patients were seen an average of 4 days after injury and were hospitalized for an average of about a week. Three patients had two separate injuries. The dorsum of the long or ring metacarpophalangeal joint was affected most often. *Streptococcus* was the most common bacterial contaminant; *Staphylococcus aureus* was found in only 5 cases. Anaerobes were isolated in 6 cases. Six patients had pure cultures of *E. corrodens*.

All patients received antibiotics intravenously and splinting of the hand, and 25 had immediate incision and débridement. Metacarpophalangeal arthrotomy was necessary in 23 of the cases. Seven patients had an osteochondral or chondral defect, and 7 had extensor tendon lacerations. Six patients required additional débridement of infected tissue. Five patients developed osteomyelitis, and, eventually, 3 needed amputation. None of these patients had débridement within 24 hours after injury, and none was given intravenous antibiotic therapy early. Four of the 12 patients who were followed up, excluding amputees, had normal findings. Six had an extensor lag between 30 and 50 degrees, and 2 had fixed flexion contractures of 30 degrees with no metacarpophalangeal joint motion. All 6 patients with pure cultures of *E. corrodens* had significant long-term complications. Four had limited joint motion, and 2 other patients developed osteomyelitis.

Deep contamination and infection with *E. corrodens* can be present in closed fist injuries. Affected patients are often unreliable, making aggressive initial treatment important. Early adequate débridement and intravenous administration of penicillin or a second-generation cephalosporin will help prevent serious long-term complications such as osteomyelitis.

▶ This article underscores the importance of aggressive treatment of penetrating injuries of the knuckle.—R.L.L.

Anthrax of the Hand: Case Report

Paul Wylock, Roger Jaeken, and Rika Deraemaecker (Brussels)
J. Hand Surg. 8:576–578, September 1983   5–4

Anthrax is a very rare infection in western countries. The authors describe a patient in whom anthrax of a finger developed after accidental injection of *Bacillus anthracis,* a gram-positive bacillus that produces spores and toxin under aerobic conditions and is relatively resistant to disinfectants and heat.

Man, 52, a technician in the bacteriology laboratory of a veterinary college, accidentally inoculated himself with *Bacillus anthracis.* A papule appeared on the dorsum of the left long finger after 3 days and was followed by a vesicle surrounded by edema and erythema and containing dark blue fluid. Fever of 39 C developed. Trimethoprim and sulfamethoxazole had been given, and cultures never were positive. The arm was swollen and edematous, with enlarged axillary nodes. The patient was given doxycycline because of allergy to penicillin. The infection was controlled, but a black eschar developed on the dorsum of the finger and was removed, with application of a split-thickness graft. Good finger function returned.

Most cases of anthrax in the United States are due to contact with animal products. Following this industrially acquired group of cases are those related to agriculture and those that are laboratory acquired. Cutaneous infection is far more frequent than the inhalational and gastrointestinal forms. It is characterized by the formation of blisters resembling a second-degree burn or erysipelas. Septicemia can occur. Up to 20% of untreated patients die, but death is rare if adequate treatment is given.

▶ Occasional cases of anthrax are still reported in industrialized countries. A high degree of suspicion is necessary to make the diagnosis. Confirmation depends on obtaining cultures or stains, or both, prior to beginning antibiotic treatment.—P.C.A.

Phialophora richardsiae in a Lesion Appearing as a Giant Cell Tumor of the Tendon Sheath

Lee B. Moskowitz, Timothy J. Cleary, Michael R. McGinnis, and Cathy B. Thomson

Arch. Pathol. Lab. Med. 107:374–376, July 1983.   5–5

A number of fungi, including the dematiacious hyphomycene *Phialo-phora richardsiae,* have been implicated as causes of phaeohyphomycosis in man. The authors report a case of subcutaneous phaeohyphomycosis caused by *P. richardsiae* in which a splinter was found in the lesion.

Man, 52, presented with a mass of 5 months' duration on the volar aspect of the left index finger. It was 1 cm in diameter and not tender or indurated when first noticed and was 2 cm in diameter at the time of examination. No fever or adenopathy was present. The patient reported having used plywood to build a structure 6 months before the mass was first noticed. A giant cell tumor of the tendon sheath was diagnosed preoperatively and also after surgery. The wound was irrigated with antibiotic solution containing bacitracin, neomycin and poly-myxin B sulfate. It healed uneventfully after 9 weeks, and complete mobility and sensation returned to the finger. No recurrence was noted 7 months later.

Examination of the specimen showed granulomatous inflammation com-pletely enclosed by a fibrous capsule, and there was a centrally located wood splinter 1.2 cm long (Fig 5–2) that was surrounded by palisading epithelioid histiocytes and eosinophilic debris. Septate hyphae were seen within the splinter, in the adjacent tissues, and in granulomas, and my-cologic study led to the identification of *P. richardsiae.*

In contrast to other cases, central necrosis and suppuration were not seen in this lesion. It is the first one known to present as a giant cell tumor

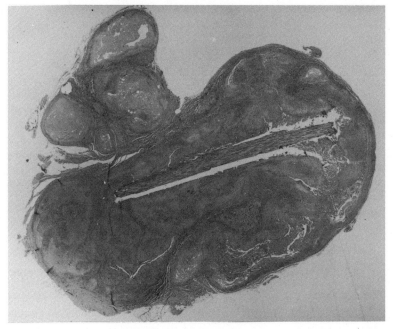

Fig 5–2.—Cross section of lesion depicting completely enclosed splinter within fibrous capsule. He-matoxylin-eosin; × 10. (Courtesy of Moskowitz, L.B., et al.: Arch. Pathol. Lab. Med. 107:374–376, July 1983; copyright 1983, American Medical Association.)

of the tendon sheath, a well-recognized clinical entity. The dematiacious nature of the fungus was apparent in culture but not in tissue sections. Excision of solitary lesions due to *P. richardsiae* is curative in the immunocompetent host.

▶ Nodular or focal tenosynovial lesions not only include the common giant cell tumor of the tendon sheath, but also a variety of infections, including not only the one mentioned in this article, but also (in certain parts of the United States) atypical mycobacteria. Because some of these infections require adjunct antibiotic therapy, special fungal and mycobacterial cultures and stains are indicated for these lesions at the time of excision.—P.C.A.

Pyoderma Gangrenosum: Successful Treatment With Intralesional Steroids
J. L. Jennings
J. Am. Acad. Dermatol. 9:575–580, October 1983.   5–6

A case of pyoderma gangrenosum (PG) involving the hand was seen at the Naval Regional Medical Center, San Diego, California. The lesion responded to intralesional steroid therapy.

Man, 52, had developed a painful ulcer at the site of an abrasion on the dorsum of the left hand a month before. The ulcer had enlarged rapidly despite treatment with dicloxacillin and hydrogen peroxide. An anaplastic carcinoma of the left lung had involuted on radiation therapy 11 years earlier. Exploration for hemoptysis 3 years before admission was followed by development of a bronchopleural fistula, which necessitated an upper lobectomy. Subsequently, chronic persistent hepatitis had developed, and *Aspergillus* was cultured from the surgical drainage tract. Investigation of rectal bleeding had shown only diverticula. The ulcer is shown in Figure 5–3. The sedimentation rate was 99 mm/hour. Inflammatory bowel disease was not documented. A biopsy specimen from the edge of the ulcer showed changes of PG (Figs 5–4 and 5–5).

The ulcer failed to respond to Burow's soaks and silver sulfadiazine cream, but it responded to injections of triamcinolone acetonide and was 80% healed after 9 days (Fig 5–6). A new lesion at the site of a previous intravenous line was noted a week after discharge. Steroid was injected into this lesion and the remaining old lesion, and both lesions responded. The original ulcer was totally healed within 6 weeks of the initial injection.

Although PG is associated with many systemic disorders, it is most commonly associated with ulcerative colitis. The present patient had chronic persistent hepatitis, radiation pneumonitis, and pulmonary aspergilloma. The etiology and pathogenesis of PG remain unclear, and treatment is empirical. Systemic steroids generally have been used in patients resistant to topical measures. Intralesional steroid was used in the present case because of relative contraindication to systemic steroid therapy. The total dosage used to treat the primary lesion was 60 mg of triamcinolone.

▶ This rare condition is easily misdiagnosed and mistreated. The details of diagnosis and treatment are important to the hand surgeon and are well covered

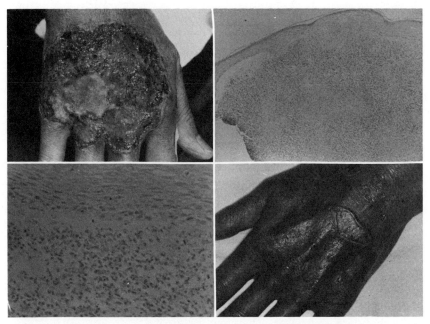

Fig 5–3 (top left).—Lesion at time of admission. Ulcer on dorsum of left hand, with shaggy, necrotic base and raised, undermined, bluish-gray margin with surrounding erythematous areola.

Fig 5–4 (top right).—Biopsy specimen from edge of ulcer demonstrated dense dermal infiltrate of leukocytes, hemorrhage, foci of necrosis, and blood vessels that were patent and those that showed fibrinoid necrosis. Innermost zone was identified by separation of overlying epidermis. Hematoxylin-eosin; × 40.

Fig 5–5 (bottom left).—High magnification of midzone where epidermal separation was beginning. Dense dermal infiltrate consisted of leukocytes and nuclear dust. Overlying keratinocytes displayed early cytologic features. Hematoxylin-eosin; × 100.

Fig 5–6 (bottom right).—Two weeks after treatment with intralesional steroid. Dusky erythematous, atrophic scar with area of ulceration and active border nearest wrist that required a second injection. (Courtesy of Jennings, J.L.: J. Am. Acad. Dermatol. 9:575–580, October 1983.)

in this article. The report by D. C. Ferlic of a similar case (*J. Hand Surg.* 8:573–575, 1983) describes the ineffectiveness of antibiotics and surgical drainage. Systemically administered steroids were of some benefit, but cure was not obtained until surgical treatment (colectomy) of an area of ulcerative colitis.—R.D.B.

Wound Botulism: Life-Threatening Complication of Hand Injuries
Frank L. Thorne and Robert J. Kropp (Univ. of Washington)
Plast. Reconstr. Surg. 71:548–551, April 1983   5–7

It is not widely known that botulism can occur in traumatic injuries. The authors report what appears to be the 24th case with typical findings of descending cranial nerve and generalized motor paralysis. The patient needed prolonged respiratory and general supportive aid, which is usually the case.

Man, 29, a farmer, caught the left hand in a potato conveyor belt and had débridement and fixation of fractured metacarpals elsewhere. The middle, ring, and little fingers were mummified from the metacarpophalangeal joint distally, and the index finger was dusky but viable. Nonviable tissue was removed, and the mummified digits were amputated. The index metacarpal had a displaced and comminuted distal fracture, and the digit was stabilized to the middle metacarpal with Kirschner wires. The volar aspect of the wound was left open for drainage and to diminish the possibility of infection. Postoperatively, the patient was treated with cephalosporins and whirlpool. Difficulty swallowing, shortness of breath, and double vision were noticed 16 days after the injury; and sudden respiratory arrest occurred 5 days later. Increasing signs of generalized paralysis of all branches of the cranial nerves ensued, with upper and lower extremity weakness, profound respiratory paralysis, and ileus. Eventually, cultures of the hand wound yielded *clostridium botulinum* type A. The serum was negative for clostridial toxin. The patient continued taking gentamicin and chloramphenicol, and the hand was débrided again to remove possible residual spores. The wound was closed by split-thickness skin grafting. Hyperalimentation was instituted, and the patient began improving neurologically 2 weeks after his collapse. Wound healing was satisfactory. The patient was working 10 months after injury, but felt much weaker than before being injured. He used the left hand to grasp small objects. The final disability rating of the hand was 72%. Cardiorespiratory capacity was essentially normal.

The clinical findings in wound botulism are the same as those in food-borne botulism poisoning. The chief distinction is from Guillain-Barré syndrome. Ventilatory support may be necessary for several months. Good general supportive nursing care is critical in these cases. There are usually no signs of residual neurologic disability after several months or years.

▶ The rarity and catastrophic consequences of this complication necessitate constant vigilance.—R.L.L.

Sarcoidosis of the Upper Extremity: Case Presentation and Literature Review.

Robert S. Adelaar (Virginia Commonwealth Univ., Richmond)
J. Hand Surg. 8:492–496, July 1983.   5–8

Osseous involvement by sarcoidosis can occur in the proximal and middle phalanges of the hands and feet, with rarefaction, cortical atrophy, and replacement of the medullary cavity by granulomatous tissue (Fig 5–7, A), and also in a sclerosing form. Two cases of sarcoidosis with involvement of the upper extremity are reported.

Black woman, 36, with biopsy-proved sarcoidosis and taking 15 mg of prednisone daily for pulmonary involvement, developed bilateral hand pain from fractures and deformities of the phalanges (Fig 5–7, B). Splinting and anti-inflammatory agents produced no improvement. A bone scan showed increased uptake in many areas, including the phalanges of the feet, which were asymptomatic and roentgenographically normal. Arteriography showed hypovascularity in the sarcoid lesions and hypervascularity in the fractures. Exploration showed total replacement

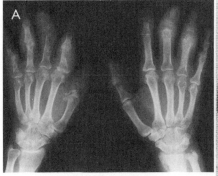
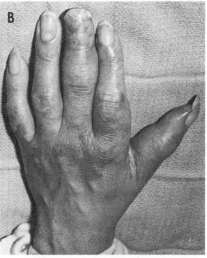

Fig 5–7.—Typist with systemic sarcoidosis who was seen with multiple painful deformities. **A,** x-ray films show typical osteolytic form of sarcoidosis, with cortical atrophy and lacy, reticular medullary pattern. **B,** clinical appearance of left hand. (Courtesy of Adelaar, R.S.: J. Hand Surg. 8:492–496, July 1983.)

of the phalanges by friable material that was both intramedullary and extraperiosteal; the subchondral bone was not penetrated. The right long middle phalanx and thumb proximal phalanx were curetted and replaced by cancellous iliac bone, and Kirschner wires were placed. No healing occurred; there was progressive resorption and collapse of the bone-grafted phalanges over 4 years of follow-up. The patient was able to work by using custom orthoplast splints. Examination of the specimen showed noncaseating granuloma with chronic inflammation.

The other patient was a black man, 19, with multisystem sarcoidosis and an olecranon fracture that did not unite after open reduction and internal fixation. A bone scan showed phalangeal involvement in the fingers and feet in this patient.

Osteolytic sarcoid of the phalanges leads to resorption and collapse, and the response to splinting or bone grafting is not good. Bone scanning is a useful diagnostic approach. Sarcoid lesions of bone have a poor blood supply. Phalangeal collapse might be managed by intramedullary cement with Kirschner wire reenforcement, though this has not been reported; bone grafts should not be used for phalangeal fractures. Sarcoid involvement of fractures can lead to nonunion. Fracture fragments should be excised where appropriate in preference to attempts at osteosynthesis.

▶ The surgical management of lesions produced by diseases of unknown cause and without satisfactory treatment is often unsatisfactory, as this article indicates. This type of problem is a well-known one, having been a feature in the past of most infections and of many diseases. It is still true of some conditions in both categories, and perhaps of most cancerous conditions. If surgery is useful at all in sarcoidosis, it apparently will be similar to cancer surgery, i.e., excision surgery, but the problem of replacement, if needed, has not yet been solved.—P.C.A.

6 Tumors

Glomus Tumor in the Hand: A Clinical and Morphological Study
T. Carlstedt and H. Lugnegård (Sabbatsberg Hosp., Stockholm)
Acta Orthop. Scand. 54:296–302, April 1983   6–1

The management of 18 cases of glomus tumor of the hand seen in 1963–1982 and followed up for 0.5–16 years was reviewed. All patients presented with intense local pain, and 70% had temperature hypersensitivity as well, usually to cold. The average duration of symptoms before correct diagnosis was 4 years. Only 1 patient had a history of trauma, and none had had frostbite. No significant occupational trauma was described. About 70% of the patients were women. The mean age at diagnosis was 47 years. Nearly all digital tumors were subungual in location.

Surgery was done in a bloodless field under magnification. The nailbed was incised longitudinally to expose a subungual tumor, and the tumor was carefully dissected and excised, then the epithelial bed was sutured with monofilament 8–0 nylon sutures. Seventeen patients were asymptomatic postoperatively. One had recurrent symptoms and was found to have new tumors. The recovery period ranged from 2 to 4 weeks.

No cause of glomus tumors of the hand was identified in this series. Glomus tumors constitute about 1% of all hand tumors. They are disabling lesions, characterized by severe pain on pressure and temperature hypersensitivity. Careful dissection and excision of the tumor yield a good outcome.

▶ The suggestion that the mast cells in glomus tumors may be responsible for the pain is intriguing and deserves further follow-up.—R.L.L.

Acquired Acro-osteolysis and Acronecrosis
Judy M. Destouet and William A. Murphy (Washington Univ.)
Arthritis Rheum. 26:1150–1154, September 1983   6–2

Acro-osteolysis (AOL) is a transverse lytic band through the distal phalangeal shaft with preservation of the tuft and base (Fig 6–1). It may be isolated or part of a more generalized skeletal disorder. Most acquired cases are due to occupational exposure to vinyl chloride monomer. The lysis of the phalangeal tuft makes the term "acronecrosis" preferable. Occupational AOL consists of Raynaud's phenomenon, sclerodermatous skin changes, and osteolysis. Its cause is unclear, but an immune complex disease leading to vascular occlusion has been suggested. The severity of AOL is not directly related to either the duration of exposure or the concentration of toxic substance. The phalangeal tuft eventually may frag-

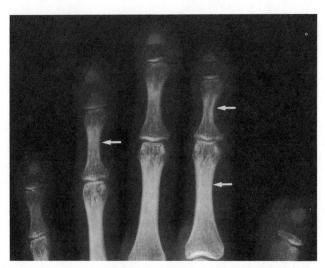

Fig 6–1.—Acro-osteolysis in woman, aged 20, with scleroderma. Linear osteolytic bands of distal phalanges are associated with soft tissue thickening of fingertips. Periosteal new bone formation is present adjacent to radial margin of several proximal and middle phalanges *(arrows)*. (Courtesy of Destouet, J.M., and Murphy, W.A.: Arthritis Rheum. 26:1150–1154, September 1983. Photograph courtesy of Louis A. Gilula, St. Louis.)

ment and resorb. If exposure ceases, the phalangeal fragments may coalesce, resulting in a shortened, "clubbed" distal phalanx. The thumb most often is affected. Preventive measures in the vinyl chloride industry have reduced the occurrence of AOL in recent years.

Transverse AOL rarely is associated with Raynaud's phenomenon, rheumatoid vasculitis, psoriasis, or scleroderma. It definitely is secondary to vascular compromise in this setting. In contrast to true clubbing, the nail bed is not elevated and the ungual angle is maintained. Thermal injuries including chemical burns can result in acronecrosis long after the initial insult, which may result from a combination of mechanical and vascular insults. Vascular impairment from local infection, hematoma, or granulation tissue can contribute to the bone defects that develop in leprosy and other disorders involving neurosensory loss. Cortical resorption of the phalangeal tuft is an early roentgenographic sign of hyperparathyroidism. Infection, tumor, gout, and other disorders can produce distal phalangeal destruction. It is likely that many forms of AOL or distal phalangeal osteonecrosis are initiated by vascular occlusion.

▶ This is a good review article that covers the differential diagnosis and pathophysiology of this interesting x-ray finding.—P.C.A.

Congenital Subungual Nevus
Ralph J. Coskey, Thomas D. Magnell, and Edward G. Bernacki, Jr.
J. Am. Acad. Dermatol. 9:747–751, November 1983   6–3

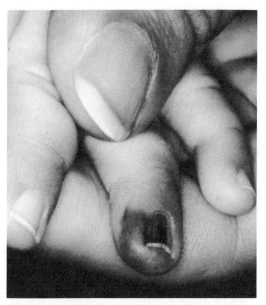

Fig 6–2.—Pigmented nevus of nail bed and periungual skin. (Courtesy of Coskey, R.J., et al.: J. Am. Acad. Dermatol. 9:747–751, November 1983.)

Proper management of small- to medium-sized congenital nevi remains controversial. The authors report data on an infant with a congenital subungual-periungual nevus, which was excised to prevent the later development of melanoma.

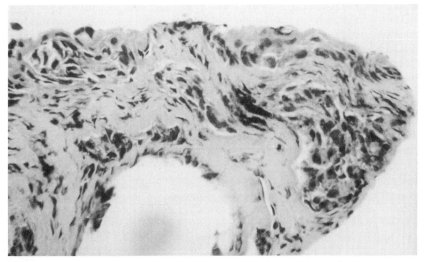

Fig 6–3.—Heavily pigmented nevus cells in nail matrix. (Courtesy of Coskey, R.J., et al.: J. Am. Acad. Dermatol. 9:747–751, November 1983.)

Infant, aged 4 months, had brown-black discoloration of the lateral half of the nail bed and nail of the right ring finger, extending from the proximal nail fold to the distal end of the nail bed and to the skin of the distal and medial aspects of the finger (Fig 6–2). Congenital subungual and periungual nevus cell nevus was diagnosed. The entire lesion was excised at age 6 months. A linear arrangement of melanin pigment was seen within the subepithelial part of the fingernail. A strip of fibrous connective tissue in the nail matrix was widely infiltrated by heavily pigmented nevus cells (Fig 6–3). Numerous nests of nevus cells were present at the dermoepidermal junction and in the papillary dermis of skin surrounding the nail.

Pigmented nevi of the nail bed and nail matrix present as pigmented bands or stripes of dark brown or black-blue hue that usually extend along the long axis of the finger. They are rarely noted at birth. The present lesion was excised because of the prevailing view that patients with congenital nevi of any size are prone to develop melanoma and because little is known of the malignant potential of subungual congenital nevi.

▶ Few hand surgeons will see congenital subungual nevi, but many will face the worrisome differential diagnosis of pigmented lesions of the nail area. Both situations are summarized nicely in this report.—J.H.D.

Pseudoclubbing in Patient With Sarcoidosis of Phalangeal Bones
Jack Lieberman and Marcel Krauthammer (Univ. of California, Los Angeles)
Arch. Intern. Med. 143:1017–1019, May 1983   6–4

Fingertip clubbing has not been described as a manifestation of sarcoidosis in major reviews. However, a patient recently was seen with apparent clubbing that proved to have resulted from inflammation associated with cystic lesions of the distal phalanges due to sarcoidosis.

Man, 25, had a history of sarcoidosis for more than 4 years, accompanied by uveitis, hepatic dysfunction, and arthritis of the hands; subsequently, mitral valve prolapse and an episode of ventricular tachycardia developed. He received steroid therapy for the sarcoidosis and later was given disopyramide phosphate. He reported two episodes of slurred speech and dizziness. Recurrent neurologic symptoms and frequent ventricular tachycardia prompted the current hospital admission. Amiodarone was used successfully in treatment. Apparent clubbing of the fingertips was noted at admission, but finger involvement was asymmetric and toe involvement was absent. The distal interphalangeal joints became painful, and the patient reported aching eyes. Prednisone was given in a dose of 60 mg daily. The roentgenographic findings are shown in Figure 6–4. Gallium activity accumulated in the distal phalanges of the left thumb and index finger. The symptoms resolved when steroid therapy was begun, and clubbing was no longer evident after 3 months, although the x-ray findings were unchanged. Lung function testing showed a mild restrictive defect.

Finger involvement in this patient appears to represent not true clubbing but, rather, phalangeal bone involvement by sarcoidosis. True clubbing can develop in patients with this disease, but pseudoclubbing also can

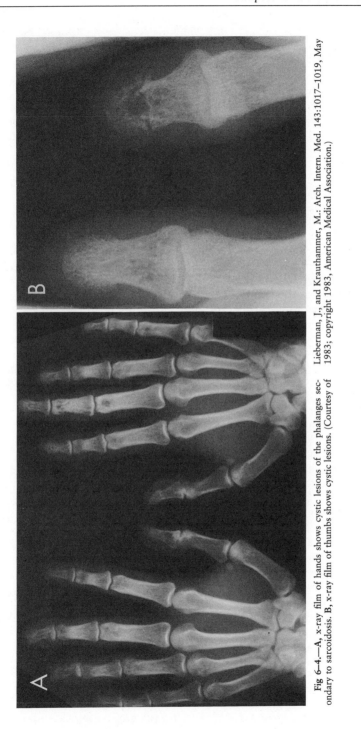

Fig 6–4.—A, x-ray film of hands shows cystic lesions of the phalanges secondary to sarcoidosis. **B,** x-ray film of thumbs shows cystic lesions. (Courtesy of Lieberman, J., and Krauthammer, M.: Arch. Intern. Med. 143:1017–1019, May 1983; copyright 1983, American Medical Association.)

occur as a manifestation of polydactylitis associated with phalangeal granulomatosis. Symmetric involvement, involvement of the toes, and persistence with treatment help distinguish true clubbing from dactylitis.

▶ A surprising number and a great variety of systemic conditions are manifest in the hands. The examiner of the hands therefore is served well by a recapitulation of the distinguishing differences between "clubbing" and "pseudoclubbing" of the digits. There are also causes of clubbing other than dactylitis, such as tumors, and causes of dactylitis other than sarcoidosis.—J.H.D.

Infantile Digital Fibromatosis: Identification of Actin Filaments in Cytoplasmic Inclusions by Heavy Meromyosin Binding
Hiroshi Iwasaki, Masahiro Kikuchi (Fukuoka Univ.), Iwao Ohtsuki, Munetomo Enjoji, Noriko Suenaga, and Ryoichi Mori (Kyushu Univ.)
Cancer 52:1653–1661, Nov. 1, 1983   6–5

Infantile digital fibromatosis, or recurring digital fibrous tumors of childhood, is a rare disorder involving the fingers or toes of infants and young children. The tumor can recur after excision but it does not metastasize, and spontaneous regression has been reported. The origin of the characteristic eosinophilic cytoplasmic inclusions in the tumor cells is unclear. The authors cultured cells from 4 cases of infantile digital fibromatosis and examined them by electron microscopic cytochemistry. Cultured cells were treated for heavy meromyosin (HMM) binding using rabbit skeletal muscle myosin.

The tumors consisted of fibroblast-like cells in an abundant collagenous matrix. Many tumor cells contained eosinophilic cytoplasmic inclusions measuring 1.5–10 μm in diameter. The inclusions in the myofibroblasts consisted chiefly of closely packed microfilaments measuring 5–7 nm in diameter. The cultured cells contained identical cytoplasmic inclusions. Cortical bundles of microfilaments, a well-developed Golgi complex, and a rich network of granular endoplasmic reticulum were observed. When the HMM binding method was applied to saponin-treated cells, the microfilaments constituting the inclusions and the cortical bundles exhibited HMM in the form of the "arrowhead complexes" specific for actin filaments. Arrowhead complexes were most apparent in the periphery of the inclusions.

The inclusions seen in tumor cells in infantile digital fibromatosis may represent the abnormal contraction of actin filaments in the myofibroblast cytoplasm. Some abnormality of regulatory proteins may be present in these cells.

▶ Infantile digital fibromatosis is a rare lesion of unknown cause. Histologically, it is characterized by the presence of the myofibroblast, a cell common to this lesion, Dupuytren's contracture, and normal contracting scar. As in Dupuytren's contracture, the problem in infantile digital fibromatosis appears to be the inappropriate stimulation to formation of these cells in the absence of a wound and the lack of a signal to turn off the cells, such as normally would occur at completion of the wound healing process.

In the past, attention has been given to possible viral stimulation for this phenomenon. Viral inclusion bodies had been described in infantile digital fibromatosis. This article is significant in that these inclusion bodies have been studied ultrastructurally and found not to be viral inclusions, but, rather, accumulations of contractile proteins associated with the myofibroblasts. Although this does not rule out a viral etiology for this condition or for Dupuytren's contracture, it makes such causation less likely. We are still far from a solution to either of these problems on a cellular basis.—P.C.A.

Cutaneous Keratotic Hemangioma
Igor A. Niechajev and Nils H. Sternby (Malmö, Sweden)
Scand. J. Plast. Reconstr. Surg. 17:153–154, 1983   6–6

Eight patients were seen since 1965 with small vascular tumors on the volar side of the fingers. The 4 men and 4 women were aged 20–66 years at the time of operation. Punctate ectasias with horny overgrowth had been present in the pulp of the finger (Fig 6–5), or, in 2 cases, at the finger base, for 1–10 years. Ten to 20 lesions were spread over a 0.5- to 2-sq cm area of slightly elevated skin. Two patients had a history of minor local trauma before the appearance of the lesion. Only 1 finger was involved in each case. Most patients had tenderness on pressure, and several had bled from minimal trauma. Microscopy showed a mixed type hemangioma involving the epidermis, dermis, and subcutaneous tissue. Capillary-like vessels usually predominated. Intraepidermal vascular spaces were present in 5 specimens.

This lesion is considered a true mixed vascular tumor. The term "cutaneous keratotic hemangioma" is suggested. The differential diagnosis includes solitary angiokeratoma and verrucous hemangioma. All patients

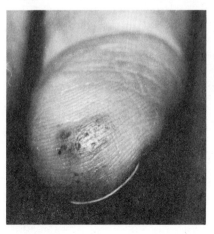

Fig 6–5.—Cutaneous keratotic hemangioma. Characteristic clinical appearance with punctate ectasias and horny overgrowth. (Courtesy of Niechajev, I.A., and Sternby, N.H.: Scand. J. Plast. Reconstr. Surg. 17:153–154, 1983.)

were treated by simple wedge excision of the affected skin and subcutaneous tissue, with excisional margins of 1–2 mm. There have been no recurrences.

▶ This brief clinical report draws our attention to a previously undescribed soft tissue lesion of the fingertip. Local excision is apparently curative.—P.C.A.

Pitfalls in the Diagnosis of the Simple Wrist Ganglion
Guy R. Fogel, Derek A. Younge, and James H. Dobyns (Mayo Clinic and Found.)
Orthopedics 6:990–992, August 1983   6–7

A wrist mass is a common clinical problem that is difficult to diagnose by physical examination alone. Although the ordinary wrist ganglion usually should be apparent when a typical mass is present in the usual site, other entities, some of them more serious, can simulate a ganglion. The most common wrist ganglion arises from the dorsal fibers of the scapholunate ligament complex. Other entities include lipoma, a posterior interosseous nerve neuroma, hamartoma, and a radial artery aneurysm. Dorsal exostoses, prominences of the proximal pole of the scaphoid, partial rupture of regional tendons, localized tenosynovitis, periarticular calcareous deposits, and various types of tumors also can be misdiagnosed as a simple wrist ganglion.

An alternative disorder can be suspected from continued growth of a lesion, an unusual pattern of pain, Tinel's sign, or unusual shape or consistency of a lesion. Transillumination may be helpful, although some ganglia may not transilluminate well. Atypical ganglia can be filled with blood, be occult, ruptured, or scarred, or be detectable only at a relatively distant site such as at a metacarpophalangeal joint. The most serious error is to fail to be prepared for proper management of a malignancy. As example, three soft tissue malignancies and two benign soft tissue tumors, all mistakenly diagnosed as ganglia, are reported in this article.

▶ From a practical standpoint, one cannot surgically perform biopsies on all dorsal wrist masses. The vast majority of them will be ganglions and need not necessarily be treated.

A history of a progressive and steady growth, a failure of the growth to transilluminate, and exceptional pain are good indications for surgery. The point of this article is well taken in that the occurrence of a dorsal wrist ganglion cannot be assumed based on the simple presence of a mass in the typical location.—R.D.B.

Giant Cell Reparative Granuloma of the Hands and Feet
Ted A. Glass, Stacey E. Mills, Robert E. Fechner, Ray Dyer, Wells Martin, III, and Peter Armstrong
Radiology 149:65–68, October 1983   6–8

Jaffe first described giant cell reparative granuloma (GCRG) as an apparently reactive intraosseous lesion of the jaw. Histologically identical lesions occasionally are seen elsewhere, particularly in the short tubular bones of the hands and feet. Five such cases are reported here in patients aged 13–53 years seen at the University of Virginia Medical Center, all presenting with swelling of an extremity. Two patients had pain as well. None had evidence of underlying disease or abnormal serum calcium, phosphate, or alkaline phosphatase levels. Four patients had a single lesion in a phalanx, metacarpal or metatarsal, and 1 had 3 lesions in the same hand. Most lesions were lytic, but only 1 appeared to be destructive. The metaphysis and diaphysis were regularly involved. Three lesions extended to the articular surface. Two recurrences were observed (Fig 6–6); 1 was managed by amputation. All the lesions contained mononuclear fibrohistiocytes and also multinucleated giant cells. Inflammatory cell infiltration was present in 4 cases.

A GCRG should be considered when a lucent, expansile lesion is present in a small tubular bone of the hand or foot, particularly in a young or

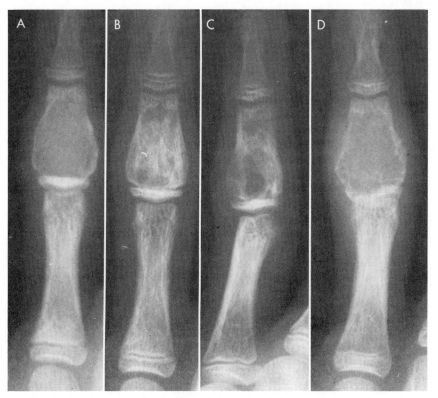

Fig 6–6.—**A,** radiograph demonstrates expansile lytic lesion of the middle phalanx of the ring finger preoperatively. **B,** postoperatively, sclerosis is from bone chips used to fill the cavity. **C,** recurrence 3 months later. Bone chips and subchondral bone have been destroyed but epiphysis is not involved. **D,** extension into epiphysis. (Courtesy of Glass, T.A., et al.: Radiology 149:65–68, October 1983.)

middle-aged person. The lesions are rarely destructive. They may recur after curettage, but total local excision is curative. The cause and pathogenesis of GCRG are unknown. Previous trauma is unusual. The histologic appearances do not suggest neoplasia. The favored view is that GCRG represents a reactive process, possibly a response to intraosseous hemorrhage.

▶ This lesion may be confused radiographically with the much more common enchondroma, as well as such lesions as giant cell tumor and aneurysmal bone cyst. This tumor may be associated with hyperparathyroidism or occur independently. Therefore, if it is diagnosed on biopsy, the patient must be evaluated for possible hyperparathyroidism. Although curettage is associated with a relatively high rate of recurrence, this lesion appears to be reactive rather than a true neoplasm. Therefore, repeated curettage, preserving digit length and function, is still acceptable. More radical excision with replacement bone graft is quite often feasible; the greater certainty of cure may make the prolonged rehabilitation time acceptable.—P.C.A.

Lymphangioma of the Forearm and Hand
William F. Blair, Joseph A. Buckwalter, Michael R. Mickelson, and George E. Omer
J. Hand Surg. 8:399–405, July 1983   6–9

The results of surgery for cavernous lymphangioma of the forearm and hand in 9 patients seen at University of Iowa Hospitals and Clinics or at Carrie Tingley Hospital, Truth or Consequences, New Mexico, in 1952–1981 were reviewed. Tumor was first noted at a median age of 2 weeks in the 5 female and 4 male patients. Tissue diagnosis was made at a median age of 17 months. Median follow-up was 11.7 years. There were 5 lesions in the forearm, 2 in the hand, 1 in the wrist, and 1 in the thumb area. All patients reported tumor-associated pain, usually occurring episodically with erythema, warmth, and systemic fever.

All patients had at least 1 operation, with a total of 18 procedures being performed. Six operations were followed by complications. Lymph vessel proliferation was a constant finding. Lymphatic cysts were present in 5 cases and lymphoid tissue in 3. In 1 case the dermis was involved to a significant degree. Proliferation of capillaries and venules was a common but not predominant feature of most cases. Lymphangioma was eliminated at final clinical examination in only 1 case. Only 2 patients were satisfied with the clinical outcome. The others complained of residual lymphangioma, tumor-associated pain, and hypertrophic scarring from the surgical incisions.

Cavernous lymphangioma usually occurs in pediatric patients. Most of the present patients had minimal functional impairment of the involved extremity, but they were bothered by exertional pain and fatigability. Surgical treatment of these lymphangiomas has generally been unsuccessful. Many adverse sequelae other than infection have occurred, most of them related in part to the unexpected accumulation of lymphatic and serous fluids. Excisional biopsy can be expected to debulk the lesion and to provide diagnostic confirmation. Primary cavernous lymphangiomas do not carry a risk of malignant transformation.

▶ Experience with this tumor, particularly in the upper extremity, is so limited that even case reports, which is what this article represents, are useful. Though management perspectives drawn from individual experiences over many years by different individuals at different institutions cannot be made completely coherent, the close corollaries between this condition and the closely related or interrelated hemangioma group is obvious. Surgery can be more useful and less harmful than this article suggests, but cures are unlikely and caution is advised.—J.H.D.

A Giant Cell Tumor in the Hand Presenting as an Expansile Diaphyseal Lesion: Case Report
James A. Shaw and John F. Mosher (Syracuse, N.Y.)
J. Bone Joint Surg. [Am.] 65-A:692–695, June 1983   6–10

The authors report a case of giant cell tumor that presented as an expansile lesion of an entire metacarpal and mistakenly was thought from radiography to be an aneurysmal bone cyst.

Woman, 58, had progressive swelling and pain in the area of the right ring finger metacarpal and was found to have an expansile osseous lesion involving the entire metacarpal. All concerned thought the lesion to be a benign tumor, probably an aneurysmal bone cyst or an enchondroma with cystic degeneration. General examination was negative. The patient insisted that the finger be salvaged. Repeat radiographs showed nearly total destruction of the osseous margins of the metacarpal, and malignancy was considered, but the patient refused primary resection of the ray. The tumor was resected completely and found to be a typical "benign" giant cell tumor, with modestly pleomorphic stromal cells and about one mitosis per high-power field. A heavy Steinmann pin was placed as a temporary strut, and later a ray resection was carried out. No disease was present a year later, and a bone scan was negative.

Both giant cell tumors and aneurysmal bone cysts are very uncommon in the hand. The present patient had no clinical evidence of other bone disease, but a bone scan was definitely indicated to exclude multicentric tumor. Giant cell tumors typically involve the epiphyseal part of a long bone, but involvement of an entire metacarpal has been described previously. Giant cell tumor cannot be ruled out by radiographic atypicality.

▶ The authors' points are important and worth emphasizing.—R.L.L.

Recurrent Giant Cell Tumor After En Bloc Excision of the Distal Radius and Fibular Autograft Replacement.
W. R. Harris (Toronto Genl. Hosp.) and E. C. H. Lehmann (St. Paul's Hosp., Vancouver, B.C.)
J. Bone Joint Surg. [Br.] 65-B:618–620, November 1983   6–11

Locally recurrent giant cell tumor after curettage, with or without bone grafting, is seen in over half of patients and is managed by en bloc excision and replacement with a large autograft. Data are reported on two patients with giant cell tumor of the distal radius who had local recurrences in a fibular autograft and adjacent soft tissues.

CASE 1.—Woman, 24, underwent en bloc excision of the distal third of the radius for giant cell tumor while pregnant and had replacement with the proximal third of the ipsilateral fibula. A lytic lesion in the distal end of the fibular graft found a year later was curetted and cauterized. The radius was fractured 6 years later at the junction with the graft, but no recurrent tumor was evident and healing was uneventful.

CASE 2.—Man, 24, was treated for recurrent giant cell tumor of the radius with en bloc excision and fibular graft. One year later he was reexplored for recurrent soft tissue and scaphoid lesions. Repeat grafting was not necessary. Radiotherapy was given postoperatively. The patient was well 6 years after initial operation, with solid fusion of the wrist.

Each of these recurrences appeared to result from tumor cells having been left in the soft tissue of the fibular autograft bed. Tumors were found at the time of revision in the soft tissues, with erosion of the adjacent fibular cortex in one case and of the scaphoid-fibular arthrodesis in the other. It is surprising that recurrences from soft tissue seeding at the time of excision and bone grafting are not more frequent. Giant cell tumors clearly can survive in soft tissue and later invade bone. Recurrences have developed at times when the autograft could not have been totally replaced by new bone and was still partly necrotic. Whether this makes the autograft more vulnerable to invasion by soft tissue seeding is not clear.

▶ This report of only two cases needs to be examined in the context of the combined experience of many authors with this problem. The points that secondary excision and curettage of recurrent tumor even after primary excision and grafting may result in long-term improvement and that surgical instruments may seed tumors in soft tissue locations are worth making. Most surgeons at this time would add copious pulsed lavage following excision to the operative procedure and use different instrument pack, gloves, gowns, etc., for the donor site.—R.L.L.

▶ One of the points the authors make in this article is that, at least in their first case, invasion of an avascular bone graft by soft tissue recurrence of the giant cell tumor appeared to have occurred. They speculate as to whether the large avascular graft had any bearing on the ability of the body to deal with soft tissue seeding at the time of original surgery. One wonders whether the use of vascularized fibular graft might alter this propensity.—P.C.A.

Closed-System Venography in the Evaluation of Angiodysplastic Lesions of the Extremities
Simon D. Braun, Arl V. Moore, Jr., Steven R. Mills, Kerry Ford, Dennis K. Heaston, G. Andrew Miller, and N. Reed Dunnick (Duke Univ.)
AJR 141:1307–1310, December 1983   6–12

Accurate delineation of the extent of angiodysplastic lesions of the extremities is mandatory when surgical removal is planned. It may be accomplished by closed-system venography, or passive filling of the vascular system after compressive exsanguination of the extremity. This approach was used by the authors to evaluate 17 consecutive patients (mean age 20.5 years) suspected of having angiodysplastic lesions of the extremities. The final diagnosis in the 13 cases operated on was cavernous hemangioma in 6 cases, arteriovenous malformation in 3, and sclerosing hemangioma, hypervascular chronic inflammatory synovitis, venous malformation, and anomalous tendinous band in 1 case each. The study was done using a 20-gauge intracath and an Esmarch bandage. Up to 125 ml of 30% iodinated contrast medium was used. Patients are premedicated with Demerol and Phenergan, and lidocaine is added to the contrast material.

Abnormalities were detected on venography in 11 cases, and surgical confirmation was obtained in all these cases. Six cavernous hemangiomas (Fig 6–7), 3 arteriovenous malformations (Fig 6–8), and 1 venous malformation were identified. The atypical homogeneous blush seen in another case proved to represent chronic inflammatory synovitis. One of the 2 patients with normal findings who were explored had a sclerosing hemangioma, and the other had an anomalous tendinous band. Standard

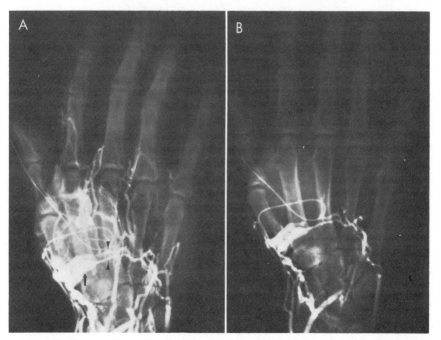

Fig 6–7.—Cavernous hemangioma in man, aged 42. A, closed system venogram. Dilated sinusoidal structure *(arrow)* over proximal part of first and second metacarpals. Two normal-sized veins *(arrowheads)* extend medially from lesion and outline smaller, partially filled normal-sized artery. Second area of abnormality over distal part of second metacarpal. B, standard venogram. Absence of retrograde flow into arterial system and total absence of filling of second area of abnormality. (Courtesy of Braun, S.D., et al.: AJR 141:1307–1310, December 1983.)

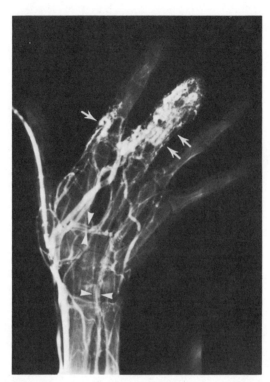

Fig 6–8.—Recurrent arteriovenous malformation in girl, aged 13. Closed-system venogram. Tangle of vessels occupies entire third digit and proximal part of second digit *(arrows)*. Third digit is hypertrophied, although distal phalanx has been amputated. Normal-sized draining veins *(arrowheads)* parallel dilated feeding arteries. Although no arterial injection was performed, there is excellent retrograde filling of arterial tree on venous side. (Courtesy of Braun, S.D., et al.: AJR 141:1307–1310, December 1983.)

venography was inadequate in 1 of 2 instances. Arteriography failed to demonstrate a cavernous hemangioma that was identified by closed-system venography.

Closed-system venography is a simple and highly accurate means of diagnosing and delineating angiodysplastic lesions of the extremity. It can be done on an outpatient basis. The only risk is related to contrast administration. The procedure should be used primarily where a cavernous hemangioma or a purely venous malformation is suspected. Arteriography remains the primary study where an arteriovenous malformation is suspected.

▶ Closed-system venography has distinct advantages over open-system venograms and arteriograms. If an arterial catheter is passed beyond the site of tourniquet application, a closed-system arteriogram might be even better. We have used this technique in cadaver arms, but have been concerned about possible endothelial damage using radiopaque compounds held static in the arteriolar system. Closed-system arteriography may have an important place in the future.—R.A.C.

Acral Melanoma in Japan

Makoto Seiji, Hideaki Takematsu, Michiko Hosokawa, Masaaki Obata, Yasushi Tomita, Taizo Kato, Masaaki Takahashi, and Martin C. Mihm, Jr.

J. Invest. Dermatol. 80:56s–60s, June 1983   6–13

Data on 81 Japanese patients seen with malignant melanoma in 1972–1982 and a total of 1,597 cases of malignant melanoma collected from the Japanese literature from 1961 to 1982 were reviewed. The annual mortality has increased nearly linearly over the past 2 decades. Mortality in 1980 was 0.21 per 100,000.

The 5-year survival in the authors' personal series was 35%. Acral melanomas (59% of the 82 melanomas) were managed by wide excision and immediate skin grafting. Subungual melanomas of the digits were managed by amputation at the metacarpophalangeal or metatarsophalangeal joint level. Node dissection was done in most cases.

Among the acral tumors, the sole and nail plate were especially frequent sites of involvement. Cutaneous melanomas in the literature series were most frequent on the lower extremity, with relative sparing of the trunk. Subungual melanomas were more frequent on the hands than the feet in both series. A preexisting pigmented skin lesion was reported by 17% of patients and trauma by 21%. Lentigo maligna melanoma and superficial spreading melanoma both were less frequent in Japan than in Caucasian series. Nodular melanomas were similarly frequent in Japanese and Caucasians. Most acral melanonas exhibited radial and vertical phases of growth. Subungual melanomas may thicken, split, or destroy the nail plate. Atypical melanocytes with heavily pigmented granules were present along the basal layer of the sweat duct epithelium in the deep dermis in some areas of plantar melanomas.

The causes of the high mortality of acral melanoma remain unclear, but intraepidermal proliferation of melanocytes in the deep dermis along the epidermal appendages and sweat ducts is a possible factor.

▶ The high incidence of acral melanoma in Japan is certainly thought provoking. In cutaneous melanomas in general, the most significant prognostic factor is the thickness of the lesion, but ulceration is another important variable. Our experience with acral melanoma likewise indicates that this is a very high-risk lesion with a high incidence of regional lymph node and systemic progression.—F.H.S.

Phalangeal Metastasis: First Clinical Sign of Bronchogenic Carcinoma

N. Khokhar and Jong D. Lee (Mason District Hosp., Havana, Ill.)

South. Med. J. 76:927, July 1983   6–14

Skeletal metastasis from bronchogenic carcinoma is common, but spread below the elbow is rare. The authors describe a patient in whom the first manifestation of bronchogenic carcinoma was metastases to the phalanges, which simulated benign disease.

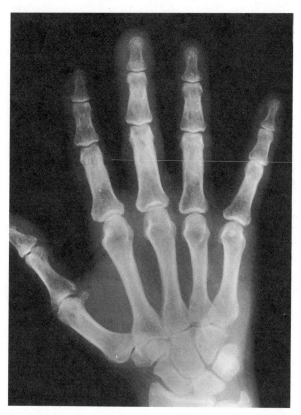

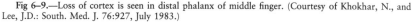

Fig 6–9.—Loss of cortex is seen in distal phalanx of middle finger. (Courtesy of Khokhar, N., and Lee, J.D.: South. Med. J. 76:927, July 1983.)

Man, 67, experienced soreness and swelling of the right middle finger for a month and reported having had a splinter removed a month earlier. He had been hypertensive for many years and was taking chlorothiazide daily; he had smoked cigarettes heavily more than 30 years. The terminal phalanx of the right middle finger was swollen, indurated, and tender. The results of systemic examination were negative. No improvement occurred when cephalosporin therapy was given for 10 days. An x-ray film showed loss of cortex at the volar aspect of the distal phalanx of the affected finger (Fig 6–9). The distal phalanx was disarticulated, and infiltrating squamous cell cancer was found. Chest radiography showed an ill-defined density in the right upper lobe; bronchoscopy indicated distortion of the carina, and bronchial washings contained malignant cells. The patient was given chemotherapy, but deteriorated gradually and died 6 months later.

Phalangeal metastasis from lung cancer can simulate inflammatory disease. The distal phalanx of the thumb is a relatively frequent site of involvement. Most patients have monostotic involvement. Other carcinomas rarely metastasize to the phalanges. Reactive bone or periosteal reaction is not seen on radiography and, despite extensive trabecular destruction, a thin margin of subchondral bone remains.

▶ The terminal segment of a digit is a common site of pathology, with the cause more likely to be systemic or from a distant source than is true of any other part of the hand.—J.H.D.

Amputation for Tumor of the Upper Arm
S. Blåder, B. Gunterberg, and G. Markhede (Univ. of Götenborg)
Acta Orthop. Scand. 54:226–229, April 1983   6–15

The authors reviewed 35 cases of proximal upper extremity amputation done for malignant tumor in a 10-year period in an orthopedic department serving a population of about 2.5 million. Eight patients had malignant bone tumors. The most common soft tissue malignancies were synovial sarcoma, malignant fibrous histiocytoma, and malignant schwannoma. One patient had a benign but locally aggressive extra-abdominal desmoid tumor. Five patients had metastatic lesions. The operations included forequarter amputation, disarticulation of the humeroscapular joint, and amputation through the humerus. The amputation was done palliatively in the 5 patients with metastatic tumor.

The average follow-up was 4½ years. Three of 10 patients followed for 5 years after forequarter amputation survived. Of 15 patients seen at follow-up at an average of 3.3 years postoperatively, 3 used a functional prosthesis and 5 used a cosmetic prosthesis sporadically. Only 1 of the 11 patients having forequarter amputation used a functional prosthesis. Five patients were doing the same work as before but were to some degree dependent on others. All the patients managed daily activities on their own. Most reported no change in social contacts. Ten patients did not seem to be adversely affected psychologically in any obvious way. One patient used analgesics daily for severe phantom limb pain. The others had only moderate phantom limb pain.

Few patients in this series used a functional prosthesis after upper extremity amputation for tumor. Several patients, however, were able to do their usual work, and activities of daily living were not a major problem. Ablative surgery should be considered only for nondisseminated disease unless a functionless and very painful arm is present. Function-preserving surgery can be considered where segmental bone resection, followed by some type of bone or joint reconstruction, is a possibility.

▶ The results of this series are similar to our own series of major amputations for tumors of the upper extremity in regard to function and survival. In recent years, increased interest has been shown in limb salvage for malignant tumors in the upper extremity, particularly when the lesion involves the shoulder girdle and proximal humerus. Improved techniques of surgical staging, particularly computed tomography scanning and angiography, help determine whether the lesion is amenable to resection. When neurovascular structures are not involved, a proximal humeral resection or interscapulohumeral resection (Tinkhoff-Lindberg) procedure can be carried out. Despite the sacrifice of shoulder function, retention of a functioning elbow and hand is extremely beneficial.—F.H.S.

▶ In selected cases, free tissue transfer can permit salvage of otherwise unreconstructable soft tissue defects, whether for tumor or trauma surgery. A case in point is reported by MacKinnon et al. (*Plast. Reconstr. Surg.* 71:706–710, 1983).—P.C.A.

7 Dupuytren's Contracture

Fasciectomy and Dupuytren's Disease: Comparison Between the Open-Palm Technique and Wound Closure
John D. Lubahn, Graham D. Lister, and Terri Wolfe
J. Hand Surg. 9A:53–58, January 1984.   7–1

The open-palm and closed-palm treatments for Dupuytren's contracture were compared in 153 patients operated on between 1976 and 1980. None had had previous operations on the involved hand or had concomitant disorders such as rheumatoid arthritis. The closed-palm technique was used in 115 patients and the open-palm method in 38. The groups were clinically comparable before operation. Follow-ups averaged 4 months in the open-palm group and 6 months in the closed-palm group. A modified Skoog incision (Fig 7–1) was used for lesions involving the palm and fingers, excluding the thumb. Z-plasties later were incorporated into the longitudinal incisions. All diseased fascia was removed. The transverse incisions were left open both in the palm and in the digital Z-plasties. Full motion was encouraged when the dorsal splint was removed 3 to 5 days after operation (Fig 7–2). A splint holding the metacarpophalangeal and interphalangeal joints in extension was used at night.

A total of 131 hands were treated by the closed-palm method and 47 by the open technique. In the closed-palm group a total of 229 rays had average preoperative and postoperative total active motions of 195 and 215 degrees, respectively, representing improvement of 10.3%. Average improvement of 17.2% occurred in 89 rays in the open-palm group. Two thirds of rays treated in the closed-palm group and 83% in the open-palm group improved. Twenty-nine percent and 8%, respectively, became worse in terms of total active motion. Full extension was present at follow-up in 45 of 78 patients in the closed-palm group and in 20 of 25 in the open-palm group. Complications occurred in 19% of closed-palm cases and in 8% of open-palm cases.

Use of the open-palm technique to treat Dupuytren's contracture may be most suited to patients with extensive disease in whom wound closure under tension would be avoided and an adequate blood supply to the wound margin insured. The open method prevents hematoma formation in the palm and permits immediate increased metacarpophalangeal joint extension.

▶ I am at least as impressed by the low incidence of reported digital hypesthesia in this series (unique in cases with significant involvement) as by the seeming superiority of open wound treatment. The discrepancy in numbers

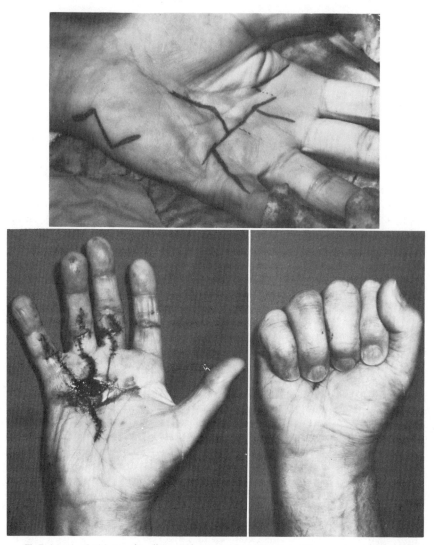

Fig 7–1 (top).—Incision used in all open palm cases. It is modification of Skoog approach with incision in distal palmar crease and longitudinal incisions extending into fingers. Where these cross flexion creases, Z-plasties are subsequently incorporated.

Fig 7–2 (bottom).—Transverse incisions at both distal palmar crease and transverse limb of Z-plasty are left open, then, at a convenient time 3 to 5 days after operation, all dressings are removed, and vigorous active range-of-motion exercises are required of patient.

(Courtesy of Lubahn, J.D., et al.: J. Hand Surg. 9A:53–58, January 1984.)

between the two series suggests a discrepancy also in time, interest, and numbers of surgeons involved; it will be a more attractive comparison when the numbers are even and standard attention has replaced attentiveness. Nevertheless, there is fire behind this smoke. The pain of too tight wound closure may be the most debilitating factor in surgery for Dupuytren's contracture, but it is almost matched by the psychic reluctance of both patient and physician to mar the symmetry of the neatly closed, slow healing, often abnormal skin margins by the apparent violence of range of motion and function.—J.H.D.

Knuckle Pads Causing Extensor Tendon Tethering
A. Addison (West Cumberland Hosp., Whitehaven, England)
J. Bone Joint Surg. [Br.] 66-B:128–130, January 1984   7–2

Knuckle pads generally are considered benign, although sometimes associated with pain and cosmetically embarrassing. A case is reported in which significant functional disability resulted from the presence of knuckle pads.

Man, 33, presented with Dupuytren's contracture of the right hand 2 years after the onset of symptoms and 18 months after the removal of a band of Dupuytren tissue from the little finger and palm. The left hand had been operated on for the same condition some years earlier. Nodules in the feet had always been asymptomatic. The patient had drunk heavily but had lessened his alcohol intake markedly in recent years. His father had had Dupuytren's tissue excised from both hands at age 50. Extensive palmar involvement by Dupuytren's tissue was noted. Knuckle pads were present over the proximal interphalangeal (PIP) joints of the middle and ring fingers, and the skin was tethered to the deep structures. The range of finger flexion and extension was grossly limited; only the little finger could be fully flexed. Partial fasciectomy and excision of Dupuytren's tissue from the palm of the right hand resulted in a significant increase in finger flexion. Subsequently, the central slip of the extensor mechanism was freed from the lateral slips, increasing passive flexion at the PIP joint. A posterior capsulotomy was required for full flexion. Biopsy specimens of the material infiltrating the skin and extensor mechanisms showed typical Dupuytren tissue. Range of motion was significantly improved 2 weeks after operation; nearly full flexion was possible at this time.

Knuckle pads are found in association with a relatively high proportion of Dupuytren's contractures, but they rarely cause significant problems. In the present patient, a relatively young man with severe disease, knuckle-pad tissue tethered the skin and the lateral extensor slips to the central slip, leading to a swan-neck type of deformity and an inability to flex the PIP joint. Dramatic improvement in movement followed operative treatment.

▶ Limited flexion of the digits in Dupuytren's disease is certainly unusual, with the exception of the distal interphalangeal joint when contractural tissue involves the oblique retinacular ligaments. The author has brought our attention to the unusual situation in which dorsal Dupuytren's tissue produced limited flexion; a positive response occurred with surgical excision. It is noteworthy that the digits involved had the appearance at rest of a swan-neck deformity variant with limited active extension of the distal joints compatible with the lateral band involvement.—R.D.B.

Microvascular Changes in Dupuytren's Contracture

Clayton Ward Kischer and Donald P. Speer (Univ. of Arizona)
J. Hand Surg. 9A:58–62, January 1984   7–3

Dupuytren's contracture is a fibrotic disorder of the palmodigital aponeurosis in which the collagenous matrix enlarges to form nodules and laminated bands. The cause is unknown, but the contraction process has been related to the presence of myofibroblasts in the nodules. The authors attempted to find occluded microvessels in fresh tissues obtained at operation from 6 patients with Dupuytren's contracture. Pervasive microvascular occlusion has been described in other fibrotic lesions such as keloids and hypertrophic scars, and lowered oxygen tension is thought to stimulate excessive collagen production. None of the patients reported specific trauma, although all had done some manual labor. One patient was alcoholic. Two patients had flexion contracture of the metacarpophalangeal and proximal interphalangeal joints exceeding 90 degrees, and the others had contracture exceeding 30 degrees.

Most sections from all patients had microvessels with occluded lumens and a great increase in, and excessive layering of, the basal laminae (Fig 7–3). The occlusion appeared to result from an increase in endothelial cell profiles, usually up to 4 or 5. Several pericytes often surrounded the microvessels. Most microvessels were oriented parallel to the long axis of

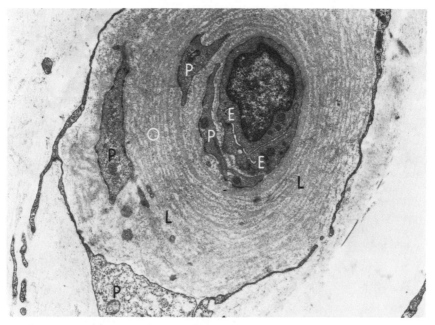

Fig 7–3.—A typical microvessel, 3 μm in diameter, from the peripheral vascular net about the body of the nodules. The lumen is occluded, and there are extreme layers of basal laminae *(L)*, endothelial cells *(E)*, and pericytes *(P)*; original magnification × 12,000. (Courtesy of Kischer, C.W., and Speer, D.P.: J. Hand Surg. 9A:58–62, January 1984.)

the contracture band. Most sections contained myofibroblasts. Polarized light microscopy showed the collagen fibers to be predominantly oriented in the longitudinal axis of the band.

The presence of occluded microvessels is a consistent finding in Dupuytren's contracture. Hypoxia from luminal occlusion may stimulate the pericytes to differentiate to myofibroblasts. The presence of pervasive microvascular occlusion, excessive pericytes, fibroblasts, and basal laminae together suggests a general pathogenesis for fibrotic disease. The microvascular changes may represent a common path through which similar fibrotic lesions can develop in trauma, diabetes, hereditary variations in vascular patterns, and alcoholic liver disease.

▶ This interesting article draws an analogy between the microvascular structures in Dupuytren's contracture and those of hypertropic scar and granulation tissue. This analogy between Dupuytren's contracture and other forms of healing wound has been made before with regard to collagen type and cell structure, particularly the presence of the myofibroblast.

Such observations are useful in shedding light on how Dupuytren's contracture develops. All the evidence indicates that this phenomenon proceeds in a manner very similar, if not identical, to that found in normal healing wounds. The difference, of course, is that in Dupuytren's contracture there is no penetrating wound, and the process is not turned off. Further investigation into signals that begin and end the wound healing-wound contracture process would be of great importance in expanding our knowledge of this condition.— P.C.A.

8 Occupational and Avocational Stress

The Jeweller's Thumb—An Occupational Neuroma: A Case Report
Ramaya Thirupathi (St. Joseph's Hosp., Denver) and Donald Forman (New Hyde Park, N.Y.)
Orthopedics 6:438–440, April 1983   8–1

Perineural fibrosis and scarring of superficial nerves can result from chronic frictional forces, as in bowler's thumb, affecting the ulna-side digital nerve of the thumb at the metacarpophalangeal joint level. The authors report data on a jeweler with perineural fibrosis of the digital branch of the thumb at the interphalangeal joint level.

Woman, 25, a right-handed jewelry worker, had had pain and swelling of the interphalangeal joint of the right thumb for a year. The patient did not respond to splints or treatment with Naprosyn and Tylenol. A 1-sq cm swelling was noted over the interphalangeal joint in the middle of its palmar surface, which was mobile at the transverse axis of the thumb and not compressible. Two-point discrimination was reduced at the tip of the volar side of the finger. Exploration showed fibrotic tissue arising from the pulp branch of the digital nerve. The fibrotic scar tissue was removed and neurolysis of the branch carried out. The histologic findings resembled scarring from trauma and also Morton's neuroma, with epineural fibrosis, mucinous endoneurial change, and distortion and degeneration of the nerve. The patient was free of symptoms postoperatively.

This traumatic neuroma involved the part of the digital nerve located in the pinching surface of the thumb. The patient held fine instruments between the thumb and index finger in the course of her work. The basic process is a proliferation of perineural fibrous elements which surround, separate, and eventually strangulate the nerve fasicles, leading to hyperesthesia and late atrophy. If the problem is discovered early, splinting of the thumb, anti-inflammatory medication, and rest may help reduce the symptoms. A change in work may be necessary to prevent the development of chronic symptoms. Excision of scar tissue around the digital nerve and neurolysis may be necessary where there is no response to conservative measures.

▶ This is another addition to the problem of chronic occupationally related perineural thickening. Conservative treatment is always tried first. This is followed by surgical exploration and perineural stripping. In established perineural fibrosis, the prognosis for cure is very poor, but however, the prognosis for improvement with protective measures or surgery or both, is good.—R.D.B.

Hand Difficulties Among Musicians

Fred H. Hochberg, Robert D. Leffert, Matthew D. Heller, and Lisle Merriman

JAMA 249:1869–1872, Apr. 8, 1983   8–2

Little attention has been given to hand difficulties of concert musicians, who have continuous strong and rapid repetitive movements. One hundred musicians were seen in a 1½-year period by the authors because of occupational difficulties. The 53 male and 47 female patients had a median age of 37.5 years. Seventy-five subjects were pianists. The musicians reported having begun playing at an average age of 8, and they practiced an average of 5 to 6 hours a day. Videotaped recordings were sometimes made of the subjects performing, and electric nerve conduction and myographic studies were done.

Usually initial complaints included pain, weakness, tightening, cramping, curling and drooping, and loss of control of the hand. Pianists had noticed loss of control and speed, but rarely noticed loss of volume. The right arm was affected twice as often as the left; the right fourth and fifth fingers were affected most often. About half the patients examined had weakness or decreased bulk or tone in the muscles, and 40% showed abnormal positioning with curling and drooping of fingers. Inflammatory disorders of tendon or synovium accounted for 42% of the cases. Tendinitis was the most common diagnosis. Also, nerve disorders were frequent. Most patients were treated with nonsteroid anti-inflammatory medications and physiotherapy. Most of those with inflammatory tendon symptoms have improved. Needle-electrode-assisted biofeedback is being tried for patients with motor control difficulties.

Tendinitis is common in musicians, usually involving the finger extensors. It may result from rapid motions and forte movements in which the thumb is fixed and the fourth finger is stretched. Many affected musicians have a good prognosis. The hand should not be used until symptoms subside, and anti-inflammatory drugs may aid the process. Splinting, followed by physical therapy, will permit more than half the patients to return to work, but recurrences are frequent. The prognosis is less hopeful at present for patients with nerve entrapment and motor control problems.

▶ These authors should be congratulated for the quality of their investigations regarding this challenging and often frustrating group of patients. Professional musicians are highly motivated people who frequently demand extreme degrees of both dexterity and endurance from their hands. As they push on to greater technical challenges, the physical disabilities described in this article may result. The problems are not unlike those encountered by physicians who treat long-distance runners, in that occasionally the patient will desire or attempt to perform at a level beyond his or her physical capabilities. Management, therefore, not only must consider the physical impairment and its treatment, but also must assist patients to accept realistic technical or performance goals based on their physical capabilities.—P.C.A.

Plasma Guanosine 3',5'-Monophosphate Responses to the Cold Pressor Test in Patients With Vibration Disease

Fumihiko Okada, Miyuki Honma, Michio Ui, and Norihiro Kiyota
Arch. Environ. Health 38:144–147, May–June 1983   8–3

Vibration disease is a traumatic vasospastic disorder of occupational origin, affecting those who use vibrating tools. The symptoms resemble those of Raynaud's disease, and animal studies have suggested increased responsiveness to norepinephrine in arterial smooth muscle after vibratory stimulation. The authors examined plasma cyclic guanosine 3',5'-monophosphate (cyclic GMP) responses to cold pressor testing in 39 men with vibration disease and 10 healthy subjects. The patients had worked with vibratory tools for a mean of 10 years. Twenty-eight had received kallidinogenase and nicametate citrate, whereas 11 were untreated. The cold pressor test was done by immersing the hand in water at 10 C for 5 minutes.

Initial plasma cyclic GMP concentrations were comparable in patients and controls. No significant increase occurred on cold pressor testing in the controls, but the untreated patients had a sharp rise in plasma cyclic GMP during and after the test. The rise was suppressed by simultaneous injection of phentolamine or atropine on repeat testing a week later. Treated patients had no significant rise in plasma cyclic GMP concentration on cold pressor testing. An untreated patient had a suppressed response on repeat testing after 2 weeks of treatment with dihydroergotamine.

The rise in plasma cyclic GMP in response to catecholamines appears to depend on stimulation of the α-adrenergic receptors. The features of vibration disease that suggest peripheral circulatory impairment may be explained by enhanced vasoconstriction resulting from an exaggerated response of α-adrenergic or cholinergic receptors in arterial smooth muscle. The hyperresponsiveness of α-adrenergic receptors may be suppressed by dihydroergotamine.

► ↓ The following epidemiologic study by Brubaker and associates points out the high incidence of Raynaud's phenomenon in workers exposed to vibrating tools or machinery. Although modern equipment is designed to dampen the vibration of this equipment, over half of all lumbermen have significant Raynaud's phenomenon. Many of them consider it a normal part of their job. The high incidence of vibration white finger disease among those who use chain saws occupationally would suggest that further efforts are necessary to lessen the vibration transmitted to the worker. The extremely high incidence of Raynaud's phenomenon in lumbermen also suggests that it is a work-related disorder in many patients.

The article by Okada and associates investigates the physiologic abnormality in these patients. It appears to be a hyperresponsiveness of the adrenergic system causing an exaggerated vasospastic response. This seems to be partly reversible with medication, although, unfortunately, only the change in GMP was investigated. There is no mention in the article regarding any clinical response of the white fingers to medical treatment. However, the study does lend a scientific rationale to the use of vasodilating agents in the management of this frequently occupationally related disorder.—P.C.A.

Vibration White Finger Disease Among Tree Fellers in British Columbia
Robert L. Brubaker, C. J. G. Mackenzie, P. R. Eng, and D. V. Bates (Univ. of British Columbia, Vancouver)
J. Occup. Med. 25:403–408, May 1983   8–4

Vibration from the use of chain saws and other vibrating hand tools can cause vibration white finger disease (VWFD), a type of secondary Raynaud's disease, which can be disabling and require a change of occupation in its advanced stages.

The occurrence of VWFD was examined in 146 tree fellers at seven lumber camps in British Columbia. The control group included 142 workers with minimal or no exposure to hand-arm or intense whole body vibration. Symptoms of Raynaud's phenomenon were reported by 51% of the tree fellers and 5% of the control subjects, a highly significant difference. More than one fifth of the tree fellers had extensive blanching of at least 4 fingers throughout the year. The median interval from the start of full-time tree felling to the onset of symptoms of VWFD was 6.2 years. Only 1 worker who had used a chain saw for less than 5 years reported Raynaud's phenomenon, whereas 82% of those working for 21 to 25 years were affected. The middle 3 digits were most often affected, and the thumb was least often affected. Cigarette smoking was comparably frequent in the feller and control groups.

Raynaud's phenomenon is a common problem in tree fellers exposed to chain saw vibration for longer than 5 years. The latency period appears to be quite variable. The condition does not seem to be related to cigarette smoking. The use of antivibration saws, as recommended, should prevent VWFD in most tree fellers.

Upper Dorsal Sympathectomy for Palmar Hyperhidrosis
A. Bass, S. Inovrotzlavski, and R. Adar (Tel Aviv Univ.)
Isr. J. Med. Sci. 19:112–115, February 1983   8–5

The results of bilateral upper dorsal sympathectomy in 133 patients with palmar hyperhidrosis (HH) were reviewed. Sixty-seven patients were followed up for 5 to 10 years (mean, 7 years). Sixty-six patients were followed up for 1 to 4 years (mean, 2 years). All the patients had plantar HH as well, and about half had excessive axillary sweating. The T-2 and T-3 ganglia on both sides were removed. All patients had failed to respond adequately to nonoperative measures.

Complete drying of both hands was achieved postoperatively in 98% of the total group. There were only a few serious complications, and none led to permanent disability. Horner's syndrome was less frequent in later cases, and fewer than 1% of all patients had persistent, severe Horner's syndrome. Some degree of compensatory HH developed in almost all patients, and in one third of the cases, this was troublesome and persisted at long-term follow-up. Gustatory phenomena were frequent but not a serious problem. Half the patients noted reduced effort tolerance for several months after the operation. Some recurrent HH was noted in the hands in 26% of the patients, usually within 3 to 12 months of the operation. The patients preferred this to completely dry skin. Moderate HH returned in 4 hands of 3 patients, and severe HH returned in 10 hands of 7 patients. Only 10 patients regretted having had the procedure; 2 others were uncertain.

Bilateral upper dorsal sympathectomy is a highly successful treatment for palmar HH and has a relatively low morbidity rate. Late failure followed 5% of the operations in the series. Severe Horner's syndrome is a cosmetic problem, especially for female patients, but it is quite uncommon. Compensatory HH is most troublesome to persons who work outdoors in hot weather. Upper dorsal sympathectomy can be recommended for properly selected patients with palmar HH.

▶ The authors have accumulated a very large series of patients with what they describe as severe disabling hyperhidrosis. In active office hand practice, I see this problem extremely infrequently. While this treatment is noted to have been reported elsewhere, this appears to be a very radical procedure for a condition that may be psychogenically based. Complication rates are high short-term, but low long-term.

It is my opinion that this procedure should be reserved for very severe cases with failure of long-term medical or biofeedback training in attempts to change sympathetic activity short of surgery.—R.D.B.

Treatment of Writers' Cramp With Sodium Valproate and Baclofen: Case Report
R. Sandyk (Johannesburg)
S. Afr. Med.J. 63:702–703, April 1983   8–6

Writers' cramp is a disorder of unknown cause characterized by muscle spasm, incoordination, and discomfort. Many physicians believe the condition represents a focal form of dystonia and, if this is true, it might result from a striatal dopaminergic predominance, secondary to disinhibition of dopamine striatal neurons. Previous treatment has been unsatisfactory. Sandyk reports a case of simple writers' cramp that remitted completely after treatment with the γ-aminobutyric and (GABA)-mimetic combination of sodium valproate and baclofen.

Man, 27, for a year had noticed arm and forearm pain, palmar perspiration, and, occasionally, tremor on writing. The symptoms had progressed during the past few months. Writing became slow and labored after 1 to 2 hours. The cramp was characterized by pressure of the adducting thumb. After that, the pen tended to roll out of the tight grip. No other abnormality was apparent. The patient tended to overflex and adduct the thumb when attempting to write. The wrist flexed and was elevated above the writing surface, and the writing was jerky. Laboratory studies, skull radiographs, an EEG, and a computed tomography study failed to show a specific cause of dystonia. Sodium valproate was given in increasing doses up to 1,200 mg daily, with baclofen given in doses up to 60 mg daily. The patient's writing gradually improved 2 weeks after the start of treatment, and significant remission was noted after 4 weeks. The condition remained in remission for 3 months. No side effects occurred.

These drugs have a synergistic action in reducing activity in the nigro-striatal dopaminergic pathway and inhibiting dopamine release from striatal terminals. Another patient with dystonic writers' cramp responded to this approach. These cases support the suggestion that writer's cramp is a form of focal dystonia in which a deficiency of GABA has an important role. Treatment with valproate and baclofen should be tried in the initial treatment of patients with writers' cramp.

▶ Writers' cramp is a difficult condition, and one for which I have found no help with any known form of therapy. The author's suggested treatment regimen is certainly enticing and apparently effective. Careful monitoring for potential drug side effects would need to be performed, and the question of duration of treatment is not clarified in this author's experience with two cases.— R.D.B.

Acupuncture Therapy for Tennis Elbow
Gunilla Brattberg
Pain 16:285–288, July 1983   8–7

Corticosteroid injections fail to provide significant relief in some patients with tennis elbow. As a result, acupuncture was evaluated in 26 male and 11 female patients, aged 30 to 60 years, with persistent epicondylitis. All but 6 patients had had symptoms for longer than 6 months. Twenty-four had had corticosteroid injections. Twenty-eight had lateral epicondylitis. Four had bilateral pain. Twenty-six other patients, 11 with symptoms for longer than 6 months, were treated solely by corticosteroid injections. Five to eight acupuncture needles were inserted in the elbow region, particularly the brachioradialis muscle, and mechanical stimulation was carried out intermittently for 15 minutes. An average of six treatments were given, usually in a 4-week period.

None of 34 evaluable patients became worse after acupuncture, and 21 reported having no pain. Eighteen of 29 patients with symptoms for longer than 6 months had no pain at follow-up. Five of 9 patients returned to work after acupuncture therapy. Acupuncture therapy appeared to be significantly better than corticosteroid therapy.

Acupuncture appears to be an effective treatment for tennis elbow. It is more time-consuming than corticosteroid injections, but it should be considered when initial corticosteroid injection fails. No side effects have been reported from acupuncture therapy, whereas several corticosteroid-treated patients have reported worsening of the condition. Most acupuncture treatments in this study were given by a nurse.

▶ This rather interesting report of 37 cases of tennis elbow treated with acupuncture does not state the exact patient selection program. In any event, the control group which had steroid injection, demonstrated consistent improvement in only 2 of 11 patients, compared to 21 of the 34 patients who were treated with acupuncture. This poor showing of the steroid injection group has not been my clinical experience. Further comparisons of patients with different levels of symptoms consistently demonstrated that acupuncture was superior to cortisone. It should be noted, however, that acupuncture requires six treatments over a 4-week period. One wonders whether acupuncture offers an alternative to routine management, whether it offers an alternative to failed steroid injections before any surgery is offered, or whether, in fact, it offers an alternative to surgery. Theoretically, steroid injection may offer some pharmacologic effect decreasing the inflammatory response. The acupuncture would seem only to affect the patient's perception of pain. In any event, this is an interesting article that offers some potential for future investigations.—B.F.M.

9 Pain and Vascular Dysfunction Syndromes

Posttraumatic Dystrophy of the Extremities: Clinical Review and Trial of Treatment
Z. J. Poplawski, A. M. Wiley, and J. F. Murray
J. Bone Joint Surg. [Am.] 65-A:642–655, June 1983   9–1

Sudeck's posttraumatic dystrophy causes much more disability than would be expected from disuse alone. It often is not diagnosed in its early stages, or it is misdiagnosed and mistreated. The authors evaluated a new treatment method in patients with established posttraumatic dystrophy. Review of 126 cases with involvement of the extremities, followed for 5 years or longer, showed that almost all patients had continued symptoms and signs. Pain was by far the most disabling symptom. Twenty-five patients had marked loss of motion. Almost half the patients complained of stiffness. Vascular instability was apparent in most of the affected hands and feet. Radiography showed patchy demineralization or generalized osteoporosis in 49 cases. Twenty-five of 55 previously employed patients remained unemployed as a direct result of the injury, and 7 others had changed to less demanding work.

Twenty-seven other patients with posttraumatic dystrophy in 28 extremities were treated by intravenous injections of steroid and lidocaine. Sixty-four blocks were produced with a lidocaine-methylprednisolone mixture. Generally, they lasted 30 minutes. Manipulation was performed if indicated. Areas of induration were massaged by the deep friction technique, and the web spaces were repeatedly stretched. The metacarpals or metatarsals were mobilized in the anteroposterior and lateral planes. Physiotherapy was continued after each block, and other treatment was given as indicated. Dynamic splints were used in patients with marked stiffness and loss of motion. All but 7 of the 28 affected extremities improved significantly, and 11 had an excellent outcome. All poor results were in patients with posttraumatic dystrophy for longer than 9 months. These patients and most of those with fair results were unemployed. Many patients required 2 or 3 blocks, and some had as many as 5. No serious or lasting complications occurred.

Intravenous regional block with steroid is an effective approach in many cases of established posttraumatic dystrophy, helping to break the pain cycle and permitting rehabilitation by conventional physical therapy. The best results are obtained when treatment begins within 6 months of the onset. The technique is simple and causes no significant complications. The steroid may somehow stabilize the cell membranes of inflamed nerve endings, thereby alleviating pain.

▶ There is almost too much in this article and one can quarrel with almost every investigational technique. Yet, the article addresses one of the major and continuing problems in the management of upper extremity rehabilitation (not just from trauma) and confirms or establishes two important points: (1) Time seldom cures these patients, and (2) all of the known useful treatments become less effective with time. Both facts indicate that early identification and treatment are vitally important. Luckily, diagnosis is easy if physicians will but "look at" and "listen to" their patients. Treatment is not so easy even utilizing the method endorsed by the authors (though it is useful). The principles are early recognition of the problem and early restoration of function. Doing this requires some assistance in control of the perceived discomfort and results in considerable improvement in the motivation, confusion, and frustration of the patient.—J.H.D.

The Seriously Uninjured Hand: Weakness of Grip
Harold M. Stokes
J. Occup. Med. 25:683–684, September 1983   9–2

Loss of grip force is a rateable factor in determining permanent disability in some states, but malingerers or persons with psychological disability can purposely record lower grip measurements in the ostensibly injured hand. The author developed an objective means of documenting true loss of grip strength. A sealed hydraulic dynamometer is used as a grip measuring device. The patient is unable to observe the distance that he has moved the handle he grasps. Grip force is recorded at each of 5 handle positions, first with the uninjured hand. A patient with true grip weakness will have a decrease in grip strength in the injured hand, but a slightly skewed bell curve will be observed. A person who tries to simulate a weak grip will apply the same minimal pressure at each position, producing a straight-line record. Variance of 5 lb or less at each position is noted in these cases.

This method of testing grip strength can show objectively whether a given subject is cooperating by applying maximal pressures, as instructed. Real, as opposed to fictitious, loss of grip strength can be documented better than by reporting simple numerical values, and subjective statements relative to a lack of cooperation can be avoided.

▶ Although it can be measured in exact numbers and thus seems to be precise and "scientific," grip measurement is truly a subjective evaluation that requires a good deal of patient cooperation.

Several factors must be taken into consideration when using the Jamar dynamometer to evaluate grip. First, clearly, finger joint excursion related to either joint or tendon injury will affect the amount of force generated at each of the five positions. Likewise, nerve or muscle damage will have a similar effect. Pain also honestly may limit power at one position more than another; however, given these caveats, knowledge of the normal bell-shaped curve for grip strength in the five dynamometer positions can be helpful in evaluation of possible malingering.—P.C.A.

Reflex Sympathetic Dystrophy (Causalgia): Treatment With Guanethidine
Takeshi Tabira, Hiroshi Shibasaki, and Yoshigoro Kuroiwa
Arch. Neurol. 40:430–432, July 1983   9–3

Orally administered guanethidine was used successfully to treat 3 patients with reflex sympathetic dystrophy associated with cervical spondylosis.

Woman, 66, had transient paresis of the right arm after slipping and striking her forehead against a rock. The patient noted extreme pain in the upper extremities an hour later, followed by marked edema in the painful areas. The pain was not relieved by conventional analgesics, and the patient could not use the upper extremities. Examination, 45 days after the onset, showed severe pitting edema of the hands and fingers and trophic changes of the skin and nails. Severe hyperalgesia was present in the C-6 to C-7 areas of the upper extremities. There was mild hyperreflexia at the knees and ankles. X-ray studies showed intervertebral and foraminal narrowing at the C-4 to C-6 level. Electromyography showed active denervation in muscles innervated by the C-6 segment. Nerve conduction velocities were normal. Interpeak latencies on somatosensory evoked potential recording were above normal. An epidural block relieved the pain for no longer than 3 hours, and a stellate ganglion block did not provide lasting relief. Oral administration of 20 to 30 mg of guanethidine sulfate reduced the pain and edema. The medication was stopped after 25 days because of orthostatic hypotension. There was no recurrence in more than 2 years of follow-up, although mild hypoesthesia and hyperalgesia persisted in the C-6 segment.

Mild orthostatic hypotension in this patient was the only side effect of guanethidine therapy. A direct effect was demonstrated by infusing guanethidine locally in 1 patient. Guanethidine blocks the release of norepinephrine from nerve terminals, suggesting that reflex sympathetic dystrophy may result from hypersensitivity to norepinephrine. More than one mechanism may be responsible for this disorder, but some cases appear to be amenable to treatment by oral administration of guanethidine.

▶ Pain dysfunction syndromes of the extremities are common and important, but still confusing because of the variable degree of reflex sympathetic dystrophy from case to case and from time to time in the same case. The suggestion by the authors that there may be more than one type of reflex sympathetic dystrophy would be almost intolerable if they did not soften the blow by (1) reviewing some instances of unique causation of the problem, (2) adding support to the reported efficacy of guanethidine as a treatment, and (3) adding support to a new mechanism for reflex sympathetic dystrophy.— J.H.D.

Treatment of Upper Extremity Reflex Sympathetic Dystrophy With Prolonged Continuous Stellate Ganglion Blockade

Mark A. Linson, Robert Leffert, and Donald P. Todd
J. Hand Surg. 8:153–159, March 1983

9–4

Reflex sympathetic dystrophy (RSD) appears to be a disordered response to trauma that far exceeds the actual structural damage to an extremity and involves varying degrees of pain, loss of joint motion and function, and trophic and vasomotor changes. The authors evaluated prolonged continuous stellate ganglion blockade with an indwelling catheter in 29 consecutive patients with RSD of the upper extremity who failed to respond to physical therapy, mild analgesic therapy, and treatment with tranquilizers. Prolonged blockade was used in all but 1 patient. An 18-gauge Teflon catheter is placed via the anterior approach close to the lateral part of the anterior surface of the body of C7 on the involved side (Fig 9–1); the response to administration of 0.5% bupivacaine and epinephrine is determined before the catheter is sewn in place. No antibiotics were used. About half of the patients required replacement of migrating catheters

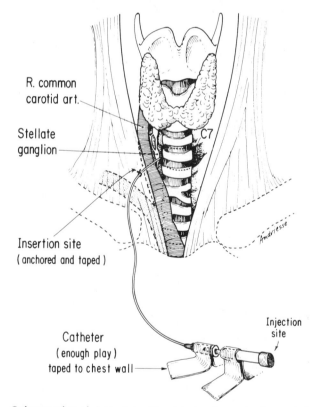

R. common
carotid art.

Stellate
ganglion

C7

Insertion site
(anchored and taped)

Injection
site

Catheter
(enough play)
taped to chest wall

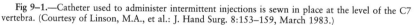

Fig 9–1.—Catheter used to administer intermittent injections is sewn in place at the level of the C7 vertebra. (Courtesy of Linson, M.A., et al.: J. Hand Surg. 8:153–159, March 1983.)

after 2–4 days. When a block was in effect, as evidenced by the Horner sign and warming of the hand, intensive physical and occupational therapy was instituted. Elevation of the hand and administration of oral nonsteroidal anti-inflammatory drugs, mild analgesics, tranquilizers, and muscle relaxants also were used, but transcutaneous electrical stimulation was not.

Most patients were aged 50–70 years. Fifteen had had fractures before onset of RSD, all of which were healed at the time of treatment. Five patients had had carpal tunnel release, and 1 had had cervical laminectomy. The average duration of disabling symptoms of RSD exceeded 1 year. Complications included cardiac ischemia from hypertension induced by anxiety in 1 patient and a limited tachyarrhythmia in another; because of these reactions, epinephrine no longer is used. The average duration of blockade was 7 days. Marked overall improvement occurred in 90% of patients, and 19 of 26 reported persistently less pain at follow-up after an average of 3 years. Trophic and vasomotor changes improved, and there was lessening of pain and improved motion. Six of 7 patients in whom improvement was not maintained had psychiatric, legal, or disability problems. Only 4 patients who responded over the long term had such problems.

A favorable response to sympathetic blockade is a helpful diagnostic feature of RSD, and prolonged, continuous stellate ganglion block appears to be a useful approach. Most of the present patients experienced long-term improvement after this procedure. Intensive physical therapy during the block is an important part of treatment.

▶ It is encouraging for the authors to confirm the reported excellent early results in treatment of reflex sympathetic dystrophy with prolonged continuous stellate ganglion blockade. It is equally heartening to note that (1) significant complications are minimal with skilled control, even though the nuisance level remains high; (2) maintained results are surprisingly good; and (3) good results can be obtained in very chronic states. Less satisfying is the concentration on patients with relatively pure reflex sympathetic dystrophy, a minority group in most pain clinics, and the discouraging results with motivationally impaired patients, a majority group in most pain clinics.—J.H.D.

Reflex Sympathetic Dystrophy in a 14-Year-Old Female
Richard M. Buchta (Univ. of California, San Diego)
J. Adolesc. Health Care 4:121–122, 1983   9–5

Reflex sympathetic dystrophy (RSD) is rare in adolescents. Sixteen cases in patients younger than age 19 years have been described. Most patients have recovered with treatment, but significant morbidity can occur. An adolescent girl with RSD who had significant sequelae despite treatment is described here.

Girl, 14, sustained minimal injury to the right elbow while playing tennis and afterward could not extend the distal phalanx of the right fifth finger. Ruptured extensor tendon was diagnosed by an orthopedist, but there was no response to immobilization, and exploration a month later showed an intact tendon. Continuous pain, edema, hypothermia and cyanosis of the extremity developed 3 months after injury, involving the hand and forearm midway to the elbow. An x-ray study was negative. Immobilization, analgesics, and a 2-week course of systemic prednisone therapy failed to help. A brachial plexus block followed by sympathectomy was only partly helpful. Pain continued on use of the hand, and immobilization of the hand led to a contracture of the fifth finger. The child had had many somatic complaints previously, and recovery from minimal injuries had tended to be prolonged.

A good outcome cannot be predicted for pediatric or adolescent patients with RSD. The cause of the disorder remains unknown. Treatment is symptomatic. Prednisone therapy often is helpful in adult patients with RSD. Local ganglionic blockade or sympathectomy can be recommended if there is no improvement in a few weeks or if severe symptoms are present. There may be a substantial psychosomatic component to the disorder, but it is not clear whether the psychopathology is primary or results from the chronic discomfort.

▶ Though the history in this case report seems incomplete, the probability of pain sources other than reflex sympathetic dystrophy seems likely, and the resort to sympathectomy seems precipitate. The reservations expressed concerning the prognosis of pediatric and adolescent patients whose pain dysfunction syndromes may be inclusive or noninclusive of reflex sympathetic dystrophy are well founded. Results range from dramatically good to tragically poor. A psychiatric survey is a useful preoperative assessment.—J.H.D.

Controlled Double-Blind Trial of Nifedipine in Treatment of Raynaud's Phenomenon

Richard J. Rodeheffer, James A. Rommer, Frederick Wigley, and Craig R. Smith (Johns Hopkins Univ.)
N. Engl. J. Med. 308:880–883, Apr. 14, 1983   9–6

The calcium-channel blocker nifedipine, which causes vascular smooth muscle relaxation and relieves arterial vasospasm, was evaluated in a double-blind crossover trial of 15 patients with symptomatic Raynaud's phenomenon related to cold or stress. The 12 female and 3 male patients had a mean age of 34 years. Nine patients had systemic sclerosis, and 1 had systemic lupus erythematosus. Seven patients had a history of digital ulcers. The mean duration of Raynaud's disease was about 6 years. Nifedipine was given in 10-mg capsules along with a placebo in a 5-week trial. A maximum of 2 capsules was ingested 3 times daily if no severe side effects occurred.

Nine patients reported moderate to marked improvement while taking nifedipine, and 2 reported improvement while taking a placebo. The mean rate of attacks fell from 15 attacks every 2 weeks with a placebo to 11 every 2 weeks with nifedipine. The effect of cold exposure on digital artery systolic pressure was attenuated by nifedipine in 4 of the 9 patients, but analysis of brachial indices suggested that nifedipine did not significantly alter the mean cold-induced fall in digital artery systolic blood pressure. Mild transient headache occurred in most patients using nifedipine, and light-headedness was experienced in one third of the patients. There were no significant changes in the erythrocyte sedimentation rate, blood counts, or electrolytes during treatment.

This study and two other double-blind controlled trials have shown nifedipine to be effective in the treatment of Raynaud's phenomenon. Two thirds of the patients had subjective symptomatic improvement when taking nifedipine. The drug is well-tolerated, but additional study of dose-response relations and effects of long-term treatment are needed.

▶ This is an excellent study that shows some improvement with the use of nifedipine in the treatment of Raynaud's phenomena. It should be noted from review of the article that the drug will not prevent attacks but will only reduce their incidence. Continued studies and better treatment modalities will be available in the future.—R.D.B.

▶ The benefit of nifedipine in Raynaud's phenomenon also has been reported by Porter and Taylor (*World J. Surg.* 7:326–333, 1983), who reviewed the available treatment modalities for Raynaud's syndrome and recommended nifedipine combined with other conservative measures such as local skin care, avoidance of cold, and avoidance of cigarette smoke. The benefit of surgical sympathectomy was questioned in their report, and there is some physiologic research supporting the hypothesis that the peripheral vasoconstriction may not be mediated through the sympathetic nervous system, as the vasoconstriction can be broken by histamine even in the presence of exogenous noradrenaline (*Clin. Sci.* 66:343–349, 1984), and is not corrected by exogenous β-sympathetic stimulation (*Microvasc. Res.* 27:110–113, 1984). The fact that histamine and nifedipine have both been shown to relieve vasospasm suggests that they or analogous drugs may prove useful in the long-term treatment of Raynaud's phenomenon and other vasospastic conditions.—P.C.A.

Vascular Participation in Deep Cold Pain
Heinrich Fruhstorfer and Ulf Lindblom
Pain 17:235–241, November 1983   9–7

Since the degree of cold pain probably depends on blood flow and therefore on internal limb temperature, the nociceptors that are activated should be close to or within the walls of veins. The authors tested this hypothesis by injecting 20-ml volumes of cold saline into an empty hand vein in 16 healthy subjects, 12 men and 4 women, aged 23–37 years. The arm veins were drained with the use of a pressure cuff before saline solution was injected at temperatures ranging from 5 C to 37 C.

Saline below 26 C elicited pure cold sensations, while at temperatures below 20 C, both cold and pain sensations occurred. The pain was described chiefly as deep and radiating along the veins. Many subjects reached their pain tolerance when saline at 5 C was injected. Pain consistently appeared after cold and disappeared either before or together with cold sensation. Paresthesias were reported toward the end of each stimulation trial, due to ischemia after inflation of the pressure cuff.

These observations can be explained on the basis of two types of vascular receptor, a sensitive specific cold receptor and a nociceptor with a threshold at about 20 C. Cold receptor neurons with delta fibers might elicit a pure cold sensation, while those with C fibers add a superimposed burning sensation. The internal tissue temperature declines because of advancing arterial constriction, stimulating the paravascular low-threshold cold receptors. Below a tissue temperature of 20 C, the deep nociceptors would be activated, leading to deep, radiating, aching pain. When activation of the low-threshold cold receptors ceases, only pain is present until the arteriospasm resolves.

The Nerve Response After Autotransplantation of the Rabbit Ear.
G. Lassmann and H. Piza (Univ. of Vienna)
J. Hand Surg. 9A:121–124, January 1984 9–8

A neurohistologic study of nerve regeneration after autotransplantation of the rabbit ear was undertaken in order to elucidate the persistent cold intolerance seen after the replantation of fingers and extremities. Studies were done on 16 autotransplants 3 weeks to 18 months after the procedure. The nerve supply to the vascular system of the rabbit ear consists chiefly of noradrenergic fibers. Histochemical methods included hematoxylin-eosin staining by cholinesterase and glyoxylic acid fluorescence; silver and osmium-zinc iodide impregnation methods also were used.

Wallerian degeneration of the central nerve and of the adventitial nerve plexus in the central vessels was noted at 3 weeks. Degeneration in the basal parts of the central nerves was complete at 4 weeks, and degeneration of the adrenergic nerves in the basal parts of the central vessels was far advanced. The adrenergic plexus of the peripheral arteries and the afferent nerve supply to the skin and adnexa were reduced. Regeneration of axons into some fascicles was noted in the basal part of the central nerve. Central nerve regeneration to the middle of the ear was nearly complete at 8 weeks. At 6 months there was regeneration of the central nerves and nerves to the central artery, peripheral arteries, and skin. The newly formed adrenergic adventitial plexus was separated from the central artery by connective tissue.

The rabbit ear appears to be useful for investigating factors that influence the outgrowth of nerves to the vascular system and skin after replantation. Defects in restoration of the adrenergic vascular plexus may be responsible for cold intolerance that persists after replantation procedures.

▶ The localization of cold and cold pain receptors is an important first step in approaching the management of problems with cold sensation. This field would include conditions such as Raynaud's phenomenon, sympathetic dystrophy, and cold intolerance such as that experienced after replantation. The localization of the receptors within the peripheral veins may help to explain why intravenous blockade with therapeutic agents such as reserpine and guanethidine is effective in treatment of cold-sensitive conditions.

The brief report by Lassmann and Piza demonstrates that the reinnervation of the perivascular sympathetic nervous system is incomplete after replantation of the rabbit ear. Presumably, this also would be true in replantation of other parts. The authors suggest that such a phenomenon may be related to the presence of cold intolerance in such replanted parts. Unfortunately, their experiment was not carried far enough to demonstrate that; blood flow and response of blood flow to cold were not investigated in their model. It would seem that such a study would be an appropriate follow-up for these authors to consider, particularly in light of the information provided by Fruhstorfer and Lindblom in the preceding article. It is conceivable that abnormal reinnervation of cold receptors in peripheral veins could play some role in the cold intolerance experienced in replanted parts. Further research into this area is clearly in order.—P.C.A.

10 Compression Neuropathies

Neuropathy After Bupivacaine (Marcaine) Wrist and Metacarpal Nerve Blocks
Gunter Born (St. Joseph's Hosp., Hamilton, Ont.)
J. Hand Surg. 9A:109–112, January 1984   10–1

The data were reviewed on 44 patients who had 49 wrist and metacarpal blocks with concentrations of 0.25% or 0.5% bupivacaine for surgical and therapeutic purposes in a 1-year period. The 0.5% concentration was used in all but 2 cases. Epinephrine was included in 3 cases. Blocks were made using a 27-gauge, 1½-in. needle. Direct infiltration of the nerves was avoided in the wrist blocks. An average of 10–15 ml of anesthetic solution was used. The digital nerves were infiltrated through the dorsal web for metacarpal block. An average of 6 ml was used. A tourniquet was employed in all but 1 case.

Surgical anesthesia developed 5–10 minutes after infiltration. Analgesia often lasted 10–12 hours and occasionally longer. The need for analgesia postoperatively was minimal. Seven patients noted hypesthesia in areas supplied by the blocked nerve. Sensibility to touch and pinprick was preserved, as was two-point discrimination. Most patients recovered from numbness to some degree in a few months. One patient had radiating pain and a positive Tinel sign in the distribution of the dorsal branch of the digital nerve that subsided gradually over 2½ months.

Anesthetic block with bupivacaine can cause a clinically significant, reversible nerve lesion in anatomically confined regions. Further study of this practice is warranted. Nerve blocks with bupivacaine in anatomically confined areas should be done cautiously, using low concentrations and small quantities.

▶ It is noteworthy that the author has identified and described complications after local peripheral nerve blocks for anesthesia in surgery. He attributes the cause of these neuropathies to the use of bupivacaine within the closed spaces. Certainly, with the techniques described one would anticipate some peripheral nerve disorders despite the medications utilized. Metacarpal blocks can be achieved more safely by the use of large-volume, low-concentration injections at the metacarpal neck level rather than in the web space where they will reach an area where the neurovascular bundles are confined within the digital space. At the wrist level, direct infiltration of the area of the nerve and direct injection into the nerve can be expected to be associated with secondary nerve paresthesias, although these are usually temporary. In my own practice, I prefer to use Xylocaine 1%, injecting approximately 20 cc for a block of the digit at the metacarpal neck level without directly injecting the nerve or a closed space, followed by wrapping with a firm Esmarch tourniquet bandage to compress the Xylocaine into the nerve tissue. The method is safe and effective although utilizing larger doses. Direct injection or compression of nerves or vessels is avoided. I personally believe that wrist-level nerve blocks with the potential risk of injection directly into the nerve are more hazardous than large-volume, low-concentration anesthetics, injected about the general area of the nerve, followed by compression wrapping.—R.D.B.

Sensibility Testing in Patients With Carpal Tunnel Syndrome
Robert M. Szabo, Richard H. Gelberman, and Mary P. Dimick (San Diego)
J. Bone Joint Surg. [Am.] 66-A:60–64, January 1984   10–2

The usefulness of the monofilament pressure and vibration threshold sensibility tests was examined in 20 patients with idiopathic carpal tunnel syndrome affecting 23 hands. The 10 men and 10 women were aged 32–81 years. All patients had proved abnormalities of median nerve conduction at the wrist. All underwent division of the transverse carpal ligament, and 5 patients with abnormal two-point discrimination had internal neurolysis as well. The patients were followed for at least 6 weeks after operation. Threshold tests were done using vibrotomy, 256-cps vibration, and the Semmes-Weinstein monofilaments. The two-point discrimination test of innervation density also was used. The wrist-flexion, nerve-percussion, and tourniquet tests were carried out preoperatively.

Preoperative sensory abnormalities were most often demonstrated by

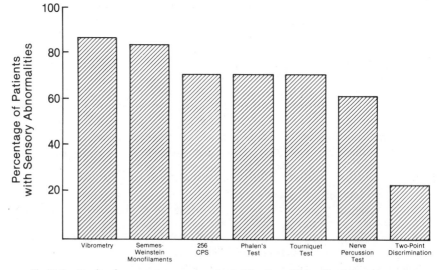

Fig 10–1.—Results of preoperative sensory testing in 20 patients (23 hands) with carpal tunnel syndrome. The percentage of patients demonstrating a specific sensory abnormality is illustrated by the bar graphs. (Courtesy of Szabo, R.M., et al.: J. Bone Joint Surg. [Am.] 66-A:60–64, January 1984.)

vibrometry testing (Fig 10–1). Abnormal vibratory thresholds were found in 87% of affected hands. All 5 hands with abnormal two-point discrimination also had markedly abnormal threshold test values. All hands showed improvement on threshold testing 6 weeks after carpal tunnel release, and two-thirds had normal findings. Two-point discrimination was normal in 3 of 5 hands that had been abnormal preoperatively. All patients were relieved of pain and paresthesias immediately after surgery.

Threshold tests are more sensitive and reliable than innervation-density tests in assessing cutaneous sensibility in patients with chronic compressive neuropathies. Sensory fibers are more sensitive than motor fibers to the early effects of compression, and they recover more slowly. Threshold tests are under study for use in a variety of spinal and lower-extremity nerve compression syndromes.

▶ This article amplifies the work pioneered by Dellon and demonstrates what appears to be a more objective method of documenting the surgical results after carpal tunnel release. The concepts of nerve threshold and innervation density should be familiar to all those dealing with disorders of peripheral nerves and specific methods of testing both should be in the armamentarium of all hand surgeons. Widespread use of more objective and more sensitive measures of sensibility can only help to increase our understanding of the pathology and treatment of peripheral nerve injury.—P.C.A.

Response of Vitamin B₆ Deficiency and Carpal Tunnel Syndrome to Pyridoxine
John M. Ellis, Karl Folkers, Moise Levy, Satoshi Shizukuishi, Jan Lewandowski, Satoshi Nishii, H. A. Schubert, and Richard Ulrich
Proc. Natl. Acad. Sci. USA 79:7494–7498, December 1982   10–3

Ellis et al. have reported that vitamin B_6 deficiency is present in patients with carpal tunnel syndrome (CTS), and pyridoxine therapy leads to neurologic improvement.

A double-blind trial of pyridoxine was carried out in 7 patients with "idiopathic" CTS, diagnosed clinically and by nerve conduction studies. Specific activity and the percentage deficiency of erythrocyte glutamic-oxaloacetic transaminase (EGOT) were determined. Tablets of 50 mg of pyridoxine hydrochloride and placebo were given for 12-week periods.

The EGOT data indicated severe vitamin B_6 deficiency in these cases. The patients, aged 43 to 77 years, had had symptoms of CTS for 3 months to 10 years. Paresthesias and finger stiffness were the most prominent features. The clinical response to pyridoxine correlated with restored EGOT levels, which presumably result from a long-term increase in the number of EGOT molecules through the correction of pyridoxal 5'-phosphate deficiency. Improvement occurred in a period of days. Two physicians identified the pyridoxine-treated patients and patients given placebo without error.

Carpal tunnel syndrome would appear to be a primary vitamin B_6 deficiency state rather than a dependency state. The clinical response to pyridoxine may preclude the need for hand surgery in many cases. Patients with symptoms of CTS for many years have improved significantly after being given pyridoxine.

▶ This is one of a series of articles from these authors regarding the use of pyridoxine in the treatment of carpal tunnel syndrome. In their studies, all patients with carpal tunnel syndrome have been found to have deficiency of vitamin B_6 by the authors' criteria and all responded to vitamin B_6 treatment.

Close evaluation, however, reveals some problem with the authors' analysis. The definition of vitamin B_6 deficiency used by the authors is a stimulation of vitamin B_6-dependent enzyme activity by the addition of vitamin B_6 in vitro. Other authorities have felt that such a stimulation is normal and should not be considered a sign of vitamin B_6 deficiency. In fact, such a stimulation is present in almost all persons not taking vitamin B_6 supplements. The authors of this article have taken such information to conclude that almost everyone is deficient in vitamin B_6. If nothing else, such a position represents a considerable departure from traditional thinking.

The second problem comes with patient selection. Patients are selected primarily on the basis of complaints, and there is little in the way of objective documentation of median neuropathy. For example, sensibility in the median nerve distribution was not documented in any patients nor was the status of the thenar muscles. Of the 5 patients who had electromyography and nerve conduction studies, only 1 was abnormal; thus, it is possible that the authors' selection criteria may include cases other than those that would be considered typical of carpal tunnel syndrome by hand surgeons.

The authors make no mention of why a vitamin deficiency, presumably present throughout the body, should affect only one peripheral nerve. The authors' findings, most particularly their claimed 100% response rate, have not been observed by others who have investigated this problem. A recent study presented to the American Association for Hand Surgery attempted to reproduce the authors' methods, but was unable to reproduce their results.

Although it would be extremely difficult, if not impossible, to show that pyridoxine is not helpful in any patient with carpal tunnel syndrome, the weight of evidence at present suggests that the vast majority of patients with significant symptoms related to carpal tunnel syndrome will continue to require surgical decompression.—P.C.A.

CT of Carpal Tunnel Syndrome
V. John, H. E. Nau, H. C. Nahser, V. Reinhardt, and K. Venjakob (Univ. of Essen, West Germany)
AJNR 4:770–772, May–June 1983   10–4

The carpal tunnel was examined by high-resolution computed tomography scanning in 2 cadavers, 2 healthy persons, and 20 patients with carpal tunnel syndrome. The muscles, ligaments, tendons, and synovial sheaths in the carpal canal were easily recognized. The median nerve is a flat hypodense structure 3 to 8 mm thick, with a density of 40 to 50

Hounsfield units. Computed tomography showed compression of the median nerve by the carpal ligament and bones and volume augmentation of the carpal tunnel contents. Postoperatively, a return to the normal biconvex form of the carpal tunnel was evident. Scar tissue was seen in the early postoperative phase, but computed tomography scanning did not show scar tissue reaction in the nerve.

Computed tomography can provide information on the pathogenesis of entrapment syndromes. An increase in the contents of the carpal tunnel and compression of the contents by surrounding structures have been observed in cases of carpal tunnel syndrome. Reformatting can provide information about joints and show degenerative "chronic traumatic" lesions of the wrist bones. If a computed tomography study is done on a patient with carpal tunnel syndrome plain radiography in standard projections is not necessary.

▶ The authors have a nice study contributing to the understanding of the etiology of carpal tunnel syndrome. It is obviously not a practical way to make this diagnosis, which can be confirmed so well electromyographically. It would be nice to be able to use postoperative computed tomography scanning to quantitate the change in the size of the carpal canal following release of the tendons. Comparing the wrists in unilateral carpal tunnel syndrome might help confirm the conclusions. The authors do not do either in this report.—R.D.B.

Pressure and Nerve Lesion in the Carpal Tunnel
Carl-Olof Werner, Dan Elmqvist and Per Ohlin (Helsingborg, Sweden)
Acta Orthop. Scand. 54:312–316, April 1983   10–5

Carpal tunnel syndrome is the most common peripheral nerve entrapment disorder. The authors recorded pressures on the median nerve beneath the carpal ligament in different positions and during muscle contraction in 16 patients with typical symptoms of carpal tunnel syndrome, 15 women and 1 man aged 25–59 years. Both motor and orthodromic sensory nerve conduction studies were carried out on the median and ulnar nerves, using surface and needle electrodes. Only patients with abnormalities restricted to the distal part of the median nerve were included in the study. Both sensory and motor conduction was abnormal in 11 patients. Pressures were recorded with a catheter (Fig 10–2) at rest, with passive volar and dorsal wrist flexion, and during elicited contraction of the wrist and finger flexor and extensor muscles.

Resting pressures between the median nerve and carpal ligament averaged 31 mm Hg. Pressure increased to 75 mm Hg on passive volar wrist flexion with the fingers straight and to 60 mm Hg with the fingers flexed. On passive dorsal wrist flexion, the pressure was 105 mm Hg with the fingers straight and 113 mm Hg with the fingers flexed. Maximum muscle contraction produced threefold to sixfold increases above resting pressure. Pressures were highest in patients with more marked electrophysiologic abnormalities.

The median nerve is subjected to rather high local pressures during

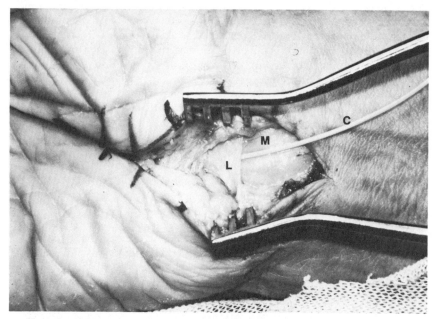

Fig 10–2.—The pressure recording catheter *(C)* in place on the volar surface of the median nerve *(M)* beneath the carpal ligament *(L)*. (Courtesy of Werner, C.-O., et al.: Acta Orthop. Scand. 54:312–316, April 1983.)

contraction of the wrist and finger muscles. Nerve compression correlated with the electrophysiologic abnormalities in the present patients with carpal tunnel syndrome. Intermittent pressure increases could lead to mechanical nerve damage through telescoping of the internodes with swelling and folding of the myelin sheets or to impairment of blood flow with protein leakage through the epineural venules, resulting in edema and epineural fibrosis.

▶ This study confirms the work of Gelberman in this area. It seems clear that increased pressure beneath the transverse carpal ligament is associated with carpal tunnel syndrome and is probably a prime etiologic agent.—P.C.A.

Carpal Tunnel Syndrome: Median Nerve Stress Test
Edgar L. Marin, Sanford Vernick, and Lawrence W. Friedmann (Nassau County Med. Center, East Meadow, N. Y.)
Arch. Phys. Med. Rehabil. 64:206–208, May 1983   10–6

Patients with carpal tunnel syndrome (CTS) report often that prolonged and strenuous use of their hands aggravates the symptoms. The effects of wrist position on distal sensory and motor latencies of the median nerve were examined in 12 female and 2 male patients (mean age, 49 years) with CTS. The mean duration of symptoms was 13 months. Twelve healthy subjects with a mean age of 30 years also were assessed. Standard electrodiagnostic studies were performed with the wrist held in extreme tolerated flexion and extension by an orthosis.

Distal latencies increased somewhat in the extreme wrist positions in the normal subjects, but remained within normal limits. Nine of the patients with presumptive CTS had increased distal latencies in neutral wrist position, and 8 also had increased distal latencies on the opposite side. All 9 of these patients had a considerable increment in distal latencies with extreme extension and flexion of the wrist. Three of the 5 patients with normal distal latencies in neutral wrist position bilaterally showed an increase in sensory latency to above normal with extreme wrist positions, especially flexion. These patients reported paresthesia in the territory of the distal median nerve. Two other patients had increases in sensory latency to the upper range of normal and also had paresthesia. The greatest increment was in sensory latency after 5 minutes of wrist flexion. The percent increment in motor latency was higher after 5 minutes of wrist flexion than when the wrist was extended.

Wrist position appears to influence distal sensory and motor latencies of the median nerve in patients with CTS. Distal latency is increased significantly after wrist flexion for 5 minutes. Patients with symptoms of CTS, but normal median nerve distal latencies, should be restudied after wrist flexion for 5 minutes. An increase in distal latency, especially sensory latency, to above the normal range will confirm the diagnosis of CTS.

▶ The authors have nicely documented with electric conduction studies the clinically established Phalen's test. It is of interest that normal subjects also had changes in conduction velocity, but not generally above normal. Phalen's test is certainly useful in demonstrating wrist etiology in suspected median neuropathies of the extremities.

I personally have found application of direct pressure over the median nerve to be the most useful test in clinical evaluation for carpal tunnel syndrome. In this test, the thumb is pressed firmly just radial to the palmaris longus tendon at the wrist flexion crease. In patients with carpal tunnel syndrome of a severe nature, numbness in the median distribution will occur generally within 15 to 30 seconds, and in those with mild carpal tunnel syndrome, numbness will occur in approximately 1 minute. In those patients without carpal tunnel syndrome, numbness rarely occurs.—R.D.B.

Median Nerve Residual Latency: Normal Value and Use in Diagnosis of Carpal Tunnel Syndrome
George H. Kraft and Glen A. Halvorson (Univ. of Washington)
Arch. Phys. Med. Rehabil. 64:221–226, May 1983   10–7

The elimination of normal variability in nerve conduction velocity from distal latency measurements would reduce the standard deviation of distal latency and narrow the normal range, which is useful in diagnosing carpal tunnel syndrome. The authors measured median motor distal latencies, sensory distal peak latencies, motor nerve conduction velocities, and motor residual latencies in 100 normal subjects of both sexes, aged 15–83 years. Residual latency was calculated by dividing the distance between the cathode and active electrode by the motor nerve conduction velocity and subtracting the quotient from the motor distal latency.

The mean motor residual latency was 1.97 msec, with a SD of 0.27 msec and normal range of 1.4–2.5 msec. Values from 98% of the subjects were within the calculated normal range. The mean motor distal latency was 3.4 msec, with a SD of 0.31 msec and a normal range of 2.8–4.0 msec. The mean sensory distal peak latency was 3.19 msec, the SD was 0.36 msec, and the normal range was 2.5–3.9 msec. The SD and normal range of the residual latency were smaller than those of the motor and sensory distal latencies. Residual latencies remained constant into the ninth decade of life, while the motor and sensory distal latencies increased with age. Three patients with recent onset of carpal tunnel syndrome had prolonged residual latencies, which were the only abnormalities.

The median motor residual latency is simple to calculate and provides a refinement to neurophysiologic evaluation of the distal nerve segment without the need for additional nerve stimulation. Normal values for residual latency have a smaller SD and a narrower normal range than do the motor or sensory distal latencies, and the values vary less with age. Determinations of residual latency may be particularly useful in confirming early or mild carpal tunnel syndrome and should be done when carpal tunnel syndrome is suspected.

▶ The authors have described a more sensitive means of detecting subclinical carpal tunnel syndrome. At our institution, palmar sensory latencies measured over shorter distances and in comparison with the ulnar palmar sensory latencies will give a test with similar sensitivity to that demonstrated by the authors. They subtract the effect of variable median nerve conduction velocity in calculating the median, motor, and sensory latencies without performing additional studies.

From a practical standpoint, the clinical history and physical findings of patients with this smaller degree of median nerve compression at the carpal canal are as useful as are the subtle electrodiagnostic studies, but as pointed out by the authors, the latter can offer some help in questionable cases.—R.D.B.

Compression of the Deep Branch of the Ulnar Nerve: A Case Report
Peter J. Stern and Marvin Vice (Univ. of Cincinnati)
J. Hand Surg. 8:72–74, January 1983   10–8

A case is reported of entrapment neuropathy of the deep motor branch of the ulnar nerve where it exits from Guyon's canal, resulting in paralysis of all the ulnar-innervated intrinsic muscles except the abductor digiti quinti without ulnar sensory loss.

Man, 36, a right-handed pipefitter, sustained blunt trauma to the ulnar aspect of the right hypothenar eminence while at work and presented 3 months later with mild pain, weak grip, and loss of key and fine pinch, but no paresthesias. Examination showed atrophy of the interossei, especially the first dorsal interosseous muscle, but no atrophy of the abductor digiti quinti or the thenar muscles. Mild clawing of the ring and small fingers was noted. A Tinel sign was positive just distal to the hook of the hamate. Tests for the Froment and Jeanne signs were positive. Pinch strength was much reduced on the right dominant side. Carpal tunnel x-ray studies were negative. Electromyography showed fibrillation potentals at rest in all the interossei and the abductor pollicis. Exploration showed constriction of the motor branch of the ulnar nerve by scar in the pisohamate canal. The branch was released by extraneurolysis and intraneurolysis with the use of the operating microscope. The claw deformity was absent 7 months postoperatively, when pinch strength had improved. All the interossei were functioning, although mild atrophy of the first dorsal interosseous persisted.

The surgical setting relevant to compression of the deep motor branch of the ulnar nerve is shown in Figure 10–3. Compression at Guyon's canal may require surgery, with division of the palmar carpal ligament and the removal of any space-occupying lesions. The present patient had a satisfactory outcome after division of the fibrous arch of the flexor digiti quinti brevis and neurolysis of the deep motor branch.

▶ Motor branch compression has been reported now for both the median and ulnar nerves in the palm. It would appear that these branches should be spe-

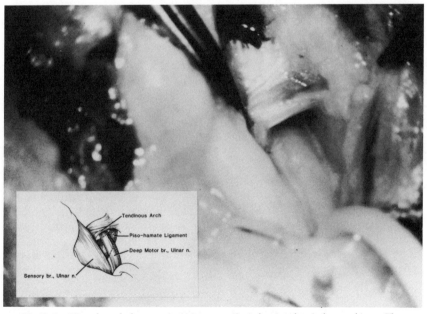

Fig 10–3.—View through the operating microscope (9×) showing the pisohamate hiatus. The tendinous arch must be divided to visualize the motor branch beyond the hiatus. The branch to abductor digiti quinti arises from the deep branch proximal to the level of this photograph. (Courtesy of Stern, P.J., and Vice, M.: J. Hand Surg. 8:72–74, January 1983.)

cifically inspected when nerve decompression is performed for carpal tunnel syndrome or ulnar nerve compression within Guyon's canal.—P.C.A.

Peripheral Neurologic Causes of Writers' Cramp: Middle Median Nerve Lesion
J. Kómár and M. Szegvári (Budapest)
Nervenarzt 54:322–325, June 1983   10–9

Writers' cramp is a rare syndrome which until 10 years ago was believed to be of psychologic origin but had no response to therapy. Some researchers tried to find organic causes, such as muscle fatigue, variations of dystonia, or organic extrapyramidal syndrome. However, corresponding therapy remained unsuccessful.

The authors report data on 3 patients in whom the syndrome could be demonstrated through the middle median nerve lesion. In all 3 cases neurolysis was performed. One of these cases is featured below.

Man, 36, had difficulties 3 years prior to hospitalization. While writing he experienced painful flexion spasms in the first and second finger of the right hand. His writing was almost illegible. Neurologic examination showed no Rask reflex. Other organic deviations could not be found. During the writing test the patient had, for a few seconds, flexion cramps in the right thumb and index finger. According to the electromyogram (EMG) the distal motor latency of the right lateral anterior interosseous nerve was 4.5 msec, that of the left lateral was 2.5 msec, and the distal motor latency of the median nerve was bilaterally 3.8 msec. Laboratory findings were normal. Under the assumption of an anterior interosseous syndrome, surgery was performed. The nerve was freed from the compression caused by a fibrous ligament. After surgery the Rask reflex returned and writing improved. Four months after surgery the patient again had complaints; the wound had healed with a keloid scar. A second operation was performed, but the patient continues to have writers' cramp.

In the other 2 patients the pathologic condition was caused by the median nerve lesion (pronator teres syndrome). In 1 of these patients a lipoma caused the nerve compression. Both had surgery and were free of complaints and without symptoms 6 to 9 months after the operation.

The diagnosis of anterior interosseous syndrome is aided if the reflex described by Rask is not present. Normally, this reflex is identified when, with the wrist bent slightly, the tendon crossing the muscle flexor pollicis longus at the lower third of the forearm is tapped and flexion of the last joint of the thumb occurs. Including the 3 cases reported here, a total of 8 writers' cramp syndromes with peripheral neural causes have been described in the world literature.

▶ The pronator teres and anterior interosseous syndrome often present in vague and unusual symptoms. To this must be added writers' cramp.—R.L.L.

Double-Entrapment Radial Tunnel Syndrome
Paul D. Sponseller and William D. Engber (Univ. of Wisconsin, Madison)

J. Hand Surg. 8:420–423, July 1983   10–10

A case of posterior interosseous nerve compression representing a "double-crush" lesion, with compression both at the arcade of Frohse and at the distal border of the supinator is reported. Only two previous lesions have been documented at the latter site.

Woman, 57, had right forearm pain after minor direct trauma to the lateral aspect of the elbow and had failed to respond to nonoperative measures. The extensor carpi radialis brevis (ECRB) had been released 2 years after injury. Pain and tenderness were present a year later both over the mobile wad of Henry and on the dorsoradial aspect of the forearm at the junction of the ECRB and the extensor digitorum communis. Nerve conduction velocities were normal. Electromyography showed polyphasic motor units in radially innervated muscles. Exploration showed the posterior interosseous branch of the radial nerve to be markedly constricted by the fibrous edge of the superficial head of the supinator on passive pronation. Pseudoneuromatous swelling of the nerve was seen just proximal to the arcade of Frohse. The arcade and the fascial covering and muscle fibers of the supinator were sequentially sectioned to free the nerve entirely. Pain persisted distally after operation, and 2 months later, exploration showed compression of the posterior interosseous nerve just proximal to its point of exit from the supinator in the forearm. Pain was improved after the point of exit was divided, and the patient was essentially free from symptoms 15 months later.

The precise causes of compression of the posterior interosseous branch of the radial nerve may be difficult to delineate. Compression can occur at the radial tunnel distal to the arcade of Frohse. A double-level entrapment should be considered if the patient has two distinct sites of pain and tenderness along the course of the posterior interosseous branch. Awareness of this possibility may permit better relief from pain at surgical decompression.

▶ The authors do a nice job of reviewing the anatomy and describing the radial tunnel syndrome. A similar situation can exist from the ulnar side of the elbow, and during cubital tunnel releases or anterior transpositions, occasionally the distal deep fascia of the flexor carpi ulnaris may be noted to be entrapping the ulnar nerve. This should be searched for during ulnar nerve transpositions.

Complete release as determined by digital palpation or direct inspection should be achieved in each of these cases.—R.D.B.

Radial Tunnel Syndrome: A Spectrum of Clinical Presentations
Steven H. Moss and Hugh E. Switzer (Univ. Hosp., Jacksonville, Fla.)
J. Hand Surg. 8:414–420, July 1983   10–11

It may be difficult to distinguish between early radial tunnel syndrome due to compression of the radial nerve and simple lateral epicondylitis due to local inflammation and trauma. The findings were reviewed in 9 men and 6 women, aged 29–63, treated for radial tunnel syndrome. The dominant hand was involved in 14 cases. Seven of the men were manual laborers, and the other 2 participated often in racquet sports. Five patients related the onset of symptoms to minor injuries. Two patients had a history of radial head or neck fracture.

Nine patients presented with resistant tennis elbow and 6 with resistant radial tunnel pain. Ten patients exhibited at least one of the following: radial paresthesia, radial paresis, or popping sensations. All had pain localized to the extensor mass of the forearm overlying the radial tunnel. The average duration of symptoms was 2.3 years. Long finger extension testing was positive in all cases. Conservative management was tried for an average of 9 months and was unsuccessful.

Fourteen patients had an excellent response to surgery on an average follow-up of 26 months. Various forms of constriction were found at surgery. Five patients required neurolysis for hourglass constriction, flattening, hyperemia, or inflammation of the radial nerve. One patient required a second release procedure. Two patients had keloid scar formation, and 1 had transient paresthesias of the lateral cutaneous nerve.

The likelihood that radial tunnel syndrome is less frequent than lateral epicondylitis emphasizes the importance of initial conservative management. Delay in diagnosing true nerve compression can, however, lead to pain and paralysis. Reported results of radial tunnel release have been satisfactory. Fourteen of the 15 patients in the present study had significant postoperative improvement.

▶ This article emphasizes the increasing recognition of the radial tunnel syndrome and its variability and sometimes bizarre presentation. The authors do not call attention to the sometimes protracted disability that occasionally is noted in patients with workmen's compensation claims.—R.L.L.

A Case of Cubital Tunnel Syndrome Caused by the Snapping of the Medial Head of the Triceps Brachii Muscle

Yasuo Hayashi, Tadao Kojima, and Toshihiko Kohno (Tokyo)
J. Hand Surg. 9A:96–99, January 1984   10–12

A case of cubital tunnel syndrome caused by snapping of the medial head of the triceps brachii is described. Only 4 similar cases previously have been reported.

Man, 20, had the right forearm squeezed in a film-processing machine. Eleven days after suture of the wound on the palmar-ulnar aspect of the middle of the forearm, he was seen with a claw deformity of the hand and hypesthesia in the ulnar distribution. Exploration showed only crush injury of the belly of the flexor digitorum superficialis; the ulnar nerve appeared normal. No improvement occurred in the next 10 weeks, and muscle atrophy progressed. The patient had had a right supracondylar fracture at age 12. A small lump was noted posteriorly in the medial epicondylar region. There was significant atrophy of the dorsal interossei, and adduction of the small finger was not possible. Electromyography showed decreased motor nerve units in the flexor carpi ulnaris and a marked reduction in the abductor digiti minimi and first dorsal interosseous.

Exploration 5 months after injury showed the lump to be the medial head of the triceps brachii, not a pseudoneuroma as was initially thought. On flexion of the right elbow joint, the muscle belly of the medial head dislocated anteriorly over the medial epicondyle, with snapping, and the ulnar nerve was strongly compressed from back to front by the muscle belly. The nerve was tethered by the tendinous arch. An epineurotomy was done after detaching the tendinous arch, and a medial epicondylectomy also was carried out. Improved muscle strength was noted a month later, and the claw deformity was absent 6 weeks postoperatively. The sensory disturbance had resolved by 3 months, when grip strength was improved. No symptoms were present 1½ years later.

Snapping of the medial head of the triceps brachii presumably is due to the slightly protruding medial epicondyle with varus deformity. Medial epicondylectomy and division of the tendinous arch removed the snapping and relieved ulnar nerve compression in the present case. This would appear to be a logical surgical approach to this rare disorder.

▶ Cases of snapping on the medial aspect of the elbow associated with ulnar paresthesias are almost routinely originally thought to be caused by subluxation of the ulnar nerve at the elbow, a known condition that can lead to chronic ulnar neuropathy. In this case, as in reported cases and cases I have seen, snapping does indeed occur as the enlarged medial head of the triceps snaps over the medial epicondyle. The authors have treated this with cubital medial epicondylectomy. I have treated it by excising the medial portion of the triceps and folding back the medial edge and suturing it onto itself rather than performing the bony procedure. I think either operation is satisfactory. The importance of the condition is the recognition of the physician that snapping on the medial side of the elbow during flexion of the elbow is not necessarily the ulnar nerve but may in fact be the triceps. Treatment should include passive mobilization of the elbow at the time of surgery to determine indeed which structure it is, so that the appropriate treatment may be undertaken.—R.D.B.

Results After Surgical Release of the Ulnar Nerve in Cubital Tunnel Syndrome
F. Chaise, T. Bouchet, L. Sedel, and J. Witvoet
J. Chir. (Paris) 120:251–255, 1983   10–13

Sixty patients (62 nerves) were treated surgically for neuropathies in the region of the elbow. Three different techniques were used: (1) neurolysis combined with longitudinal epineurotomy, which stabilized or improved 24 of 25 cases; (2) subcutaneous anterior transposition of the nerve, which stabilized or improved 21 of 26 cases (78% good results); and (3) endofascicular neurolysis, a procedure that caused an aggravation of the disorder in 2 of 11 patients and should therefore be abandoned. The condition of the nerve as observed during surgery is emphasized: a tight stricture in 15 cases, perineural hemorrhagic suffusion in 2, and a laminated, flattened appearance in 4. The most frequently encountered picture was one of swelling in the retroepitrochlean groove, evoking a "continuous neuroma." In 10 cases the nerve was of fibrous, dull appearance, adhering to the walls of the tunnel; in 10 others no lesion whatever was found.

Such factors as patient age, duration of neuropathy and degree of paralysis, which theoretically might be expected to influence the results, are of little consequence. The technical factor dominates all others, assuming that the functional potential of the ulnar nerve is present.

Subjective symptoms of pain and paresthesia disappeared consistently as a consequence of the first two procedures, and simple neurolysis combined with longitudinal epineurotomy seems to be the treatment of choice for cubital tunnel syndrome.

▶ These results are interesting, although somewhat disparate from other reports in the literature. Longitudinal epineurotomy has been less successful in our experience.—R.L.L.

The Treatment of the Cubital Tunnel Syndrome
Robert S. Adelaar, William C. Foster, and Charles McDowell (Med. College of Virginia)
J. Hand Surg. 9A:90–95, January 1984   10–14

Recommended treatments for ulnar neuropathy secondary to cubital tunnel syndrome have included in situ release, submuscular transposition, and anterior subcutaneous transposition. A prospective study was undertaken of 32 patients having 37 procedures for cubital tunnel syndrome. All were followed for at least 9 months after operation. The average age of patients was 50 years, and the average duration of symptoms was 15 months. The average follow-up after surgery was 13 months. Seven release procedures, 8 submuscular transpositions, and 22 subcutaneous transpositions were carried out.

Good results, with complete resolution of symptoms and no motor or sensory deficit, were obtained in 1 case of release, 2 cases of submuscular transposition, and 5 of subcutaneous transposition. Three release operations, 3 submuscular transpositions, and 4 subcutaneous transpositions yielded poor results. The only significant preoperative clinical prognostic feature was intrinsic atrophy. Evoked sensory potentials were absent preoperatively in patients with poor operative results. A high proportion of patients with poor results had fibrillations before and after surgery. All 5 alcoholic patients without electromyographic or clinical evidence of neuropathy had fair and poor results.

Good surgical results can be expected in patients with cubital tunnel syndrome who lack intrinsic atrophy and fibrillation potentials and who have evoked sensory potentials preoperatively. Transposition has given slightly better results than the in situ release procedure, but the preoperative status appears to be more important than the type of surgery used. Alcoholic patients have not done well. The outcome has not been related to patient age or the duration of symptoms of cubital tunnel syndrome.

▶ The authors have identified very little difference in various types of surgical management of cubital tunnel syndrome (ulnar neuropathy at the elbow in the absence of bony or structural abnormalities). They do point out quite appropriately, however, that early operative intervention is associated with best results. The presence of muscle atrophy (a sign of late disease) is associated with poorer results. This is the way I would interpret the data, although the authors have pointed out specifically that the period of preoperative symptoms did not affect the results. Certainly the severity of them did. Therefore, one would be inclined to treat the condition with operative intervention as soon as it is recognized. The average follow-up period was less than 2 years, and recent information has indicated that there may be a progressive recovery of ulnar nerve function after deep anterior transposition for up to 6 years following surgery and surgical repairs. Therefore, it would seem to me that this same study could be repeated at a period of 4 to 6 years postoperatively to see if indeed the authors' conclusion that the technique of surgery itself does not affect the clinical results is correct. It is not mentioned whether or not any of the patients suffered from a postoperative positional cubital tunnel syndrome. In these patients, surgical treatment of all varieties has been of less success in my hands.—R.D.B.

Motor and Sensory Ulnar Nerve Conduction Velocities: Effect of Elbow Position
Catherine Harding and Eugen Halar (Univ. of Washington)
Arch. Phys. Med. Rehabil. 64:227–232, May 1983   10–15

Measurements of ulnar nerve conduction velocity (NCV) often are used to localize sites of compression neuropathy in the elbow region, but variance in measurement of skin distance over the ulnar nerve with elbow flexion can create a problem. The authors measured ulnar motor and sensory NCV bilaterally in 20 healthy subjects, 12 men and 8 women aged 21 to 68 years. Below-elbow (BE) and across-elbow (AE) segments were studied in four different elbow positions, 0, 45, 90, and 135 degrees of flexion, to assess the effect on NCV. Subjects were tested supine with the shoulder abducted to 45 degrees, forearm supinated, and wrist in neutral position. Studies also were done on four cadaver ulnar nerves.

Although constant skin stimulation marker points were used, the length of the AE segment became progressively greater with increasing elbow flexion. At zero flexion the motor NCV of the AE segment was slower than the NCV of the BE segment and at 45 degrees of flexion it was faster. At further elbow flexion there was an erroneous increase in motor and sensory NCV values for the AE segments, chiefly due to stretching of the skin over the flexed elbow. The cadaver dissections showed that the nerve slid distally with respect to an above-elbow skin marker.

Values of motor NCV for the AE and BE segments varied least with 45 degrees of elbow flexion in this study, and this would appear to be the optimal position for recording. Short AE segments are associated with increased variation in NCV, but long segments may lead to failure to detect the pathologic slowing of NCV that occurs over only a short portion of the nerve. Optimal length of an AE segment for evaluating patients for compressive neuropathy at the elbow is about 12 to 14 cm.

▶ This article nicely demonstrates the value of performing ulnar nerve conduction studies with the elbow flexed. Spurious apparent localized slowing of conduction may be obtained in other positions. The article suffers only from the absence of measurements of motor evoked response amplitude, which is sometimes the only criterion of a localized ulnar neuropathy.—J.R.D.

Clinical Electrophysiologic Assessment of Ulnar Nerve Transposition in Tuberculoid Leprosy
Mohamed A. Amer, Hassan H. A. Gawish, Abd El Samed I. El Hawala, Samih A. Amer, and Kawther Amer (Zagazig Univ., Egypt)
Int. J. Dermatol. 22:481–484, October 1983   10–16

The findings with regard to ulnar nerve involvement were reviewed in 54 patients, 42 men and 12 women with an average age of 30 years, attending a leprosy outpatient clinic. Twenty-four patients were operated on, 3 of them bilaterally, while 30 were managed conservatively. The ulnar nerve was mobilized under general anesthesia and transposed in front of the medial epicondyle.

All patients had sensory change and thickening of the ulnar nerve preoperatively. Muscle wasting and deformities ensued. Local tenderness behind the medial epicondyle and distal pain in the distribution of the ulnar nerve were consistent findings. The sensory changes ranged from hypoathesia to pinprick to complete anesthesia. Postoperative recovery was more apparent in patients with a shorter history, mild nerve thickening, and minimal sensorimotor changes. Thickening of the ulnar nerve and epineural adhesions were found at operation in all cases. *Mycobacterium leprae* were identified in 3 of 10 specimens of medial cutaneous nerve. All patients were relieved of pain after operation. Sensory changes resolved faster than the motor impairment.

Ulnar nerve transposition can give excellent clinical results in leprosy patients seen early in the course with minimal electromyographic changes, but late cases have not improved after operation. The procedure is based on shortening the course of the nerve to eliminate mechanical factors, removing epineural adhesions, and providing a healthy bed to encourage healthy vascular granulation.

▶ Although hand surgeons in the United States are not likely to see many patients with leprosy, the basic surgical principle elaborated in this article bears emphasis. Patients with generalized peripheral neuropathic processes, be they due to leprosy, diabetes, or some other condition, are not immune from local compressive changes related to mechanical factors. Such patients may respond quite favorably to ulnar nerve transposition, carpal tunnel release, and the like and should not be excluded from consideration merely because, in addition to their local symptoms, a generalized process is present. If physical examination and electric testing point to a superimposed focal lesion, then this can be addressed surgically, with a reasonable likelihood of symptomatic relief.—P.C.A.

Thoracic Outlet Syndrome
C. V. Ruckley (Royal Infirm., Edinburgh)
Br. Med. J. 287:447–448, Aug. 13, 1983   10–17

The thoracic outlet compression syndrome involves compression of nerves, vessels, or both in the root of the neck or axilla and involves such pathologic conditions as a cervical rib, the scalenus anterior syndrome, and abnormalities of the clavicle. Patients are difficult to evaluate and are apt to be seen by many different specialists, including psychiatrists. Up to 90% of patients have neurologic types of thoracic outlet syndrome, which are most frequent in slender women with drooping shoulders. Vascular compression is seen more often in men.

Patients with vascular symptoms should be evaluated rapidly because subclavian artery lesions can produce microemboli that cause irreversible damage or can thrombose completely, endangering the entire extremity. Venous thrombosis can cause long-term morbidity. Angiograms should be obtained in the 90-degree abducted position when vascular embarrassment is a possibility. If venous occlusion is present, phlebography should be performed bilaterally. Neurologic symptoms, in contrast, call for assessment over a period of time. The differential diagnosis includes cervical disk disease, osteoarthritis, and carpal tunnel syndrome. Long-standing neurologic compression can cause wasting of the interossei. A complete series of cervical spine x-ray films should be obtained in all cases. The value of nerve conduction studies and electromyography is uncertain.

Patients with arterial compression should be managed by early operation, and some authorities have suggested early operation for acute venous thrombosis. Patients with neurologic symptoms should be managed conservatively if at all possible. Minor nerve injuries usually resolve over time. Operation should be reserved for the minority of patients who have troublesome symptoms for a prolonged period.

▶ This brief article summarizes current knowledge of this frequently confusing condition. It emphasizes the importance of differentiating the classic, but much less common, vascular compression syndrome, which usually requires surgical treatment, from the much more common, more difficult to diagnose nerve compression syndrome that may or may not respond to surgical decompression and that frequently may be treated successfully by nonsurgical means.

The neurologic subtype of thoracic outlet syndrome may be present in a variety of upper extremity conditions, including its secondary development in painful or disabling disorders involving the hand or distal extremity that cause the patient to modify the posture or mobility of the shoulder girdle. A high degree of suspicion is necessary to make the diagnosis in these cases, but early diagnosis can be rewarding because conservative treatment may be sufficient to eliminate the need for surgical decompression.—P.C.A.

Somatosensory Evoked Responses as a Diagnostic Aid in Thoracic Outlet Syndrome: Postoperative Study
J. Siivola, R. Pokela, and I. Sulg (Oulu Univ., Oulu, Finland)
Acta Chir. Scand. 149:147–150, 1983   10–18

Clinical diagnosis of the thoracic outlet syndrome is often difficult, and routine electroneurography is usually not specifically diagnostic in this disease. The authors recorded evoked responses in the supraclavicular fossa (Erb's point) after stimulation of the median and ulnar nerves in 13 patients with unilateral symptoms and signs that are typical of thoracic outlet syndrome and in 20 healthy adults of similar age. The patients had subtotal resection of the first rib via the transaxillary approach after not responding well to physiotherapy. Abnormalities, such as scalene muscle anomalies, fibrotic bands, and clear narrowing of the thoracic outlet, were found in 12 of the 13 patients.

Nine of the 13 patients had abnormal preoperative Erb's point recordings and definitive operative findings. All had abnormal amplitudes. One patient had no clear response to ulnar nerve stimulation. Conduction velocities were abnormal in only 2 cases. Postoperative recordings made 2 months after the procedure showed normal findings in 3 cases. Four of the other 6 patients had persistent abnormalities 1 to 2 years postoperatively. Good clinical recovery was apparent in 11 patients 2 months after the operation. All 3 patients with normal Erb's point recordings at this time had a good clinical recovery.

Erb's point recordings appear to be useful in the diagnosis of thoracic outlet syndrome. The preliminary findings suggest that the recordings correlate with clinical recovery after the first rib resection. Amplitude deformities are the chief abnormality. The stimulus intensity should be adjusted to twice the threshold level causing muscle contraction in the hand.

▶ This carefully done study nicely identifies somatosensory evoked potentials as an additional study that may be of benefit in evaluation of patients with brachial plexopathy due to compression in the thoracic outlet. It is important to note that abnormalities were found only in association with a neurologic deficit, and then primarily in amplitude, a difficult parameter to quantitate reliably. It is surprising that these authors did not find the peripheral electrophysiologic abnormalities that most authors have found in patients with neurologic deficit due to thoracic outlet syndrome.—J.R.D.

A Chronic and Painless Form of Idiopathic Brachial Plexus Neuropathy
G. D. Schott (Natl. Hosp. for Nervous Diseases, London)
J. Neurol. Neurosurg. Psychiatry 46:555–557, June 1983   10–19

Idiopathic brachial plexus neuropathy is typically characterized by severe shoulder girdle pain and subacute development of weakness and wasting of the periscapular muscles. The prognosis is generally good, but recovery may be protracted. Schott reports data on 3 patients in whom localized weakness and atrophy of muscles developed around one shoulder girdle in the absence of any pain. The weakness and wasting developed very gradually. Complete recovery occurred within several months.

Girl, 15, had progressive difficulty lifting the left arm for 2 months, but no pain or sensory symptoms. Marked wasting and weakness of the left spinati and deltoid muscles were observed, with no fasciculation. There was questionable weakness of the left triceps and small muscles of the hand, and a small patch of impaired cutaneous sensation was noticed in the lateral aspect of the left upper arm. Tendon reflexes were absent in the left arm. Electromyography showed denervation in the left deltoid muscle and similar, but less marked, changes in the left brachioradialis and triceps muscles. Nerve conduction studies had normal results. Strength was normal 2 months later, and all reflexes were elicited. There were no abnormal signs at this time.

Pain was completely absent in these cases, and the muscle weakness and wasting developed very slowly. There were no features suggesting an inflammatory cause at any time, and there was no evidence of a compressive condition, such as cervical disk protrusion. These patients may have an unusual, chronic, painless variant of idiopathic brachial plexus neuropathy. If the condition is recognized, studies such as myelography can be avoided. With additional experience, it may be possible to give a more reassuring prognosis at an earlier stage.

▶ One of the more frustrating situations for the surgeon who operates on the upper extremity is deciding that a nerve lesion, particularly a proximal nerve lesion, is one that can be helped by surgical intervention. This report makes the problem even more frustrating, because it suggests that even lack of pain and slow progression are not necessarily compression lesions nor is the prognosis necessarily poor. On the other hand, this may be good news for some of our patients.—P.C.A.

11 Muscle and Tendon

A Staged Technique for the Repair of the Traumatic Boutonnière Deformity
Raymond M. Curtis, Robert L. Reid, and John M. Provost
J. Hand Surg. 8:167–171, March 1983   11–1

Twenty-three patients, aged 17–57 years, who had chronic traumatic boutonnière deformities were treated with the use of a staged technique. All the injuries originally were open and generally had been caused by laceration with a sharp instrument. Several patients had had splinting in flexion for 4–6 weeks. Seventeen patients who lacked an average of 41 degrees of extension of the affected digit at the proximal interphalangeal (PIP) joint received stage I–III treatment, while 6 who lacked 55 degrees of extension at the PIP joint had stage I, II, and IV treatment.

Before treatment begins, splinting is required to stretch out the contracted palmar capsule of the stiff PIP joint. Full passive extension is a prerequisite for surgery. In stage I a dorsal incision is made. The transverse retinacular ligament is freed by a blunt probe, and a tendolysis of the extensor tendon is performed. Stage II is used if full extension is not present after stage I and involves sectioning the transverse retinacular ligament throughout its length on both sides of the finger. Patients who fall 20 degrees short of a straight line in extending the finger at the PIP joint require stage III treatment, a modified Fowler tenotomy. If after stages I and II, the gap in the central tendon is too large to be corrected by stage III, stage IV is carried out following stage II. The central tendon is separated from the lateral bands. Either the central tendon is advanced 4–6 mm into a drill hole in the dorsal base of the middle phalanx or the extensor tendon is sutured to its remnant left at the base of the middle phalanx. The lateral bands are loosely sutured to the central tendon.

The 17 patients having stage I–III treatment lacked an average of 10 degrees of extension at the PIP joint postoperatively. The 6 having stage IV surgery lacked an average of 17 degrees of extension postoperatively. All but 3 patients had an improved ability to touch or approximate the distal palmar crease. The inability to touch the distal palmar crease was by an average of 1 cm.

▶ The authors present a progressive approach to boutonnière deformity that depends on attempting to correct the deformity with the simplest measures first, while using active patient extension of the finger during surgery to predict success. One would wish that the authors would mention the possible surgical importance of the spiral fibers originally described by Gaul and VanZweiten, as these may play a critical role in control of the descent of the lateral bands, relative to the central slip.—R.L.L.

Locomotor System Disorders in Diabetes Mellitus: Increased Prevalence of Palmar Flexortenosynovitis

Ido Leden, Bengt Scherstén, Björn Svensson, and Madeleine Svensson
Scand. J. Rheumatol. 12:260–262, 1983   11–2

A variety of locomotor system disorders are associated with diabetes mellitus, and Mackenzie reported a possible association with palmar flexor tenosynovitis (FTS). Leden et al. determined the prevalence of FTS in 122 consecutive diabetic patients, 19 with type I and 103 with type II diabetes, and in 150 patients of similar age and sex without diabetes or inflammatory rheumatic disorders. Palmar flexor tenosynovitis was diagnosed in 13 (10.9%) of the diabetics and in 1 control subject (0.7%). Seven of the 13 affected diabetics had involvement of more than 1 tendon. The first, fourth, and third flexor tendons were most often affected, in that order. Diabetic complications were more prevalent in patients with FTS, and the duration of disease was twice as long as in patients without FTS. No significant treatment differences were apparent.

This disorder is significantly more prevalent in diabetics than in other patients. Surgery was indicated in 4 patients who had severe symptoms. Musculoskeletal disorders are produced in diabetics by means not well understood. Microangiopathy and hyperglycemia-induced changes in collagen metabolism have been proposed as factors causing connective tissue alteration.

▶ Patients with diabetes mellitus and inflammatory hand synovitis are seen commonly in hand practice. As the authors point out the relationship is little understood. This occurrence is well known to hand surgeons. From a therapeutic standpoint I have found that utilization of steroid injections and conservative measures is less helpful in patients with inflammatory synovitis of the hands and diabetes mellitus, particularly if there is a co-existent Dupuytren's contracture. In these instances, surgical treatment is necessary to relieve symptoms of flexor tenosynovitis including carpal tunnel syndrome. However, the patient must be cautioned and examined carefully following surgery because there is a definite tendency for these individuals to develop hypertrophic scarring, thickness and dystrophic changes of the hand, which respond slowly even with an aggressive hand therapy program postoperatively.—R.D.B.

Early Mobilization of Repaired Flexor Tendons Within Digital Sheath Using an Internal Profundus Splint: Experimental and Clinical Data

T. Roderick Hester, Jr., Louis Hill, and Foad Nahai (Emory Univ.)
Ann. Plast. Surg. 12:187–198, February 1984   11–3

The method of repair of severed flexor tendons within zone II was modified because of poor clinical results. The proximal profundus tendon now is pulled into the wound as far as possible, and a 2-0 Prolene splint is placed through the tendon proximally and passed back through it 1 cm distally in a figure-of-eight arrangement. The proximal tendon then is

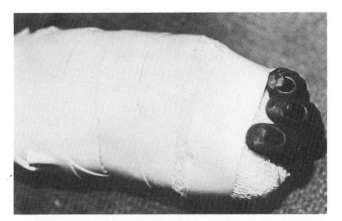

Fig 11–1.—Splint used to immobilize small finger and allow motion in index, long, and ring fingers in rhesus monkey. (Courtesy of Hester, T.R., Jr., et al.: Ann. Plast. Surg. 12:187–198, February 1984.)

allowed to retract back into its sheath. The ends of the splint are passed distally around the distal phalanx and through the nail base, and the tendon then is repaired with 6-0 nylon sutures. The splint is adjusted to insure that tension from proximal pull will not disrupt the repair.

Studies in rhesus monkeys to determine whether the severed profundus tendon had sufficient inherent healing capacity showed adequate healing at 4 to 5 weeks when the profundus was divided at the wrist to prevent disruption. The method of splinting then investigated is shown in Figure 11–1. All but 1 of 6 repairs that were splinted but not immobilized were intact 4 to 5 weeks after operation, whereas most nonsplinted, nonimmobilized repairs avulsed.

Thirty-three patients with 35 flexor tendon injuries in zone II were managed by the internal splint method and followed for 3 weeks to 40 months. All procedures but 1 were done primarily or within 10 days after injury. Physical therapy involved gradually increasing active motion starting on the third postoperative day (Fig 11–2). Emphasis was placed on blocking exercises to encourage proximal and distal interphalangeal joint pull-through. The splint was easily removed 5 weeks after operation. Over 70% of the repairs were last recorded at 2 cm or less to the distal palmar crease without significant loss of proximal interphalangeal joint extension, and 83% were within 3 cm of the distal palmar crease. Some patients were still in physical therapy when last evaluated. One failure resulted from disruption of the repair when the splint was removed at 3 weeks. Two patients had secondary procedures.

It is hoped that the results of internal splinting of repaired flexor tendons will improve as more experience is gained with the technique. A prospective study comparing the method with more traditional techniques is planned.

▶ This is an interesting report both of an experimental study of tendon healing in primates, of which there are all too few, and a clinical study of an internal suture splint in a series of 35 cases in 33 patients.

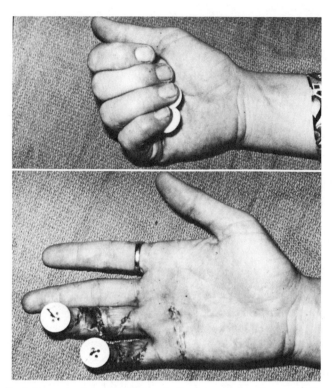

Fig 11–2.—Active motion is encouraged immediately after operation. (Courtesy of Hester, T.R., et al.: Ann. Plast. Surg. 12:187–198, February 1984.)

The experimental study is similar to work on flexor tendon healing in primates reported recently by Schepel, of the Netherlands. Unfortunately, his work is not available in English, but it agrees remarkably well with the data reported by Hester et al. Both of these primate studies are consistent with a large body of clinical and experimental data that demonstrates minimal or no adhesions following direct repair of flexor tendons with intact circulation treated with sheath closure and early mobilization.

The clinical data are interesting. The internal profundus splint suture is identical to that reported by Brunelli recently. Apparently the method is capable of permitting early active motion without tendon rupture, as Brunelli reported ruptures in only 3 of 98 cases and in this article by Hester et al., rupture occurred in only 1 of 35. Surprisingly, the results in this study are not all that good. Only 40% of patients were able to flex to within 2 cm of the distal palmar crease. These results are not as good as those reported by Kleinert and others for early *passive* mobilization. Nevertheless, I believe this work should be studied by all ·those interested in flexor tendon surgery, and I believe that the suture technique described deserves further investigation. Perhaps modifications in the postoperative therapy protocol might be helpful in improving the final results. This technique might find special application in those patients where poorer results are predictable, namely, those with multiple injuries, older patients, those unable to cooperate with the usual postoperative therapy program, and possibly those patients with damage to the vincular blood supply.—P.C.A.

Blood Supply of the Flexor Pollicis Longus Tendon
Carlos A. Azar, James E. Culver, and Earl J. Fleegler (Cleveland Clinic)
J. Hand Surg. 8:471–475, July 1983   11–4

The origin, anatomical relationships, and intratendinous pattern of the blood supply of the flexor pollicis longus tendon were examined in 15 fresh adult cadaver extremities. Dilute India ink-latex-barium solution was injected at different arterial levels, including the median nerve artery. Vascularity in the digital area was via two vincula (Fig 11–3). One of them, V_1, located just proximal to the metacarpophalangeal joint and the A_1 pulley, arose either from both digital arteries or from the princeps pollicis artery alone. The other, V_2, located at the interphalangeal joint level under the A_2 pulley, arose from both digital arteries. In the predigital region, branches of the median nerve artery supplied the area from the thumb base to the musculotendinous junction. The microvascular network of the mesotendon also made a contribution. Intratendinous vascularization was more abundant in the predigital area. Several zones of sparse intratendinous vascularization were present, including the areas between V_1 and V_2 and between V_2 and the tendon insertion.

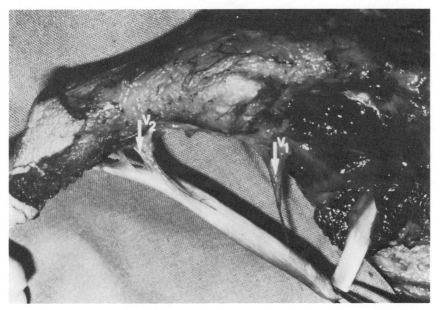

Fig 11–3.—Vincular system of the flexor pollicis longus tendon: V_1 and V_2. (Courtesy of Azar, C.A., et al.: J. Hand Surg. 8:471–475, July 1983.)

The flexor pollicis longus tendon has a segmental vascular supply. The intradigital area is supplied by vincula from both digital arteries or from the princeps pollicis artery alone. Sparse intratendinous vascularization is observed between each of the segmental arteries.

▶ Like the finger flexors, the flexor pollicis longus has a segmental blood supply. There are also some palmar hypovascular areas, suggesting that synovial nutrition may be important for this tendon as well. Understanding the sources of tendon nutrition and their potential for injury is likely to be important in future understanding of the biology of tendon healing.—P.C.A.

Restoration of Flexor Pollicis Longus Function by Flexor Digitorum Superficialis Transfer.

Lawrence H. Schneider (Thomas Jefferson Univ.) and David Wiltshire (Pointe-Claire, Que.)

J. Hand Surg. 8:98–101, January 1983   11–5

A flexor digitorum superficialis transfer was performed in 14 patients with unrepairable flexor pollicis longus (FPL) lesions. Twelve patients had tendon rupture or laceration, and 2 had anterior interosseous nerve damage. The injuries were presented late and direct repair of the tendon or nerve was not possible. None of the patients had significant scarring. The flexor digitorum superficialis was transferred to the distal phalanx of the thumb with the thumb metacarpal in abduction and in line with the index metacarpal from the palmar view and at an angle of 35 degrees to the index metacarpal in the lateral view. The thumb interphalangeal joint is flexed 30 degrees after the transfer juncture is secured.

Eight patients had 60 degrees or more of active motion from neutral position on follow-up at ½ to 11 years, and 4 had 30 to 60 degrees of active motion. One patient had less than 30 degrees of active motion, representing a fair result, and 1 had no active motion. Side pinch exceeded that in the opposite hand in 4 cases and equaled it in 4 other cases. Side pinch was stronger than tip pinch. Complications included a hyperextension deformity and rupture of the juncture at the wrist requiring resuturing. No carpal tunnel syndrome developed.

Loss of FPL function impedes precision pinch activities. The ring finger flexor digitorum superficialis can be used to restore active motion of the thumb interphalangeal joint after FPL disruption if a Boyes grade I or II injury is present. The procedure has been used successfully as an alternative to tendon grafting in patients who have lost FPL motion and desire a return of interphalangeal motion.

▶ The transfer of the flexor digitorum superficialis of the ring finger to the flexor pollicis longus is an excellent tendon transfer. It is easy to reeducate, easy to attach, and very functional in its use. Minor complications are encountered by the authors. If a satisfactory proximal muscle is present, however, I believe that it is preferable to utilize a tendon graft to restore more functional anatomy.

Interphalangeal motion of the thumb is not necessary for most functional activities, but the power of the thumb adduction contributed by the flexor pollicis longus is certainly significant. The powerful superficialis is also a good muscle to achieve this.—R.D.B.

Adduction Contracture of the Thumb in Cerebral Palsy: A Preoperative Electromyographic Study
M. Mark Hoffer, Jacquelin Perry, Manual Garcia, and Daniel Bullock (Rancho Los Amigos Hosp., Downey, Calif.)
J. Bone Joint Surg. [Am.] 65-A:755–759, July 1983   11–6

A tight thenar cleft in children with cerebral palsy traditionally is managed by a Z-plasty of the web and total release of the adductor origin, combined with capsulodesis of the metacarpophalangeal joint where required. Grasp of large objects was generally satisfactory in 21 patients who were previously operated on, but 2 children with voluntary adductor brevis electromyogram (EMG) activity during grasp and no activity on release of grasp lost some pinch ability after total muscle release. Twenty-three subsequent surgical candidates with spastic hemiplegia had preoperative EMG evaluation. Recordings were made with wire electrodes in the adductor muscle as the patient grasped and released a cylinder.

Two patients had complete selective control of the extrinsic muscles. Ten had patterned control only during release and 2 only during grasp. Nine patients had patterned control during both grasp and release. Clinical indications for surgery included at least some selective control of the hand and reasonable cognition. Eight patients with intermittent EMG activity in the adductor muscle had a partial release (Fig. 11–4). Two patients with nearly continuous activity (Fig 11–5) and the 2 original patients had a total release of the adductor insertion. Other procedures were done as well in all 12 surgically treated patients. Eleven had a flexor carpi ulnaris transfer to the extensor digitorum communis, and 7 had a transfer of the palmaris longus to the radially transposed extensor pollicis longus. The width of grasp was increased in all cases on follow-up 2 years or more after operation. New two-handed activities had become possible. The patients having partial transverse myotomy had lost no pinch activity clinically.

A combination of thumb release and appropriate tendon transfers can give quite predictable and satisfactory results in children with cerebral palsy who have adduction contracture of the thumb. Preoperative EMG analysis can help determine whether a partial or a total release of the adductor muscle should be performed.

▶ This report from the Rancho Los Amigos Hospital group points out once again the utility of kinesiologic studies coupled with electromyography for sur-

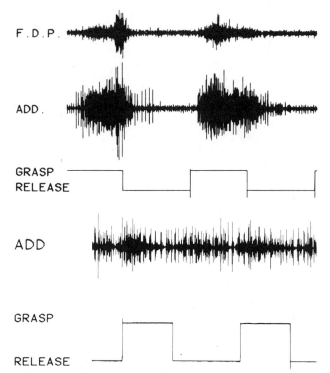

Fig 11–4 (top).—An electromyogram of the thenar adductor shows selective activity during grasp. Thus, partial release was performed.

Fig 11–5 (bottom).—A photograph after partial adductor release shows adequate prehension with no loss of pinch.

(Courtesy of Hoffer, M.M., et al.: J. Bone Joint Surg. [Am.] 65-A:755–759, July 1983.)

gical decision making in cerebral palsy. This technique has the advantage of identifying muscles that are under voluntary control and those that are not under voluntary control and function continuously during agonistic and antagonistic movements. Muscles in the former group may be lengthened or transferred; those in the latter group should be released, because transfer merely moves the deforming force from one side of the joint to the other.

In this particular study the adductor muscles of the thumb were investigated. In 17 of 23 patients voluntary control of these muscles was identified. This information suggests that in the majority of such patients, partial rather than complete release would be appropriate, and this actually was the procedure carried out for the authors' patients with good success. In fact, when complete release was carried out for voluntarily controlled muscles, function was actually lost, in that pinch was weakened.

Studies such as this are important in helping the surgeon improve the predictability of surgery in cerebral palsy. Hopefully, more centers similar to the one utilized by the authors will become available around the United States in the near future.—P.C.A.

Comparative Study of EFMT and Sublimis Transfer Operations in Claw Hand

Gabriel D. Sundaraj, Ambrose J. Selvapandian, and Kandasamy Mani (Tamil Nadu, South India)

Int. J. Lepr. 51:197–202, June 1983   11–7

Two hundred cases each of extensor flexor many-tailed transfer extensor carpi radialis longus (EFMT)—motor palmaris longus tendon—graft and sublimis transfer for claw hand deformity resulting from leprosy were reviewed. Littler's modification of the sublimis transfer and Brand's EFMT operation were used. Reclawing was most frequent in the little and ring fingers. The incidence in the EFMT series was considerably greater than in the sublimis series. Intrinsic plus deformity was infrequent in both series, but it was more frequent in the EFMT group. Sublimis minus deformity was more frequent in the sublimis group, especially in the long finger.

Good or fair results were obtained in over 95% of hands, with a significant improvement in hand function and an effective motor transfer. The good results are attributed to the use of a standard frame for positioning, proper adjustment of tension, and adequate physiotherapy. Either of these procedures seems to be applicable in selected cases of claw hand due to leprosy, provided preoperative and postoperative management is closely supervised. Technical errors and postoperative complications have been more frequent with the EFMT operation than with the sublimis procedure.

▶ This study is important because of the large size of the population receiving the two most popular and well-defined operations for claw hand. This is likely to remain the definitive reference, as the population at risk appears to be decreasing.—R.L.L.

Correction of Intrinsic-Minus Hands Associated With Reversal of the Transverse Metacarpal Arch

Dinkar D. Palande (Sacred Heart Leprosy Centre, Kumbakonam, India)

J. Bone Joint Surg. [Am.] 65-A:514–521, April 1983   11–8

Paralysis of the intrinsic hand muscles leads to finger clawing, abnormal digitopalmar grasp, and deformity of the distal transverse metacarpal arch. The author found that although the Brand transfer of the extensor carpi radialis longus to the lateral bands via the flexor route usually corrects the appearance of the fingers and the pattern of grasp, restoration of the arch sometimes is inadequate (Fig 11–6). A flexor force acting on the carpometacarpal joints seemed necessary, along with a reduction in the extensor force acting on the distal joints in some fingers, and the Brand operation was modified accordingly. Either the radial wrist extensor or the palmaris longus is transferred. Surgery is done with the patient under axillary block anesthesia. The surgery in the interdigital space is illustrated in Figure 11–7. The graft is divided into five slips rather than four, and

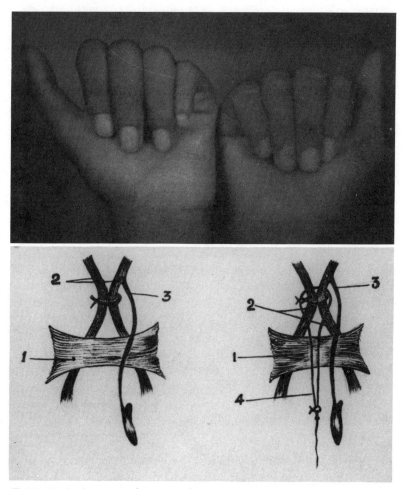

Fig 11–6 (top).—Appearance of converging fingers 1 year after surgery. Both hands had reversal of metacarpal arch preoperatively. Hand on left had Brand operation; hand on right had Palande operative procedure, with all fingers pointing toward trapezial ridge.

Fig 11–7 (bottom).—Operative steps in interdigital space (*1*, deep transverse metacarpal ligament; *2*, one palmar and one dorsal interosseous tendon; *3*, lumbrical tendon; *4*, transferred slip). *Left*, two interosseous tendons are tied. *Right*, transferred slip is tied to interosseous tendon, and folded-back slip is sutured to itself proximally. Slip passes in front of deep transverse metacarpal ligament.

(Courtesy of Palande, D.D.: J. Bone Joint Surg. [Am.] 65-A:514–521, April 1983.)

these are tunneled dorsally and sutured to the interosseous muscle tendons, the first dorsal interosseus muscle and tendon, and the hypothenar muscle-tendon mass.

Sixteen hands were operated on using this approach. High ulnar paralysis was present in 9 hands and ulnar-median paralysis in 7. Leprosy was responsible in 14 cases and motor neuron disease in 2. The hands had been paralyzed for an average of 3½ years. The radial wrist extensor was used for transfer in 10 hands and the palmaris longus in 6. Adequate

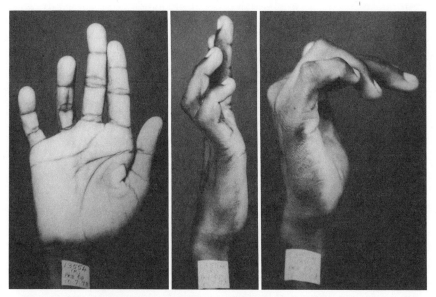

Fig 11–8 (left).—Preoperative photograph showing clawing, mainly of little and ring fingers, as well as thumb, of ulnar-median paralysis.

Fig 11–9 (center).—Clawing and reversal of metacarpal arch.

Fig 11–10 (right).—Marked flexion of interphalangeal joints of ring and little fingers is seen in attempted lumbrical position.

(Courtesy of Palande, D.D.: J. Bone Joint Surg. [Am.] 65-A:514–521, April 1983.)

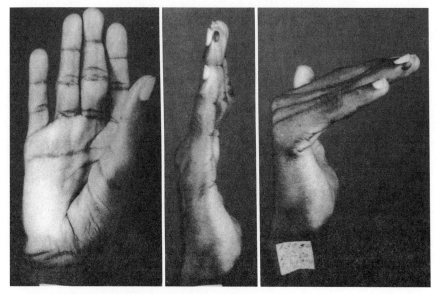

Fig 11–11 (left).—Appearance 2 years postoperatively.

Fig 11–12 (center).—Restoration of metacarpal arch.

Fig 11–13 (right).—Achievement of normal lumbrical position.

(Courtesy of Palande, D.D.: J. Bone Joint Surg. [Am.] 65-A:514–521, April 1983.)

restoration of the arch was achieved in all hands, and deformity and disability were corrected in 85% of the affected fingers. The outcome in 1 case is shown in Figures 11–8 to 11–13. Poor results were attributed to faulty technique or to inadequate protection of the hand in the postoperative period.

The lateral and medial transfers tend to deepen the hollow of the palm after this operation, and the converging pull of all the slips on the fingers adds to the flexion-rotation effect and tends to further restore the metacarpal arch. Attachment of the slips close to the phalangeal insertions of the hypothenar muscles and interossei effectively transmits the flexor force acting on the metacarpophalangeal joints and nearly always prevents hyperextension. The hand must be adequately protected and trained in the postoperative period.

Extensor Carpi Radialis Brevis Tendon Transfer for Thumb Adduction: Study of Power Pinch
Richard J. Smith (Massachusetts Genl. Hosp.)
J. Hand Surg. 8:4–15, January 1983   11–9

In 18 male patients disabled by weak thumb adduction, an attempt was made to improve power grip by transferring the extensor carpi radialis brevis (ECRB) to the tendon of the adductor pollicis. The ECRB was lengthened with a tendon graft and passed through the second intermetacarpal space, as shown in Figure 11–14. A palmaris longus tendon graft was used in most instances; it was sutured to the adductor pollicis tendon, and its proximal end then was passed subcutaneously to the most proximal incision and joined to the ECRB, taking up slack with no tension. The patients, aged 16–50 years, had lost adductor pollicis function through ulnar nerve injury, peripheral neuropathy, local muscle avulsion, partial amputation, or aplasia. Eight patients had a tendon transfer for abduction of the index finger at the same time as the adductor plasty.

One patient had synovectomy for synovitis about the tendon graft 6 months after operation. Another patient was operated on for de Quervain's tenosynovitis that was not directly related to the adductor plasty. One patient believed he was worse after operation, but all the others noticed significant improvement in ability to use the thumb for pinch and grasp. Most returned to their previous work. Only 2 patients had permanent loss of abduction; both had had opposition transfers initially. All 3 patients who had adductor plasty for conditions other than paralysis or avulsion had useful results.

Transfer of the ECRB to the adductor pollicis tendon in patients with weak thumb adduction may restore pinch strength to 50% of normal. Overcorrection is a possibility in patients who also have weak thumb opposition. Wrist function is not compromised by the ECRB transfer.

▶ The desirability of establishing a substitute for the adductor pollicis is now well established. The original concern voiced by many that wrist extension

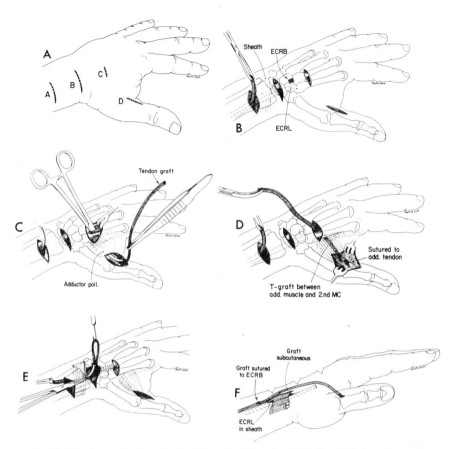

Fig 11–14.—A, usual incisions for detaching and withdrawing ECRB *(A and B),* channeling tendon graft through second interspace *(C),* and attaching graft to tendon of adductor pollicis *(D).* **B,** ECRB is transected distally and withdrawn proximal to dorsal retinacular ligament *(Sheath).* **C,** tendon graft (palmaris longus or plantaris) is passed deep to adductor pollicis and between second and third metacarpals. **D,** tendon graft is sutured to adductor tendon. **E,** proximal end of tendon graft is passed subcutaneously to proximal incision. **F,** tendon graft is sutured proximally to ECRB with thumb adducted and wrist at 0 degrees extension. The ECRB is at resting length. Graft is made slightly longer if thenars are paralyzed. (Courtesy of Smith, R.J.: J. Hand Surg. 8:4–15, January 1983.)

would be weakened appears to be answered by the author's statistics. This transfer appears to offer good synergy and force equivalents.—R.L.L.

Surgical Reconstruction of the Upper Limb in Traumatic Tetraplegia: A Review of 41 Patients
Douglas W. Lamb and K. M. Chan (Princess Margaret Rose Orthopaedic Hosp., Edinburgh)
J. Bone Joint Surg. [Br.] 65-B:291–298, May 1983   11–10

The prevailing attitude toward surgical reconstruction of the upper extremity in tetraplegics has been negative. The results of such surgery performed on 41 tetraplegic subjects during a 20-year period were reviewed. The 38 men and 3 women had an average age of 29 years. All patients had at least wrist dorsiflexion, pronation, and supination. Threee had flexor carpi radialis function, 16 had elbow extension, and 5 had finger extension.

The posterior third of the deltoid was transferred to motor the triceps in 16 limbs of 10 patients. Thirty-one patients (45 hands) had an extensor carpi radialis longus transfer to the flexor digitorum profundus and a brachioradialis transfer to the flexor pollicis longus. Six patients (7 hands) had a flexor pollicis longus tenodesis. Four patients (5 hands) had a flexor pollicis longus tenodesis plus an extensor carpi radialis longus to flexor digitorum profundus transfer.

The average follow-up after surgery was 7 years 5 months. Active elbow extension against gravity was restored in all patients, and 10 of 16 elbows had full restoration of extension. Functional testing of 48 hands operated on in 27 patients revealed excellent results in 10% of cases, good results in 58%, fair results in 23%, and poor results in 9%. All poor results were in early cases. In no patient was hand function impaired by operation. Most of the 29 patients evaluated claimed significant improvement in basic activities of daily living. Improved self-care was very beneficial psychologically to the patients. Improved upper extremity function had facilitated personal interests and hobbies. Eight patients had returned to employment, and 3 others were actively engaged in voluntary work.

Restoration of both elbow and hand function can be very useful to tetraplegic patients. Most patients have been very satisfied with the results, but the prospect of useful function being restored should not be exaggerated. It is useful for surgical candidates to see patients who have had successful surgical results.

▶ This demonstrates that experience and careful assessment and follow-up are keys to the treatment of the tetraplegic patient.—R.L.L.

Upper Limb Reconstruction in Quadriplegia: Functional Assessment and Proposed Treatment Modifications
Vincent R. Hentz, Margaret Brown, and Leo A. Keoshian
J. Hand Surg. 8:119–131, March 1983   11–11

The functional results of upper extremity reconstruction in higher spinal level quadriplegic patients were reviewed. Key grip was reconstructed in 40 extremities of 30 patients and active elbow extension was achieved in 14 extremities of 9 patients. Nearly 60% of patients had sufficient resources to allow reconstruction of key pinch activated by moderate to strong wrist extension and reconstruction of active elbow extension, or at least resources for some active digital flexion. Orthoses remained necessary for another 20% of patients; the remainder were able to have reconstruction of active digital extension and flexion, including some independent thumb flexion and more refined pinch.

Good functional results were obtained in 18 (55%) extremities operated on, fair in 10 (30%), and poor in 5 (15%). Patients in the last group were the weakest before operation or had the longest intervals from injury to surgery. Functionally active elbow extension was achieved in 10 of 14 extremities, but the convalescence time was prolonged.

"Weaker" patients should have reconstruction only if highly motivated. A satisfactory outcome is less predictable when the postinjury interval exceeds 5 years. Apart from lengthening the tenodesis, patient dissatisfaction is most closely related to poor index finger positioning before and during pinch and an unstable thumb metacarpophalangeal (MP) joint during key pinch.

The key grip procedure was modified to eliminate these problems. If the thumb MP joint has more than 45 degrees of passive flexion, a tenodesis of the extensor tendons into gouge holes in the thumb metacarpal is done just proximal to the MP joint, using a pullout wire technique. A wide strip of fascia lata is used in place of the long toe extensors to bridge the gap between the deltoid and triceps. Immobilization has been prolonged to 6 weeks. Frequent functional evaluation after operation is important.

It is concluded that more than three fourths of quadriplegic patients can benefit from reconstructive surgery on the upper extremity.

▶ The authors have developed a refinement of the surgical procedures described by Moberg in 1975. We have found the deltoid to triceps transfers to be very acceptable and useful in patients and have had some problems with pullout of transfers. I have modified these by utilizing all toe extensors and in some instances the anterior tibial tendon woven in a shoestring fashion through the proximal deltoid and distally through the triceps tendon. The authors feel that utilization of fascia provides them with an easier and more reliable technique with earlier mobilization, but I think longer-term follow-up will have to be obtained before the potential benefits of this alteration in the technique can be assessed. Our success and patient satisfaction, like the authors', have been much less in thumb procedures, but the modifications that they have suggested seem outstanding and should be considered strongly.—R.D.B.

Compartment Syndrome of the Arm: Complication of the Pneumatic Tourniquet; Case Report
Thomas L. Greene and Dean S. Louis (Univ. of Michigan)
J. Bone Joint Surg. [Am.] 65-A:270–273, February 1983   11–12

A localized compartment syndrome developed in the arm of a patient after a prolonged operation on the forearm and hand performed with pneumatic tourniquet control.

Woman, 29, with a slowly enlarging right palmar mass for 15 years and increasing median nerve symptoms, underwent dissection of the nerve and complete removal of a fibrofatty tumor with a single-cuff pneumatic tourniquet inflated to 250 mm Hg at the midarm. The tourniquet was inflated for a total of 655 minutes during the 12½-hour operation and deflated for 60 minutes. Marked pain in the right arm was reported 12 hours after operation, and a tense circumferential swelling was apparent from the elbow to the shoulder. Passive elbow extension produced severe arm pain. Pressures were 70 mm Hg in the anterior compartment and 50 mm Hg in the posterior compartment of the arm. Fasciotomy was carried out and the wound left open. Pain resolved immediately, and all swelling disappeared within a week of the procedure. No subsequent loss of neuromuscular function was observed. The pathologic diagnosis was lipofibroma of the median nerve.

Compartment syndrome in the upper extremity due to prolonged external compression is most often seen in drug abusers. Direct external pressure can have a localized ischemic effect on the compartment contents, and the duration of ischemia directly influences the extent of edema and subsequent muscle fiber necrosis. In the authors' patient the syndrome appears to have been caused by the local compressive effects of the tourniquet, added to the effects of continued reinflation. When the arm muscles were unable to recover adequately from postischemic edema, a cycle of edema and ischemia was initiated. Muscle necrosis was prevented by the intervals of tourniquet deflation.

▶ The authors have brought to light a significant complication of prolonged use of the tourniquet in operative procedures. Certainly, excessive tourniquet time can contribute to swelling and a secondary compartment syndrome, as in the authors' case. One also must be entirely aware of the actual pressures within the tourniquet during its elevation, particularly in operations over 1 hour in duration (Aho et al.: *J. Bone Joint Surg.* [*Br.*] 65-B:441–443, 1983). Gauge pressures may be inaccurate if they are not checked regularly (Hallett: *Br. Med. J.* 286:1267–1268, 1983).—R.D.B.

An Exercise-Induced Compartment Syndrome of the Dorsal Forearm: A Case Report
Joseph E. Imbriglia and David M. Boland (Allegheny Genl. Hosp., Pittsburgh)
J. Hand Surg. 9A:142–143, January 1984   11–13

The second known case of exercise-induced compartment syndrome of the forearm extensor muscles is reported.

Man, 46, had gradual onset of pain in the dorsal part of the left forearm several hours after using a manual boring tool. A potent oral analgesic failed to relieve the pain. Intense pain was described 48 hours after the onset. The dorsal part of the forearm was moderately swollen and very tender to palpation, especially over the muscle belly of the extensor carpi ulnaris. Passive wrist flexion greatly increased the pain. No sensory deficit was noted. There was no evidence of increased pressure in the flexor compartment. The intracompartmental pressure was 45 mm Hg. The extensor carpi ulnaris was markedly swollen and discolored, but appeared to be viable. An epimysiotomy of the individual extensor muscles was performed. The pain was much reduced postoperatively, and the patient recovered completely after delayed wound closure on the third postoperative day.

The diagnosis was missed initially in this case despite the presence of findings typical for compartment syndrome. A sensory deficit is consistently absent in compartment syndromes of the dorsal forearm. Complete recovery followed decompressive fasciotomy, which was carried out 48 hours after the onset of symptoms. The term "exercise-induced compartment syndrome" is proposed for this entity.

▶ Just when it seems that the work of Whitesides, Mubarak, and others have called so much attention to compartment syndromes that surely none will ever be missed again, a case like this is reported. This particular patient was sent home twice from a local emergency room despite what appear from the description to be classic physical findings. It behooves us all not only to remain vigilant in our own practices, but also to educate others to the early diagnosis of this condition for which early treatment is so straightforward, but for which the consequences of failure of early diagnosis are so tragic.—P.C.A.

12 Degenerative Arthritis and Related Diseases

Myxoid Cysts of the Finger: Treatment by Liquid Nitrogen Spray Cryosurgery
R. P. R. Dawber, T. Sonnex, J. Leonard, and I. Ralfs
Clin. Exp. Dermatol. 8:153–157, March 1983   12–1

Myxoid cysts arising from the dorsal surface of the terminal phalanx rarely resolve spontaneously and can cause disability through nail distortion, pain, and secondary bacterial infection. Radical excision may produce joint limitation and permanent scarring of the nail matrix. Dawber et al. used liquid nitrogen cryosurgery to treat 14 patients with single myxoid cysts of the fingers. Eight cysts were on the index finger and 4 were on the thumb. Four cysts were discharging constantly at presentation. Nine subjects had clinical and x-ray evidence of terminal interphalangeal joint osteoarthritis.

The cyst and proximal tissue up to the transverse skin crease (Fig 12–1) were treated with two freeze-thaw cycles, each freeze lasting 30 seconds. Aspirin was taken for 3–4 days after treatment. Twelve of the 14 lesions remitted, while 2 remained active. One of the latter lesions failed to respond to repeated treatment. The time to crust formation ranged from 14 to 29 days. Three patients had a hemorrhagic blister at the treatment site. Only 3 patients had discomfort. The successfully treated patients have been followed for up to 3½ years without recurrences.

A cure rate of 86% has been obtained with this regimen of liquid nitrogen cryosurgery. More prolonged cryosurgery in 2 cases resulted in residual scarring of the nail matrix (Fig 12–2). Intact myxoid cysts should first be needled, and cryosurgery should be used for failures. If both methods fail, radical local surgery can be undertaken. Cryosurgery is the appropriate initial treatment of cysts that present with persistent or recurrent spontaneous discharge.

▶ This article purports to demonstrate the benefits of cryosurgery in the treatment of myxoid cysts. The field treated is indicated in Figure 12–1. After freezing, an open wound develops that requires about 1 month to heal. Of 14 patients, 2 had recurrences after treatment and 2 had permanent nail deformity as indicated in Figure 12–2, which also indicates the appearance of the cyst after "cure."

Compared to the risks and known benefits of surgical treatment of this condition, cryosurgery does not appear to offer special advantages in terms of speed of healing postoperatively, risk of injury to the nail, or risk of recurrence. In addition, it has the disadvantage of not addressing the principal cause of

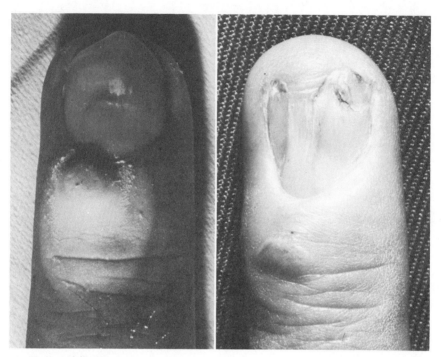

Fig 12–1 (left).—An intact myxoid cysts showing the associated field of ice formed during each treatment.

Fig 12–2 (right).—A nodular scar over the interphalangeal joint associated with nail dystrophy due to nail-matrix scarring following cryosurgery.

(Courtesy of Dawber, R.P.R., et al.: Clin. Exp. Dermatol. 8:153–157, March 1983.)

myxoid cysts, namely, osteophytes at the distal interphalangeal joint level. That these persist after this sort of treatment and may be associated with recurring myxoid cysts is indicated in Figure 12–2, which demonstrates continued prominence of the dorsal aspect of the distal interphalangeal joint after treatment.

In my opinion, surgical treatment under local anesthesia remains the treatment of choice for this condition in symptomatic patients.—P.C.A.

Gouty Involvement of a Flexor Tendon in the Hand
Dan D. Primm, Jr., and John R. Allen (Univ. of Kentucky)
J. Hand Surg. 8:863–865, November 1983

12–2

Gouty involvement of the tendons and synovial tissue at the wrist is recognized now as a cause of carpal tunnel syndrome. An unusual case is reported in which a localized deposit of urate crystals in a flexor tendon appeared as a discrete palmar mass.

Woman, 19, had first noticed a small mass in the right palm 3 years previously. It has enlarged in the past few months. A firm, nontender, 1 × 1.5-cm nodule underlay the midpalmar crease over the index metacarpal; it appeared to be confluent with the flexor tendon to the index finger. The patient was receiving 300 mg of allopurinol daily for diagnosed primary gout. The serum uric acid concentration was 13.4 mg/100 ml. The involved section of the flexor digitorum superficialis tendon was excised, and a primary palmaris longus tendon graft was carried out. Dynamic traction was maintained for 6 weeks, after which the patient had 10–70 degrees of metacarpophalangeal joint motion, 0–90 degrees of proximal interphalangeal joint motion, and 0–35 degrees of distal interphalangeal joint motion. Deposits of urate crystals were found in the surgical specimen.

Most previously described patients with gouty involvement of the flexor tendons and synovium in the carpal tunnel have had diffuse disease. The patient had a localized deposit of urate crystals in a single flexor tendon of the hand.

▶ Gouty deposits of flexor tendons are neither as unusual (in the presence of gouty disease) nor as simple, in most instances, as the case reported here. Fortunately, flexor tendon dysfunction is a rare manifestation, with the usual indications for surgery being carpal tunnel syndrome or the presence of a mass. Excision with tendon graft replacement or simply with tenodesis to adjacent functioning tendons is appropriate when severe tendon involvement is discovered and a small number of tendons are involved. However, when all tendons are significantly involved, the preferable approach is to achieve external decompression by carpal tunnel release and only sufficient internal decompression to remove large asymmetric masses. Luckily, rupture is infrequent and some help can be anticipated from adequate medical control.— P.C.A.

Perichondrial Arthroplasty in the Hand: A Case Report

George Wu and Don E. Johnson (Lackland AFB, Texas)
J. Hand Surg. 8:446–453, July 1983   12–3

Perichondrial arthroplasty requires minimal joint resection and helps preserve both bone length and ligamentous stability of a joint. A two-stage arthroplasty method was used to treat an isolated fibrous ankylosis that developed in the index metacarpophalangeal (MCP) joint after a rattlesnake bite.

Boy, 14, was envenomed by a rattlesnake over the dorsum of the left index MCP joint and developed immediate swelling. Fasciotomies were carried out, but no antivenom was given. Wound closure was attempted 5 and 10 days later. Narrowing of the index MCP joint space was noted a month after injury. At 8 months the patient had an ankylosed, painful finger with obliteration of the MCP joint space and loss of the epiphyseal plates of both bones. Joint motion was limited to 10 degrees. Exploration showed total articular destruction and fibrous ankylosis. A joint space was recreated by excising scar tissue and cartilage remnants and by contouring with a bur. A palmar pouch was restored in the retrocondylar recess of the metacarpal head, and a perichondrial graft of costal cartilage was split in two parts and secured with polyglycolic acid sutures to the lateral margins of the metacarpal head and the base of the proximal phalanx. A silicone rubber sheet was placed between the grafts. The ulnar collateral ligament and the ulnar sagittal fibers of the extensor hood were repaired. A capsulotomy was done 5 months later with removal of the silicone membrane. Biopsy of the joint surfaces showed hyaline-like cartilage. Nearly normal pain-free motion was restored 30 months after the initial operation. The most recent radiographs showed a well-defined joint space but persistent subchondrial irregularities.

Perichondrial arthroplasty offers a means of restoring motion in a joint through regeneration of a neocartilaginous lining. Motion can be preserved without the risk of prosthetic failure. If the arthroplasty fails or the results deteriorate, prosthetic replacement or arthrodesis can be carried out. This approach seems most appropriate for patients with limited joint destruction after trauma or sepsis. It should not be used in rheumatoid patients unless the disease is extremely limited and totallly inactive.

▶ Though only a single case report, this represents a unique example of the use of perichondrial arthroplasty. The necessity of releasing a collateral ligament and shortening and altering the contour of the articular surfaces seems likely to set the stage for late degeneration regardless of the success of the perichondrial grafting itself. The development of swan-neck deformity and increasing irregularity of the joint spaces shown on the 26-month film is indicative of problems that, from a biomechanical standpoint, would appear to be insurmountable with present techniques.—R.L.L.

Compression Arthrodesis of the Thumb
Donald C. Ferlic, Barry D. Turner, and Mack L. Clayton (Denver Orthopedic Clinic)
J. Hand Surg. 8:207–210, March 1983   12–4

The results of 82 thumb arthrodeses in 66 patients operated on since 1972 for pain, instability, or collapse-type thumb deformity were reviewed. The Micks External Compression Fixator was used (Figs 12–3 and 12–4). Average patient age was 44 years. Sixty-nine metacarpophalangeal (MP) joint fusions and 13 interphalangeal (IP) joint fusions were carried out. A large majority of the patients had rheumatoid disease. A Kirschner wire usually was passed across the joint to prevent angulation. The compression clamp was removed when bony union was present, usually at 6 weeks. The IP joint was placed in 0 to 15 degrees of flexion and the MP joint in 0 to 40 degrees of flexion.

Solid bony fusion occurred in all instances but 1, but 3 patients required a second operation. One patient with rheumatoid disease developed a pseudoarthrosis, despite 12 weeks of fixation, because the compression pin was too close to the joint, allowing the wire to cut into the joint and loosen the fixation. A pain-free, functionally placed fibrous ankylosis resulted. All patients used their thumbs satisfactorily. All pin track drainage resolved when the fixation device was removed. Antimicrobial therapy was

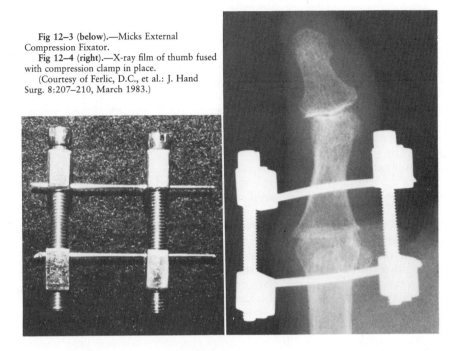

Fig 12–3 (below).—Micks External Compression Fixator.
Fig 12–4 (right).—X-ray film of thumb fused with compression clamp in place.
(Courtesy of Ferlic, D.C., et al.: J. Hand Surg. 8:207–210, March 1983.)

used in 1 case when culture yielded *Staphylococcus aureus*. One patient had delayed union of the MP joint.

Joints arthrodesed wtih external compression unite in about half the time required for union after Kirschner wire fixation. All the patients in this study were satisfied with the outcome. Proper pin placement may preclude the need for a stabilizing Kirschner wire, but a wire is useful in preventing angulation in extremely small bones and in patients with rheumatoid arthritis.

▶ Crossed Kirschner wires have worked extremely well in our hands (36 arthrodeses with 100% union, noted by Beckenbaugh). Internal fixation with a small ASIF plate similarly provides rigid fixation and permits early thumb function without the need for cast immobilization. Compression arthrodesis is a proved technique but should probably be reserved for difficult cases with reduced bone stock, failed previous arthrodesis, or infected joints.—W.P.C.

Osteotomy in the Treatment of Osteoarthritis of the First Carpometacarpal Joint
J. N. Wilson (Royal Natl. Orthopaedic Hosp., London) and C. J. Bossley (Lower Hutt, New Zealand)
J. Bone Joint Surg. [Br.] 65-B:179–181, March 1983   12–5

An abduction wedge osteotomy of the base of the first metacarpal can relieve symptoms in patients with degenerative changes of the first carpometacarpal joint who fail to respond adequately to conservative measures. The results of 23 osteotomies in 21 patients followed up for 2–17 years were reviewed. The 20 women and 1 man had an average age of 48 years. All had a diagnosis of osteoarthritis and presented with pain, usually produced by prolonged use of the hand. All patients had crepitus, local tenderness, thenar wasting, and decreased pinch grip. A closing wedge osteotomy is made at the proximal end of the metacarpal with the base of the wedge directed radially (Fig 12–5). The osteotomy is about 1 cm from the joint. Wire to be used for fixation is inserted before removing the wedge. A forearm plaster is used for 6 weeks postoperatively.

The 3 patients who were not completely relieved of pain have only slight pain and are extremely satisfied with the outcome. Symptomatic relief occurred slowly in 3 cases. Two patients have had the operation on the other side. No relapses have occurred, and no secondary operations have been required. Powerful grasp and spread of the hand were restored, allowing the patients to grip large objects readily. Three patients had pain relief despite failure to correct the adduction deformity. No radiologic improvement in the joint was observed, although further deterioration has not been seen. All the osteotomies united by bone within 3 months postoperatively. One patient had minor loss of sensation at the tip of the thumb. Breakage of the wire loop in 1 case did not produce disability.

Basal osteotomy of the first metacarpal appears to be a very satisfactory approach to osteoarthritis of the carpometacarpal joint. It is an easy procedure and has had no serious complications. All patients have had substantial pain relief and good thumb function. Care is needed to avoid extensive stripping of soft tissue. A wire loop is not necessary unless the osteotomy is unstable.

▶ This is a biomechanically sound operation and tends to correct the thrust of the first metacarpal toward the ulnar shoulder of the trapezium, reducing the

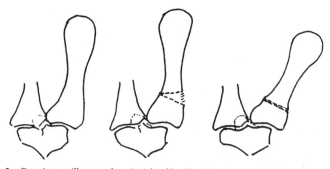

Fig 12–5.—Drawings to illustrate the principle of basal wedge osteotomy in the treatment of osteoarthritis of the first carpometacarpal joint. To avoid instability, it is important that the apex of the wedge should coincide accurately with the ulnar cortex of the metacarpal. The width of the base varies with the amount of adduction deformity to be corrected. (Courtesy of Wilson, J.N., and Bossley, C.J.: J. Bone Joint Surg. [Br.] 65-B:179–181, March 1983.)

tendency to exacerbate the radial subluxation further. It would seem likely also to change the articular bearing surface and the pattern of shear stress on the deteriorating cartilage. It would seem best directed at patients with stage I or stage II disease.—R.L.L.

Silicone Rubber Implants for Arthrosis of the Scaphotrapezial Trapezoidal Joint
Oddvar Eiken and Lars Eric Necking
Scand. J. Plast. Reconstr. Surg. 17:253–255, 1983   12–6

The scaphotrapezial trapezoidal (ST) joint may be part of a pantrapezial process and also the site of isolated arthrosis that causes pain and weakness. Interposition hemiarthroplasty appears to be a promising approach to this disorder. High-performance Silastic was used for interposition hemiarthroplasty of the ST joint in 10 patients seen since 1980, 8 women and 2 men aged 51–70 years. Isolated degenerative changes were present in all cases. Nine patients had primary arthrosis, and 1 had changes after an unhealed distal scaphoid fracture. Pain at the thumb base and weakness were the chief complaints. The operation is designed to replace the scaphoid articular surface with a spacer. The plane of transection should be at a right angle to the longidudinal axis of the ST joint. The implant stem is shortened to 4 mm. The thumb and wrist are immobilized for 3 weeks after the operation.

All patients were completely relieved of pain after the operation. Two responded slowly, with 1 patient taking 9 months to become free of pain. No patient has exhibited implant dislocation, stem fracture, fragmentation, or an untoward bone reaction to the prosthesis. Powerful grip was restored, allowing the patients to grasp large objects without difficulty. There were no complications. The average follow-up was 15 months.

Consistently good results have been obtained using silicone rubber implants to treat arthrosis of the ST joint. Implant hemiarthroplasty is indicated only when degenerative changes are confined to the ST joint. The long-term outcome is unknown, but good long-term results have been obtained from trapezium replacement using high-performance Silastic substitutes.

▶ The authors have shown that in the short term of 36 months or less, the operative procedure of excision of the distal pole of the scaphoid with insertion of a stemmed condylar Silastic implant is successful in relieving pain. I see potential problems with the operative procedure. If there is further deterioration of the carpometacarpal joint, a routine trapezial implant replacement will not be possible. I have used excision of the scaphotrapezial joint with a great toe implant with the stem inserted into the trapezium and obtained a similar successful early result. Recent information does indicate that there may be long-term potential problems with silicone rubber implants in articulating surfaces, and the authors' conclusion that they will be safe in the long run is not valid. The technique does relieve pain, however, and in elderly patients is certainly an appropriate treatment option, preferable and more easy to achieve than arthrodesis.—R.D.B.

Development of Carpal Bone Cysts as Revealed by Radiography
K. Jonsson and O. Eiken
Acta Radiol [Diagn.] (Stockh.) 24:231–233, 1983   12–7

Carpal bone cysts are often encountered, both in assocation with disabling wrist pain and as an incidental finding. Roentgenographic findings were reviewed in 7 women and 4 men, aged 29 to 70, who had intraosseous carpal bone cysts without associated inflammatory or degenerative disease. Mean follow-up was 15 years. The scaphoid and lunate were involved in 4 instances. Early roentgenograms showed an area of sparse spongiose trabeculae with a decreased mineral content. Well-defined cystic changes ensued, in 2 cases with a surrounding zone of sclerosis. Tomography showed fractures of the cyst wall in 1 case. In 2 cases the lytic process led to breakdown of the articular surface and wide communication with the joint (Figs 12–6 and 12–7).

These cysts appear to develop without symptoms and to be distinct from solitary bone cyst or juvenile unicameral bone cyst. Their pathogenesis is unknown. As osteolytic process was apparent in all cases in this study. Most of the lesions have produced no symptoms. Mechanical stress and repeated trauma may lead to intramedullary vascular changes and resultant osteolysis in affected patients. Most cysts are in the scaphoid and lunate, both of which are exposed to considerable loads during power grip. Breakdown of the subchondral layers of the affected bone can lead to communication with the adjacent joint space. The term "intraosseous ganglion" should be avoided.

▶ The authors make a good but not compelling case for the development of carpal bone cysts as being intraosseous. Unfortunately, tomography and ar-

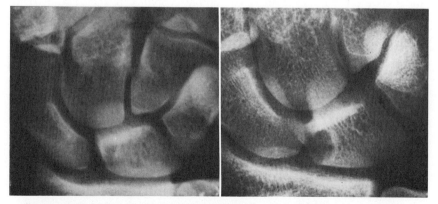

Fig 12–6 (left).—Sparse trabeculae in radial part of lunate, in man, aged 34.
Fig 12–7 (right).—Breakdown of radial wall of lunate and sclerosis of ulnar wall 4 years later. (Courtesy of Jonsson, K., and Eiken, O.: Acta Radiol. [Diagn.] (Stockh.) 24:231–233, 1983.)

thrography as determinates of articular connection are lacking. There seems little doubt that trabeculae erode under the effects of pulsatile hydraulic forces with intra-articular connections. The question of etiology should remain open.—R.L.L.

Destructive Arthritis due to Silicone: Foreign Body Reaction

Daniel I. Rosenthal, Andrew E. Rosenberg, Alan L. Schiller, and Richard J. Smith
Radiology 149:69–72, October 1983   12–8

Subcutaneous silicone implants have been widely used with good overall results in reconstructive and orthopedic surgery, but severe reactive synovitis and lymphadenitis have been caused by shedding of silicone particles. Three cases of erosive arthritis resulting from a foreign body reaction to a silicone implant in the wrist are reported.

Woman, 17, had pain and morning stiffness in the left wrist associated with Kienböck's disease. A lunate implant of high-performance silicone was placed without complications, but symptoms began to develop 4 years later, with pain near the ulnar styloid and clicking sounds on flexion and extension. Radiographs showed flattening of the implant and multiple small lucent defects with thin, sclerotic margins in the carpal bones, radial and ulnar styloid processes, and proximal metacarpals. Early changes were apparent on review of radiographs taken the year after implantation, and additional fragmentation of the implant was evident 6 years after surgery.

Exploration showed marked synovial hypertrophy with invasion of the scaphoid, capitate, and triquetrum. The scaphoid was in two pieces. The implant was deformed, flattened, and a deep yellow color. It was removed along with the proximal carpals and synovium of the wrist. The specimen exhibited fibrotic and hyperplastic papillary synovium and multinucleated giant cells containing pale yellow foreign bodies that were consistent with silicone. Large extracellular aggregates of silicone particles were embedded in fibrous tissue or fibrin. The cortical and medullary bone and articular cartilage were extensively permeated and destroyed by subarticular extension of the foreign body reaction and pannus formation.

Eleven other cases of foreign body giant cell reactive synovitis have been reported. The destructive arthritis is characterized radiographically by well-defined lytic areas, sometimes with thin, sclerotic walls. The lytic lesions are filled with hyperplastic synovial tissue. Giant cells containing phagocytized Silastic particles are abundant in the lesions, as are large extracelluluar collections of particles. Particles also may be found in regional nodes and remote intraosseous sites.

▶ The authors show three disturbing cases of synovitis of the wrist of an advanced degree with destructive changes involving all of the carpals following silicone rubber lunate arthroplasty. I have seen several identical cases. Most patients with silicone lunate replacements for Kienböck's disease have seemed to do quite well. It has been suggested by some that the insertion of a very tight implant or other load alteration factors may increase the likelihood of development of collapse deformities, fragmentation of the silicone, and so-called silicone synovitis. Because of the development of this type of synovitis in treated patients with Kienböck's disease, we are now (at least in young patients) utilizing alternative procedures, such as excisional arthroplasty with fibrous interposition, ulnar lengthening, or radial shortening. It would appear to me that, at this time, silicone implant arthroplasty should no longer be considered a primary treatment of choice but, rather, as a late reconstructive procedure, for a young patient with Kienböck's disease.—R.D.B.

Bone Cysts Containing Silicone Particles in Bones Adjacent to a Carpal Silastic Implant

Timo Telaranta, Kauko A. Solonen, Kaj Tallroth, and Juha Nickels
Skeletal Radiol. 10:247–249, November 1983   12–9

The use of silicone rubber implants in augmentation mammaplasty has been complicated by constrictive fibrosis due to contamination by silicone, and silicone has been found in lymphomatous tissue from patients with Silastic tendon prostheses. Eight patients who had 9 Silastic carpal bone implants, used as spacers, and were followed for over 2 years were studied. Bone cysts were seen in the carpal bones of 5 wrists in 4 patients, mostly in the capitate and scaphoid bones. In the most advanced case the cysts formed a halo about the implant (Fig 12–8). Three implants were definitely smaller than immediately after operation.

The patients with the most advanced findings, a man aged 43 with the lunate replaced 2 years earlier, underwent wrist arthrodesis for pain, swelling, and limited motion. Biopsy of the bone cyst showed hypertrophic villi in a pseudosynovial membrane and slightly birefringent material in the synovial interstitium and intracellularly in foreign body giant cells. Electron probe microanalysis of the implant showed silicone, which was also present in the synovial tissue from the bone cyst.

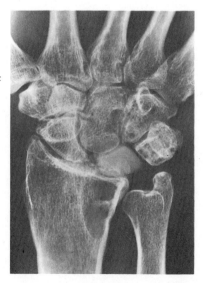

Fig 12–8.—Two years after implant into lunate, roentgenogram shows cysts in radius, capitate, hamate, and triquetral bones. Lunate implant has become slightly smaller. (Courtesy of Telaranta, T., et al.: Skeletal Radiol. 10:247–249, November 1983; Berlin-Heidelberg-New York: Springer.)

A drill hole in the triquetral bone was necessary in these cases to stabilize the lunate implant. Bone cysts developed in adjacent carpal bones, and in the radius and ulna in several cases, and the size of the implants was sometimes reduced on follow-up roentgenograms. Silicone was identified within pseudosynovial tissue of a bone cyst in 1 instance. Presumably, silicone particles migrate from the implant to the surrounding tissues, including bone, in these cases. The implants should be used cautiously and the patients followed closely for prolonged periods.

▶ Fretting of silicone implants has been recognized increasingly. Whether these shards of material are of primary consequence when found in the intracarpal cysts or are merely carried passively by hydraulic pulsations of synovial fluid is yet to be established. Intracarpal ganglions at times obviously give rise to intracarpal cysts, and if the cortex of carpal bone is broached either by insertion of the Silastic stem or through wear-contact, the same type of trabecular erosions may be possible. The effect of altered stress concentration through and around the implant must also be considered with regard to cyst formation.—R.L.L.

Long-term Silicone Implant Arthroplasty: Implications of Animal and Human Autopsy Findings
Robert M. Nalbandian, Alfred B. Swanson, and B. Kent Maupin (Grand Rapids, Mich.)
JAMA 250:1195–1198, Sept. 2, 1983   12–10

Host tissue responses to implanted material were examined in both dogs and human beings as part of a program of studying low-modulus-of-elasticity silicone implants for use in small-joint arthroplasty. Material was obtained at autopsy from 3 dogs more than 10 years after placement of silicone implants in the extremities. One arthritic patient was evaluated 12 years after hand reconstruction with silicone finger joint implants, and the subsequent placement of great toe implants.

Tissue responses to the implants were benign in both the dogs and the clinical case. Macrophages and giant cells were present in the canine tissues and in the medullary cavity of bone adjacent to the implant. No evidence of silicone material was found in the regional nodes or systemically. The patient exhibited a foreign body giant cell tissue reaction to silicone and a similar reaction to silicone particles in a lymph node. No evidence of systemic dissemination of silicone particles was obtained. Silicone particles were present without inflammation in subsynovial connective tissue.

The relatively trivial tissue response to silicone arthroplasty implants, contrasting with the reactions to other types of surgery, strongly supports the continued use of silicone in implant arthroplasty.

▶ Despite the pejorative presentation of this material, the additional data supporting the benign interaction of silicone implant material and body tissues are welcome to the hand surgeon whose use of this substance is still frequent.—J.H.D.

Hand and Wrist Arthropathies of Hemochromatosis and Calcium Pyrophosphate Deposition Disease: Distinct Radiographic Features

Thomas C. Adamson III, Charles S. Resnik, Jose Guerra, Jr., Vinton C. Vint, Michael H. Weisman, and Donald Resnick

Radiology 147:377–381, May 1983   12–11

An attempt was made to identify radiographic features that distinguish between the arthropathy of hemochromatosis and idiopathic calcium pyrophosphate dihydrate (CPPD) crystal deposition disease. Posteroanterior hand and wrist radiographs of 26 patients with each disorder were com-

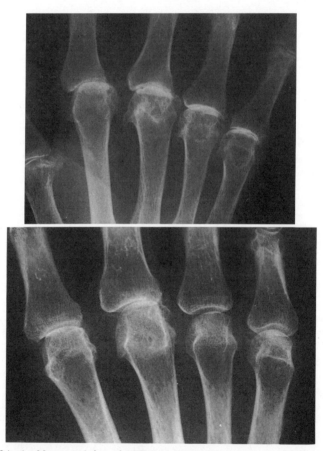

Fig 12–9 (top).—Metacarpophalangeal (MCP) joint abnormalities in hemochromatosis. Note uniform loss of joint space at all MCP articulations. Significant "crumbling" of metacarpal heads is evident, especially in third digit. Beaklike osseous excrescences arise from radial aspect of metacarpal heads, particularly third and fourth. Abnormal calcification is not present.

Fig 12–10 (bottom).—Metacarpophalangeal joint abnormalities in idiopathic calcium pyrophosphate dihydrate crystal deposition disease. Loss of joint space is evident in second and third MCP articulations, with relative sparing of those in fourth and fifth digits. Slight flattening of metacarpal heads and abnormal calcification around MCP joints are seen. Small osteophytes arise from radial aspect of second and third metacarpal heads, but they are not nearly as apparent as in Figure 12–9.

(Courtesy of Adamson, T.C. III, et al.: Radiology 147:377–381, May 1983.)

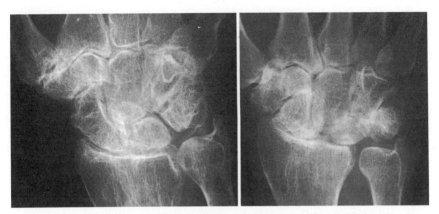

Fig 12–11 (left).—Wrist arthropathy in hemochromatosis. Note loss of joint space in many compartments of wrist, including radiocarpal, midcarpal, common carpometacarpal, and first carpometacarpal compartments. Calcification of triangular fibrocartilage adjacent to distal aspect of ulna and space between lunate and triquetrum is seen. There is no abnormal separation between scaphoid and lunate.

Fig 12–12 (right).—Wrist arthropathy in idiopathic calcium pyrophosphate dihydrate crystal deposition disease. Joint space narrowing is evident in radiocarpal, midcarpal, and common carpometacarpal joints. Abnormal calcification is evident around distal ulna. Note abnormal separation between scaphoid and lunate, with narrowing of radioscaphoid and lunate-capitate spaces.

(Courtesy of Adamson, T.C. III, et al.: Radiology 147:377–381, May 1983.)

pared. Hemochromatosis was confirmed by liver biopsy in all but 2 cases. The patients with idiopathic CPPD crystal deposition disease had typical chondrocalcinosis, as well as monoclinic and triclinic crystals in joint aspirates, which showed absent or weak birefringence on compensated polarized light microscopy. Eleven patients had a definite diagnosis of CPPD crystal deposition disease; 15 had a probable diagnosis of the disease.

Most of both groups had symmetric arthropathic changes. Narrowing at the metacarpophalangeal articulations was significantly more frequent in the cases of hemochromatosis, particularly at the fourth and fifth joints (Figs 12–9 and 12–10). Exuberant osteophyte formation was much more frequent in the group with hemochromatosis. When wrist arthropathy was present, the radiocarpal compartment was most markedly affected in patients in both groups (Fig 12–11). Scapholunate separation, or dissociation, was more characteristic of idiopathic CPPD crystal deposition disease (Fig 12–12). Metacarpophalangeal narrowing without radiocarpal joint space narrowing was more frequent in patients with hemochromatosis. Calcification at the first carpometacarpal joint was more prevalent in patients with idiopathic CPPD crystal deposition disease.

There are definite differences in radiographic abnormalities of the hand and wrist between hemochromatosis and idiopathic CPPD crystal deposition disease. Though not definitive, the differences allow a bias toward one diagnosis over the other and can suggest that iron metabolic studies be done in appropriate cases. The pathogenesis of the arthropathy of hemochromatosis apparently involves factors other than the presence of CPPD crystals.

▶ The subtle differences between the hand and wrist arthropathy changes of hemochromatosis and crystalline deposition disease may be more important to the rheumatologist, but the everyday business of the hand surgeon will involve a good many of these patients and, in a certain percentage, surgical management will be considered. Furthermore, the hand surgeon's experience with subtle x-ray changes, upon which this differential primarily is based, is extensive, and it should be within our diagnositic acumen to select those patients in whom iron metabolism studies should be performed.—P.C.A.

Hand and Wrist Involvement in Calcium Pyrophosphate Dihydrate Crystal Deposition Disease

Charles S. Resnik, Brent W. Miller, Richard H. Gelberman, and Donald Resnick

J. Hand Surg. 8:856–863, November 1983   12–12

The findings were reviewed on 51 patients who fulfulled clinical and roentgenographic criteria for calcium pyrophosphate dihydrate (CPPD) crystal deposition disease. Twelve of them had a definite diagnosis based on the identification of CPPD crystals in aspirated fluid or a tissue biopsy sample. There were 41 men, with an average age of 74 years, and 10 women, with an average age of 72, in the series. The average follow-up period was 2.4 years. The most common symptoms were pain, swelling, and stiffness in the hands and wrists. No patient had a strong family history of rheumatoid arthritis or a personal history of rheumatoid symptoms.

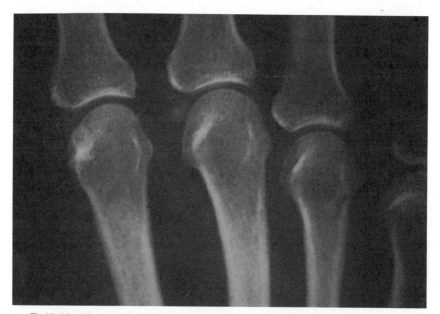

Fig 12–13.—Metacarpophalangeal joint calcifications. Synovial calcification is seen, especially in second, third, and fifth articulations. Minimal joint space narrowing is apparent. (Courtesy of Resnik, C.S., et al.: J. Hand Surg. 8:856–863, November 1983.)

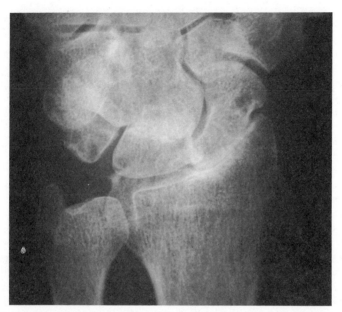

Fig 12–14.—Wrist arthropathy. Note narrowing of radioscaphoid and lunate-capitate spaces. Calcification is seen adjacent to lunate and triquetrum. (Courtesy of Resnik, C.S., et al.: J. Hand Surg. 8:856–863, November 1983.)

Twelve patients had pseudogout, 12 had pseudo-osteoarthritis with acute episodes, 23 had pseudo-osteoarthritis without acute episodes, and 4 were asymptomatic. Calcification, where present (Fig 12–13), usually was bilaterally symmetric, as was joint space narrowing (Fig 12–14). Scapholunate dissociation was evident in 9 wrists and produced symptoms in 4 instances. The presence of radiocarpal joint space narrowing was not associated with wrist symptoms. Most patients received anti-inflammatory medication. Forty-three percent were asymptomatic at last follow-up, and another 35% were improved. Nine patients were unchanged, and 2 were lost to follow-up.

Characteristic roentgenographic findings in patients with definite or probable CPPD crystal deposition disease include cartilage and synovial calcification and arthropathy of the metacarpophalangeal and radiocarpal joints. Scapholunate dissociation may be observed. The clinical symptoms do not always correlate with the radiographic findings, and many asymptomatic cases are discovered roentgenographically.

▶ As an explanation for abnormal x-ray findings in the wrist and hand, or for unusual pain syndromes, crystalline deposition disease is still taken far too lightly. As this article indicates, it is indeed quite common. The article leaves a sense of false security, however, in giving an average age of 72 years for patients with this condition. It is also quite common in the 40- to 50-year-old group and may be seen even in childhood. Furthermore, acute severe episodes are sometimes very difficult to distinguish from joint infection. Finally, the deposits may be seen anywhere in the distal forearm, wrist or hand, intra-articularly or extra-articularly. This is, therefore, one of those conditions to keep constantly in mind in the differential diagnosis of pain syndromes in this area, particularly when there are associated calcium deposits.—P.C.A.

Fascial Arthroplasty for Elbow Ankylosis
G. A. A. Oyemade (Univ. College Hosp., Ibadan, Nigeria)
Int. Surg. 68:81–84, Jan.–Mar. 1983   12–13

Ankylosis of the elbow is common in Nigeria because of the delayed diagnosis and treatment of elbow injuries and improper management of fractures of the elbow bones. The results of fascial arthroplasty were reviewed in 51 patients with elbow ankylosis who were operated on in 1968–1977. Over two thirds of patients were aged 10–30 years. Ankylosis was due to untreated elbow dislocation in 24 cases and to fracture in 14 cases. There were 8 infective lesions. Arthroplasty was done where very little movement was possible and there was severe pain or in cases of complete or bony ankylosis where the patient required elbow motion in his work or to dress and feed himself. Acute infection and recent injury were contraindications to elbow arthroplasty. Fascial arthroplasty was done except in 1 patient who had excision of a congenital humeroradial synostosis. The modified Campbell technique was used, with a fascia lata graft. If pronation-supination was absent, most of the radial head was removed with the annular ligament.

Seventeen patients had a good outcome, with movement against gravity beyond 90 degrees postoperatively. These patients were able to carry out normal activities, but had some reduction in muscle strength. Twenty-two other patients had fair results, with 45–90 degrees of movement against gravity. Eight patients had very little elbow function, and 4 were not appreciably changed after operation. Elbow joint stability was maintained in all patients.

These results warrant the use of fascial elbow arthroplasty to treat elbow ankylosis caused by trauma or localized disorders. Elbow ankylosis due to rheumatoid arthritis, however, responds poorly to nonprosthetic arthroplasty.

▶ This is an important contribution to furthering our knowledge of results to be expected with reconstructive procedures about the elbow. The report includes a younger age group, and 85% of the procedures are for posttraumatic arthritis, which is the opposite of the experience with total elbow arthroplasties, where 85% are being performed for rheumatoid arthritis. In this regard, one should recognize that less strict criteria are applied for a good result; the elbow is often weak with variable degrees of instability. In spite of this, a 75% satisfactory rate in a group largely composed of posttraumatic conditions in young people is noteworthy. The average and range of follow-up are, unfortunately, not clearly stated, but this study does cover a 10-year period. Finally, it should be noted that the posttraumatic conditions for which this procedure is recommended and was performed represent those not often encountered in the United States, for example, unreduced elbow dislocation and tuberculous arthritis. The major strength of this article consists of additional data demonstrating what might be expected from nonreplacement joint reconstruction for non-rheumatoid arthritic conditions.—B.F.M.

Massive Intrasynovial Deposition of Calcium Pyrophosphate in The Elbow: A Case Report

Cline D. Hensley and Joe J. Lin (St. Francis Regional Med. Center, Wichita, Kan.)
J. Bone Joint Surg. [Am:] 66-A:133–136, January 1983   12–14

A case of dystrophic calcinosis, first thought to represent tumoral calcinosis, is reported.

Man, 72, had had a mass at the anterior left elbow for 4 years with occasional discomfort and some pain on motion. The mass had enlarged and become more painful 2 weeks before admission. A stroke occurring 4 years before had resulted in residual right hemiparesis and dysphasia. The firm 4-cm mass, which involved the antecubital fossa, restricted flexion-extension motion of the elbow. A slight decrease in the level of serum phosphorus was noted, but the calcium level was normal. An arthrogram failed to show the origin of the mass. Arthrotomy revealed a 4-cm mass apparently arising from the synovial tissue and capsule, which was removed piecemeal. Additional pockets of calcification were noted adhering to synovial membrane. About a third of the material was collagenous tissue, and the rest was pure calcium pyrophosphate dihydrate. Pain was absent postoperatively. The density had recurred 3 years later with similar physical findings except that there was little pain and tenderness. No calcium deposition was evident in the knees or pubic symphysis.

Tumoral calcinosis typically occurs in normocalcemic young persons, predominantly blacks. A familial tendency has been noted. The present patient was an elderly white man with a lesion consisting of pyrophosphate, not calcium carbonate or phosphate as occurs in tumoral calcinosis. Large deposits of pyrophosphate are unusual. The pathogenesis of calcium pyrophosphate deposition requires further study. Articular or periarticular structures are consistently involved. Within joints the process may arise within the synovial fluid or inside cartilage, or it may be related to a systemic abnormality in calcium or phosphorus metabolism. Dystrophic calcinosis is an uncommon disorder that may be difficult to diagnose.

▶ This report provides a concise discussion of so-called tumoral calcinosis and places this case report of an intra-articular calcification involving calcium pyrophosphate in perspective. It is worthwhile to recognize the distinction that tumoral calcinosis generally is considered to exist outside the joint while calcium pyrophosphate deposition is an intra-articular process. This report simply enhances, to some extent, our understanding of the curious phenomenon of calcification and crystalline deposition about the elbow.—B.F.M.

Operative Treatment of Chronic Ruptures of the Rotator Cuff of the Shoulder

N. P. Packer, P. T. Calvert, J. I. L. Bayley, and Lipmann Kessel
J. Bone Joint Surg. [Br.] 65-B:171–175, March 1983   12–15

The results of 63 operative repairs of chronic rotator cuff tears in 61 patients treated in 1974–1980 were reviewed. The 43 male and 18 female patients had an average age of 58 years. The dominant side was involved in 70% of the cases. Only 6 patients reported significant trauma in relation to the onset of symptoms. Conservative measures had failed in all cases, and 5 patients had had previous operations. The average duration of symptoms was 41 months. Nine patients needed manipulation under anesthesia because of restricted passive movement. A transacromial approach was used in most cases. In 31 operations, measures were taken to prevent subacromial impingement.

The results were good in 71% of the 56 shoulders operated on because of pain. There was more relief of pain when subacromial space was decompressed. Function was full or adequate for most activities in 39 shoulders and improved in 5 others. It was unchanged in 16 joints and worse in 3. Fifteen of 25 patients returned to heavy manual work after the procedure, and 4 did lighter work. All but 3 of 19 sedentary workers returned to previous employment. Complications included 1 wound infection. Staples had to be removed in 4 early cases. Eleven patients had a second operation. Two of the 6 who had not had decompression initially had a good outcome. All 5 patients who had had decompression at the time of the initial operation had a poor result after a repeat operation.

Repair of the torn rotator cuff is worthwhile when symptoms persist with conservative therapy. The patients were very pleased with the outcome, particularly with regard to relief of pain. Adequate subacromial decompression is an important part of the procedure, and it appears to be the only secondary procedure worth attempting if initial surgery was inadequate.

▶ It is important to recognize that there is considerable heterogeneity within this patient series as to method of repair and apparently as to tendon pathology. In 20 shoulders, almost one third of the series, direct tendon suture alone was possible, suggesting that these tears were quite small or at least quite mobile. These shoulders are then grouped with shoulders that required the usual suture plus reinsertion of the tendon into bone and a heterogeneous group of other repairs, including the use of the long head of the biceps, heterologous fascia, or carbon fiber reinforcement. With the pathology being so different and methods of treatment varying, one wonders if the overall results can be accepted and whether it might not have been better to have presented them in relation to the pathology existing at operation. Interesting clinical impressions are supported in this study. Staples are no longer used because removal was almost inevitable, poorer results are obtained in those patients who have shoulder dislocations in association with rotator cuff tears, and reoperations for failure of a second rotator cuff repair lead to a dramatically poorer group of results than is obtained after a primary repair.—R.H.C.

Dislocation Arthropathy of Shoulder

Robert L. Samilson and Victor Prieto (Children's and Adult Med. Center, San Francisco)
J. Bone Joint Surg. [Am.] 65-A:456–460, April 1983   12–16

The findings were reviewed in 70 patients with a history of single or multiple shoulder dislocations and radiographic evidence of glenohumeral arthropathy in 74 shoulders. Sixty-two dislocations were anterior, 11 were posterior, and 1 was multidirectional. Twenty-one shoulders had dislocated only once. Severe trauma was implicated in the initial dislocation in 42 instances. No defect was observed initially in the humeral head or glenoid rim in 24 shoulders. Twenty-nine joints were not operated on.

Postdislocation arthrosis was considered severe in 15 shoulders, moderate in 14, and mild in 45. All patients with moderate and severe arthrosis were symptomatic, with pain, crepitus, and limited motion in the affected shoulder. Posterior dislocations were overrepresented among patients with moderate and severe arthrosis, but the number of dislocations was not related to the severity of arthrosis. Fifty-five percent of the shoulders not treated surgically had moderate to severe arthrosis, as did 29% of the surgically treated shoulders. Limited external rotation correlated with the severity of arthrosis. Patients who were older at the time of initial dislocation tended to have more marked arthrosis. A defect of the humeral head or glenoid rim could not be related to the severity of arthrosis.

Arthrosis appears to be more frequent after shoulder dislocation than has been thought. The higher rate of moderate and severe arthrosis in patients with posterior dislocations probably reflects diagnostic delay. Operations in which internal fixation devices intrude on the joint cartilage frequently result in the development of moderate to severe arthrosis.

▶ Arthritis of the shoulder is rare. When it does occur, a history of instability is a very commonly found historical point. That this should be recognized as a fact is the important statement of this article. It is important also to recognize that arthritis is more frequent with posterior instability problems and in patients who have had surgery with the use of internal fixation. The incidence of arthrosis after shoulder dislocation cannot be gleaned from this report; however, the instance of significant shoulder arthritis after the usual traumatic anterior dislocation of the shoulder with continuing anterior instability must be quite uncommon, as is suggested by the numbers in this report and the scarcity of other reports on this subject.—R.H.C.

Degeneration of the Glenohumeral Joint: An Anatomical Study

Claes J. Petersson (Univ. of Lund)
Acta Orthop. Scand. 54:277–283, April 1983   12–17

One hundred fifty-one shoulder dissections were performed on 41 male and 35 female cadavers, aged 18 to 92 years (average age, 68 years), to assess the relation between cartilaginous degeneration of the glenohumeral joint and degeneration of the rotator cuff. Degeneration and full-thickness rupture of the rotator cuff, cartilage degeneration, and degeneration and rupture of the long biceps tendon appeared with increasing frequency after age 60 years. There was a highly significant relationship between rotator cuff degeneration and cartilage degeneration. The degenerative changes often were most marked in the glenoid cavity. Osteophytes were found most frequently near the tubercles and sulcus. Glenohumeral degeneration was bilateral in 82% of the cases and was more frequent in women. The thickness of normal joint cartilage of the humeral head did not change with advancing age.

Although age is an important factor in degenerative joint disease, the findings suggest that the cartilage of an otherwise normal glenohumeral joint does not deteriorate over time. Occupation does not seem to be an important factor, because cartilage degeneration usually was bilateral, and both rotator cuff ruptures and cartilage degeneration were more frequent in women. Whether rotator cuff degeneration and cartilage degeneration have a causative relationship or are expressions of a common degenerative glenohumeral joint disorder remains to be determined. Cuff degeneration appears to precede cartilage degeneration. It might cause leakage of synovial fluid and impair the nutrition of the articular cartilage. Mechanical imbalance from a full-thickness rupture might lead to a displaced articulation and increased wear of the cartilage.

▶ Studies in the past on cadaver specimens have tended to focus on a limited number of anatomical structures. This study attempts to study many of the structures in the area and relate changes one to the other. Straightforward, useful information has resulted, such as the lack of cartilage degeneration with aging and the increase in frequency of rotator cuff tears with aging. Because of the thoroughness of the investigators, additional information can be gleaned, including the bilaterality of conditions in better than 80%, suggesting a strong component of anatomical predisposition; the high association of rotator cuff disease and cartilage degeneration, with rotator cuff disease being found in excess of cartilage degeneration; and the virtual absence of biceps tendon disease in the absence of significant rotator cuff disease. These findings correlate well with present thoughts regarding the importance of rotator cuff syndromes, the lesser importance of bicipital tendon syndromes, and the relationship of arthritis to severe rotator cuff disease.—R.H.C.

Cementless Total Shoulder Arthroplasty: Preliminary Experience With 13 Cases
D. Dennis Faludi and Andrew J. Weiland (Johns Hopkins Univ.)
Orthopedics 6:431–437, April 1983   12–18

Thirteen shoulder arthroplasties using the English-McNab cementless, semiconstrained implant were performed in 12 patients between 1978 and 1981. This prosthesis has a cobalt-chrome humeral component with a sintered stem and a metal-backed, high-density polyethylene glenoid component, also with a sintered back. Cancellous screws are used to fix the glenoid component in place. All but two humeral components were implanted without cement. The average patient age at the time of surgery was 62 years. The diagnosis was rheumatoid arthritis in 4 patients, post-traumatic arthritis in 3, and primary osteoarthritis, avascular necrosis of the humeral head, and failed hemiarthroplasty in 2 patients each. Criteria for shoulder replacement included intractable pain, night pain, limited motion during daily activities, and dependency on narcotic medication.

Two patients sustained humeral fractures during insertion of the humeral component that healed uneventfully after being wired. An obese patient had perforation of the humeral shaft and postoperative dislocation. One late deep *Staphylococcus aureus* infection necessitated removal of the prosthesis. Pain was relieved by the procedure, although patients with traumatic arthritis did less well than the others in this regard. Function improved in all groups of patients, and active range of motion improved to a modest degree. Muscle power did not increase significantly. No evidence of bone resorption was observed on follow-up x-ray studies in the 8 shoulders examined.

Shoulder arthroplasty with the English-McNab prosthesis relieved pain to a significant extent in all diagnostic groups of patients. Improved motion and function appear to depend on the primary glenohumeral pathology. Loosening of the components was not observed on follow-up radiography. Significant complications can occur. The procedure is not yet a reliable means of completely restoring shoulder function and motion and should be used only by experienced surgeons in carefully selected patients.

▶ The importance of this study is the presentation of a cementless, bone in-growth type of shoulder prosthesis that has not exhibited loosening over the follow-up period. One should recognize that the patient population is quite heterogeneous regarding diagnosis. Concerning results, the pain relief is satisfactory, as one would expect with total joint replacement unless a complication arises. The results regarding motion are quite poor with this series of patients, with postoperative active abduction only averaging 75 degrees, along with a decline in the average amount of external rotation to 25 degrees. The complications also were frequent and significant, including two humeral fractures, a dislocation, and an infection—indicating the complexity of this surgery. Although this prosthesis is interesting because it is an example of a cementless type of shoulder arthroplasty, it quite likely will not be used as the implant for most patients who might be candidates for shoulder arthroplasty. It seems too constrained by surface shape; furthermore, the ingrowth material extends along the entire humeral stem (there were two patients who showed proximal humeral bone resorption in the series).—R.H.C.

13 Rheumatoid Arthritis and Related Diseases

Treatment of Ischemic Digital Ulcers With Nitroglycerin Ointment
Ronald G. Wheeland, Ronald W. Gilchrist, Jr., and C. Jack Young, Jr. (Univ. of Oklahoma)
J. Dermatol. Surg. 9:548–551, July 1983   13–1

Evaluation was made of topical nitroglycerin treatment of peripheral ischemia manifested by digital ulceration in three patients. The cutaneous and muscle circulation often is affected by the same process that leads to angina pectoris.

Man, 60, with digital ulcers on all fingers, precipitated by cold weather, had a positive antinuclear antibody test and a diagnosis of drug-induced lupus erythematosus (SLE). Many antihypertensive medications had been used for some years. The biopsy findings were consistent with SLE. Silver sulfadiazine cream was ineffective, but 2% nitroglycerin ointment, used at 4-hour intervals, led to the complete resolution of all ulcers within 4 weeks. Both hydralazine therapy and smoking have continued.

Nitroglycerin was also effective in a woman, aged 68, with liver cancer and a digital ulceration and in a man, aged 63, with coronary heart disease and ulcerations of two digits. Healing began within a few weeks of the start of treatment in all cases.

Two of these patients presumably had digital ulceration due to arteriosclerotic vascular disease; the other appeared to have an underlying connective tissue disorder. The response in the last was most gratifying in view of the severity of involvement. The efficacy of topical nitroglycerin application in this limited series compares favorably with the results reported with internal medications, hyperbaric oxygenation, collagenase, dextranomer, benzoyl peroxide, and sympathectomy. Nitroglycerin can be used on an outpatient basis at low cost, and the potential for side effects from systemic absorption would seem to be low. Further controlled clinical trials are indicated. Topical nitroglycerin therapy should be considered for digital ulcers.

▶ The hand surgeon is frequently consulted to treat the patient with persistent digital ischemia after failed medical management. Topical nitroglycerin ointment, as this series of case reports by Wheeland, Gilchrist, and Young suggests, can be effective in increasing local vascular supply and providing the "environment" for open wound healing. Unfortunately, we more commonly find "resistant" cases that require amputation at a proximal, better vascularized level. Nitroglycerin paste can be helpful postoperatively in selected cases if wound healing is delayed, but its overall effectiveness is limited. It is important, however, to be aware of the potential benefit of local vasodilators such as nitroglycerin and aqua vera, as their use may salvage marginally perfused tissues.—W.P.C.

Digitalgia Paresthetica With Digital Neuropathy in Rheumatoid Arthritis
E. Wayne Massey (Duke Univ.)
South. Med. J. 76:923–925, July 1983   13–2

Digital neuropathy, or isolated finger neuritis, is a pure sensory neuropathy of a digital nerve caused by acute or chronic local trauma or pressure or associated with systemic disease. The term "digitalgia paresthetica" is used when hyperpathia is prominent. Two patients who had

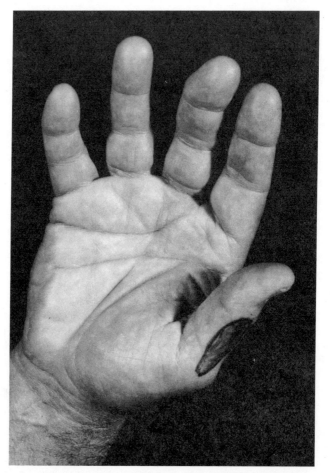

Fig 13–1.—Area of thenar hyperesthesia and associated sensory loss reported by patient with digitalgia paresthetica. (Courtesy of Massey, E.W.: South. Med. J. 76:923–925, July 1983.)

digitalgia paresthetica as the presenting feature of rheumatoid disease are described.

Man, 43, with seropositive rheumatoid arthritis, was hospitalized with progressive motor disability after treatment with aspirin, prednisone, and intra-articular steroids. Burning hyperesthesia was described on the thenar eminence. Subcutaneous nodules and ankle ulcers were noted. Depressed muscle stretch reflexes and stocking anesthesia of the feet were observed, with normal muscle strength. Sensory loss was present in the area of thenar hyperesthesia (Fig 13–1). Digital vasculitis was not evident. The erythrocyte sedimentation rate was 58 mm/hour, and the latex titer exceeded 5,120. The antinuclear antibody value was 4+. Electrophysiologic study showed absent sural responses bilaterally but normal peroneal, tibial, and median nerve conduction velocities and normal motor and sensory latencies. Use of a higher steroid dose and physiotherapy were of some help. The hyperesthesia resolved over 3 months, but the sensory loss persisted.

The second patient had some evidence of digital vasculitis, but not in the exact site of the digital neuropathy; a role for vasculitis in this neuropathy has not been established. Digital neuropathy of rheumatoid arthritis with hyperpathia is seen in patients with asymmetric random involvement of the digital nerves, usually with symmetric distal sensory loss in the legs as well, and also in patients with distal, symmetric sensory polyneuropathy, which usually is purely sensory in nature.

▶ This condition must be distinguished from peripheral nerve entrapment neuropathy. Clinical features that help in making the differentiation include the burning pain of digitalgia paresthetica, which is not commonly seen in peripheral nerve entrapment, and the fact that the nerve conduction studies at the wrist and forearm are typically normal with this condition. In the presence of such physical findings, the diagnosis of digitalgia paresthetica should be considered and high-dose steroid treatment may be helpful.—P.C.A.

Treatment of Finger Joints With Local Steroids: A Double-Blind Study
S. Jalava and R. Saario (Paimio Hosp., Preitilä, Finland)
Scand. J. Rheumatol. 12:12–14, 1983   13–3

The effects and side effects of triamcinolone hexacetonide (TH) and methylprednisolone acetate (MP) were compared in 12 male and 12 female patients (mean age, 49) with rheumatoid disease and swollen finger joints. Each patient served as his or her own control. The inflamed interphalangeal joints of one hand were injected with TH or MP in a double-blind manner, and the joints of the other hand were treated with the other agent. A total of 120 affected finger joints were injected, 59 with TH and 61 with MP. Splinting was not used after injection.

The two groups were clinically comparable at the outset. Joint circumference decreased significantly after injection of both steroids, but the reduction remained significant at 6 months only in the TH group. A tendency to relapse was noted in the MP group. At 6 months, benefit was apparent in 75.5% of TH-injected joints and in 58% of MP-injected joints.

Worsening had occurred in 3.5% and 10% of joints, respectively. Five patients had adverse reactions consisting of skin and soft tissue atrophy, 4 after TH injection and 1 after MP injection.

Injection of swollen rheumatoid finger joints with TH appeared to give better results than injection with MP in this study, but skin and soft tissue atrophy was more frequent after TH injection. Steroid should be injected only into finger joints with evidence of hydropsy, because it is easier to avoid depositing steroid outside the joint in these cases.

▶ The authors have pointed out that steroids given by injection are of benefit in the treatment of rheumatoid synovitis in the metacarpophalangeal and proximal interphalangeal joints. The duration of benefit is limited and this study demonstrated that triamcinolone was superior to methylprednisolone. I am sure that over a longer period of evaluation, there would be very little difference. The numbers of joints involved are not adequate to suggest statistically that one steroid is more likely to cause atrophy than another. But, as the authors point out, care must be taken in achieving accurate insertion of the material into the joints. In my own practice, I prefer to dilute the steroids with a 3:1 solution of 1% Xylocaine and I feel that cutaneous, ligament, or cartilage complications are not as likely to occur with this reduced concentration.— R.D.B.

Palmar Arthroplasty for Treatment of Stiff Swan-Neck Deformity
Frank A. Scott and John A. Boswick, Jr. (Univ. of Colorado)
J. Hand Surg. 8:267–272, May 1983   13–4

Proximal interphalangeal (PIP) joint stiffness in extension severely limits grasping ability of the hand. The authors have used a palmar approach to arthroplasty that is designed to correct the mechanical block to flexion caused by palmar plate adhesions and collateral ligament contracture and adhesions. The operation can be done at the same time as correction of the primary cause of PIP joint hyperextension and can be supplemented by superficialis tenodesis to minimize recurrent hyperextension. Release of adhesions is illustrated in Figure 13–2. The sheath need not be closed, but a rectangular flap, if intact, can be laid across the defect. Flexor dynamic traction is begun 24–48 hours postoperatively and continued for at least 3–4 weeks.

Arthroplasty was done in 47 stiff, extended PIP joints in 14 hands of 9 rheumatoid patients. Eight patients had previously had metacarpophalangeal joint arthroplasty with ulnar intrinsic release. The average patient age was 56 years. The average range of motion on an average follow-up of 2 years was − 7 degrees of extension to 72 degrees of flexion. Fifteen joints showed hyperextension postoperatively, mostly in the first 3 patients. This was minimized in later cases. The total arc of motion improved from 29.5 degrees to 65 degrees postoperatively, and the arc was adjusted from an attitude of hyperextension to one of flexion, resulting in a more functional range of motion.

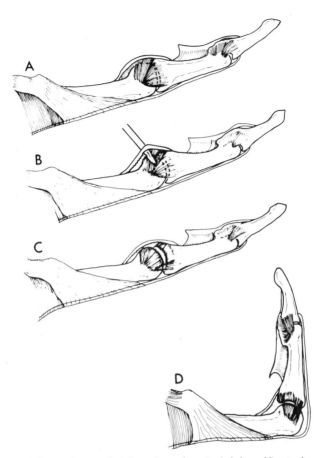

Fig 13–2.—A, adhesions between the palmar plate and proximal phalanx obliterate the retrocondylar recess. **B,** retrocondylar recess adhesions are released with bilateral incisions on each lateral edge of the palmar plate and blunt dissection beneath the plate. **C,** collateral ligament contracture is incised sequentially until full passive motion is obtained. **D,** manipulation will stretch remaining dorsal contractures. (Courtesy of Scott, F.A., and Boswick, J.A., Jr.: J. Hand Surg. 8:267–272, May 1983.)

Increased function is gained from palmar arthroplasty of the PIP joint in patients with rheumatoid stiff swan-neck deformity. Both increased motion and a more functional arc result. Motion must be monitored postoperatively in order to obtain optimal results. This approach also has been used with good results in patients with fracture, tendon injury, and replantation. In posttraumatic cases it is often necessary to supplement the palmar release with an extensor tenolysis.

▶ The authors make a good case for palmar exploration of the stiff swan-neck PIP joint. Their technique allows a logical progression of increasing release. This approach inherently allows for increased bowstringing of the flexor tendons across the PIP joint during full palmar flexion, but in this condition this is unlikely to result in a flexion contracture of the joint at a later date, particularly as long as the distal aspect of the A-2 pulley is left intact. Little or no attention is directed to the frequent concomitant palmar subluxation of the base of the proximal phalanx on the metacarpal head, which may be the initiating factor in swan-neck deformity and in provoking the so-called intrinsic contracture. Use of a slip of the flexor superficialis both to decompress the flexor tendon sheath and to use as an extension limiting ligament, as previously proposed by Ferlic and Clayton, is worth emphasizing.—R.L.L.

Preliminary Experience With a Noncemented Nonconstrained Total Joint Arthroplasty for the Metacarpophalangeal Joints
Robert D. Beckenbaugh (Mayo Clinic)
Orthopedics 6:962–965, August 1983   13–5

A review was made of initial experience with a simple, nonconstrained, stemmed resurfacing prosthesis of the ball-and-socket type, made of Pyrolite carbon, developed for use in the metacarpophalangeal joint. After evaluation in baboons, 43 arthroplasties were done in 15 patients, 13 with rheumatoid arthritis and 2 with osteoarthritis. A total bone resection of 2–3 mm is carried out at the base of the proximal phalanx. Protuberant bone is removed to obtain full gliding of the distal component to 90 degrees of flexion without abutment. The capsule and radial collateral ligament are repaired as necessary, and the extensor tendons are centralized over the metacarpophalangeal joint. Splint support for the digits is continued for 3 months postoperatively.

The average follow-up has been 1 year. The overall range of flexion increased from 33 to 47 degrees after operation. The average motion of the index finger was 19–63 degrees postoperatively, and the small finger had +10 degrees of extension to 30 degrees of flexion. One patient may have had a fracture of the distal stem, but remained asymptomatic. Another with radiographic evidence of loosening also was asymptomatic. All patients appeared to have bony fixation at follow-up. Dislocation has occurred in 5 joints, and was operated on in 4 cases. One dislocation was treated closed, with a good outcome.

The use of a pyrolytic carbon prosthesis in the metacarpophalangeal joint position has been followed by relief of pain and increased motion. Biologic fixation appears to occur in bone. Recurrent deformity and subluxation, however, are possibilities. The concept of the self-fixing carbon prosthesis is being applied to nonconstrained or semiconstrained prostheses for the carpometacarpal joint of the thumb, the digital interphalangeal joints, and the wrist.

▶ The author cautions us that the report is preliminary and points out that trouble with subluxation and ulnar drift is a function of soft tissue reconstruction when the joint offers no inherent stability. The goal of eventually having a satisfactory surface type of replacement arthroplasty available for the metacarpophalangeal joint requires work of this nature.—R.L.L.

Clinical Synovitis and Radiologic Lesions in Rheumatoid Arthritis: A Prospective Study of 25 Patients During Treatment With Remission-Inducing Drugs
Margrethe Ingeman-Nielsen, Ole Halskov, Troels Mørk Hansen, Poul Halberg, Poul Stage, and Ib Lorenzen (Univ. of Copenhagen)
Scand. J. Rheum. 12:237–240, 1983   13–6

A total of 1,150 joints in the hands and feet of 25 patients with definite or classic rheumatoid arthritis, initially active, were monitored during 2 years of treatment with remission-inducing drugs. All were aged 16 years or older. None received gold salts, penicillamine, levamisole, chloroquine, glucocorticoids, or cytostatic agents within the 3 months preceding entry into the study. The 17 women and 8 men had a mean age of 60 years. The mean duration of disease was 8.5 years. Ten patients were in functional class III at the outset. Fifteen were in functional class I or II. Three patients were treated with levamisole, 13 with penicillamine, and 9 with azathioprine.

Synovitis improved in all patients during the 2 years of observation, but some patients had exacerbations in 1 or more joints. The proportion of joints with signs of synovitis declined from 47% to 17% during the study period, while the percentage of joints with radiologic damage rose from 23% to 27%. Radiologic progression was seen in 7.2% of the joints that showed regression of clinical synovitis. Radiologic progression was more frequent in swollen joints than in tender joints without swelling. Twenty-three percent of joints with progressive bone lesions showed no clinical evidence of synovitis during the observation period. Joints in which signs of synovitis disappeared had a significantly smaller risk of radiologic progression than those in which clinical synovitis persisted.

Clinical synovitis correlated with the progression of bone lesions in patients with rheumatoid arthritis in this study. Marked individual variation in the number of joints with radiologic progression was noted, however, and it may be misleading to use the number of patients with radiologic progression as an indicator of radiologic joint deterioration.

▶ These data, showing that joints with rheumatoid synovitis not responding to remission-inducing drugs are more likely to progress to overt bony changes than those without synovitis or those that respond to drugs, lend support to the concept of early synovectomy in this disease for nonresponding joints or to the use of ancillary intra-articular medication.—P.C.A.

Role of Telethermography and Arthrography in Rheumatoid Wrist
N. Colavita, C. Orazi, and A. Fusco
Diagn. Imaging 52:189–196, July–Aug. 1983   13–7

The roles of telethermography and contrast arthrography of the wrist in assessing synovial involvement were evaluated in 40 patients with rheumatoid arthritis. Eleven patients had both studies. Thermography showed obvious hyperthermia, whereas arthrography showed a fading of outlines that reflected multiple communications between the synovial compartments and the lymphatics and tendon sheaths. Tendon sheaths were filled at arthrography in 7 of 35 cases. Interphalangeal arthrography yielded abnormal results in both patients in whom it was performed. All 16 patients who underwent telethermography had abnormal findings, although only 4 had previously had abnormal radiologic findings. Carpal temperature was increased in most cases, and 10 patients had prominent digital hypothermia. Some patients who had abnormal thermographic findings but normal standard x-ray films also had normal arthrograms.

Telethermography and arthrography are complementary in the evaluation of patients with possible early rheumatoid arthritis. Thermography is indicated after standard roentgenography in patients with hand pain not related to trauma in whom rheumatoid disease is suspected. If the results indicate synovial involvement, contrast arthrography should be done to determine the distribution of lesions and select appropriate treatment. Telethermography is helpful in following these patients. The findings are more objective and reliable than are biochemical data.

▶ The use of thermography and arthrography in the diagnosis and follow-up of rheumatoid arthritis in the wrist and hand is certainly interesting, but one wonders about the practical utility. The authors make no indication as to whether changes in the thermographic or arthrographic appearance can be correlated with clinical changes afer therapy or whether these have any prognostic value with regard to future joint injury or destruction. With regard to diagnosis, surely increased joint temperature and the demonstration of synovitis on arthrography are not sufficient criteria to make a diagnosis of rheumatoid arthritis. Perhaps in that regard, arthroscopic synovial biopsy might be a more efficient tool. I doubt that these techniques will find much utility in the future for the practicing hand surgeon.—P.C.A.

Synovectomy With Resection of the Distal Ulna in Rheumatoid Arthritis of the Wrist
Claus Munk Jensen (Univ. of Copenhagen)
Acta Orthop. Scand. 54:754–759, October 1983   13–8

Review was made of the results of wrist synovectomy with resection of the distal ulna in 47 extremities with "caput ulnae syndrome" in 36 patients with rheumatoid disease. The average patient age was 61 years; most patients were female. A majority of patients had classic seropositive rheumatoid arthritis. The average duration of wrist involvement was 7 years, and the mean follow-up postoperatively was 33 months. Indications for surgery included capsular swelling or dorsal tenosynovitis, or both, pain during rest or during wrist motion, and failure to respond to at least 6 months of medical therapy. Subperiosteal resection of the distal ulna was performed, and then as much of the diseased synovium as possible was removed. Eight patients had tenosynovectomy of the extensor tendons.

Pain was absent at follow-up in 31 wrists and was moderately relieved in 8 others. In 8 cases, pain on wrist motion was unchanged at follow-up. Range of both supination-pronation and volar-and dorsiflexion was significantly improved. Subjective assessments of function also indicated improvement. Radiography showed progression in most cases. Deviation at the wrist was unchanged at follow-up. Three patients were reoperated on. One patient had spontaneous rupture of two extensor tendons a month postoperatively. Stability was good in all cases. There were no serious complications. In several cases, the extensor carpi ulnaris tendon appeared to be dislocated volarward by rotational movement, but this did not cause discomfort or pain.

Synovectomy of the wrist with resection of the distal ulna can be recommended for rheumatoid involvement causing pain and synovitis where regular medical treatment has been ineffective for 6 months or longer. Pain is relieved, the range of motion improves, and wrist joint stability is maintained. Radiographic progression of disease, however, is not prevented by the operation.

▶ The authors have pointed out that within a 33-month follow-up, wrist synovectomy will produce pain relief and stability in most patients. Inevitably after wrist synovectomy in rheumatoid patients, there will be progression of destructive arthrosis and the potential for the return of pain. Therefore, this particular procedure, without implant arthroplasty, I believe is indicated in those patients at risk for extensor tendon ruptures who are young with arthroplasty not indicated but with pain that demands relief. One must anticipate, however, that, in the long run, additional reconstructive surgery may very well be necessary.—R.D.B.

Long-term Effects of Excision of the Radial Head in Rheumatoid Arthritis
L. A. Rymaszewski, I. Mackay, A. A. Amis, and J. H. Miller (Glasgow Royal Infirm.)
J. Bone Joint Surg. [Br.] 66-B:109–113, January 1984   13–9

Most authors have recommended excision of the radial head at the time of synovectomy of the elbow joint, particularly in late cases with marked radiohumeral joint degeneration. There is biomechanical evidence suggesting that radial head excision may have adverse effects, such as proximal migration of the radius, valgus deformity, and traction lesions of the medial soft tissues. A review was done of the results of synovectomy and radial head excision in 37 patients having 40 elbows operated on in 1972–1980. Follow-up after operation averaged 6 years. The average age was 56 years. All but 2 patients had classic features of rheumatoid arthritis. Most had received or were still receiving gold, penicillamine, or steroids. The average duration of elbow involvement was 12 years. An average of 3 other operations had been done for rheumatoid arthritis. Silastic sheeting had been interposed in 15 elbows. The ulnar nerve had been transposed in only 2 cases.

Eighteen elbows were free of pain and often functionally improved after surgery, but pain had remained the same or become worse in 12 elbows and, in 10, initial relief was followed by deterioration. Stability was much better in patients who were satisfied with the outcome. Placement of Silastic sheeting did not significantly influence the clinical findings at follow-up. The effects of surgery on the wrist were unclear because of frequent wrist involvement by rheumatoid disease. The radiologic findings correlated poorly with the clinical outcome, but radiologic improvement after surgery was not documented in any case. Most of the elbows exhibited medial displacement of the radius toward the ulna, and radical resection of the radial head and neck had been done in several of these cases.

Clinical deterioration after initially satisfactory results was not infrequent in this series. The axial load on the radius in lifting objects is transferred to the ulna after radial head excision, and considerable tension on the medial ligament results, adding to the humeroulnar force. Osteoarthritic effects can be seen at the predicted site of maximal loading. Radial head replacement should be done at the time of resection if possible. If painful instability develops after radial head excision, the subsequent insertion of a radial head prosthesis may prove very difficult.

▶ This study presents additional and significant information on 40 elbows with a mean of 6 years' follow-up. The objective follow-up assessment is as good, or better, than in most other such series in the literature. A significant finding is that 18 of the 40 patients, or 45%, were not pleased or had "deteriorated" at long-term follow-up of the procedure. This percentage of "unsatisfactory" results may be slightly deceptive in order to make the point that, functionally, these elbows were not doing as well as is suggested by the subjective response or as indicated in the literature. The emphasis of medial joint symptoms secondary to ulnar collateral ligament overload is noteworthy. Although recurrent synovitis is certainly a factor in late deterioration, these authors emphasize the mechanical aspects of the operation, which is a significant contribution to our understanding of radial head resection and synovectomy for rheumatoid arthritis.—B.F.M.

14 Congenital and Pediatric

Congenital Malposition of Flexor Pollicis Longus: Anatomy Note
William F. Blair and Joseph A. Buckwalter (Univ. of Iowa)
J. Hand Surg. 8:93–94, January 1983   14–1

Congenital malposition of the flexor pollicis longus (FPL) and the associated abduction deformity of the thumb metacarpophalangeal joint are being increasingly recognized. A patient with significant abnormalities in the more proximal part of the hand recently was seen.

Boy, 5, had clinically apparent malposition of the FPL in the right hand. The FPL and extensor pollicis longus (EPL) were interconnected on the radial aspect of the thumb at the midproximal phalangeal level by a tendinous band extending from the FPL distally and dorsally to the EPL. The FPL had no flexor tendon sheath or pulleys. Its tendon passed superficially to the thenar muscles, with fine tendinous insertions into the deeper muscle fascia. The abductor pollicis brevis was absent, and the opponens pollicis brevis and flexor pollicis brevis were hypoplastic. The FPL entered the thenar eminence after passing through the transverse carpal ligament. The tendons of the FPL and the flexor digitorum profundus to the index finger had a common muscle belly. A large ulnar sensory branch from the median nerve to the thumb traversed the palmar aspect of the thumb parallel to the FPL. A single, small recurrent median nerve entered the hypoplastic thenar muscles. A single digital artery, a branch of the superficial arch, accompanied the ulnar sensory branch from the median nerve to the thumb.

This disorder is distinct from syndromes of absent thenar intrinsics. Distal reconstruction alone is unlikely to provide optimum clinical results in cases of anomalous insertion of the FPL where significant proximal abnormalities may be present.

▶ The authors properly infer that the multiple changes in both extrinsic and intrinsic musculotendinous units, as seen in their case, suggest radial dysplasia. Such radial dysplasia, although with much variation in its manifestations, is a much more common problem than the sparse reports about flexor tendon anomalies would indicate. Not only are variations seen throughout the spectrum of radial dysplasia to hypoplasia, but similar anomalies are seen in defects of failure of formation, defects of failure of differentiation, and even duplication defects. As properly noted by the authors, reconstruction must take into account the full gamut of deficits present.—R.D.B.

Treatment of Monodactyly by the Distraction-Lengthening Principle: A Case Report

Avraham D. Baruch and Otto A. Hecht (Kaplan Hosp., Rehovot, Israel)
J. Hand Surg. 8(Pt. 1):604–606, September 1983   14–2

An unusual deformity of the upper extremity was seen that consisted of a deformed radius, short ulna, and single digital ray in continuity with the ulna. The functional capacity of the hand was significantly improved by reconstructing the post with a distraction-lengthening procedure.

Man, 25, had been born with a hypoplastic left upper extremity and a mono-digital hand, which he had used only as a hook. The left arm was 6 cm shorter than the right (Fig 14–1). Active motion of the forearm was from neutral position to full supination; there was no wrist motion. The digit corresponded to the small finger. The hand stump was well padded with soft tissue and had normal sensibility. The digit had limited flexion-extension motion and strong adduction-abduction, activated by some intrinsic muscles. Films showed a bowed radius and a hypoplastic ulna articulated with one metacarpal and two phalanges (Fig 14–2).

The radius was osteotomized 5 cm proximal to its distal end and a distraction apparatus was inserted. A 3-cm gap was present after 12 days, when a bone graft from the olecranon was interposed and fixed with two Kirschner wires. This two-stage procedure was repeated to gain another 4 cm. A decubitus over the lengthened radius was covered by a local rotation flap, and the bone was shortened 6–7 mm. The radial post then was 2 cm shorter than the solitary digit side. A Z-plasty was used to deepen the digit-post web. The patient was very satisfied with the outcome.

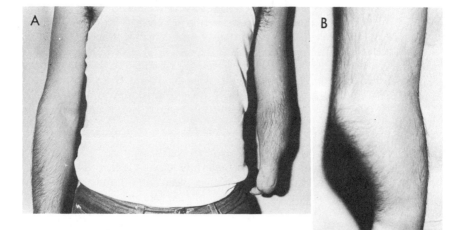

Fig 14–1.—Clinical appearance of deformity. **A,** entire extremity. **B,** monodigital hand. (Courtesy of Baruch, A.D., and Hecht, O.A.: J. Hand Surg. 8(Pt. 1):604–606, September 1983.)

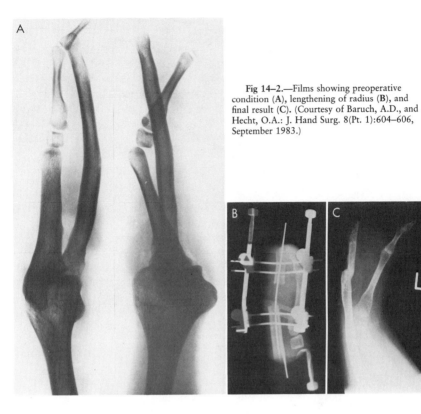

Fig 14–2.—Films showing preoperative condition (**A**), lengthening of radius (**B**), and final result (**C**). (Courtesy of Baruch, A.D., and Hecht, O.A.: J. Hand Surg. 8(Pt. 1):604–606, September 1983.)

He could hold small- and medium-sized objects (Fig 14–3), and sensibility was preserved. Pinch strength improved to 9 lb. The patient is now able to work as a bank clerk, holding papers, booklets and pencils.

No identical case of congenital monodactyly of an upper extremity could be found in the English literature. The present patient rejected a prosthesis and the Krukenberg operation, and the toe-to-hand transfer carried a significant risk of failure because of possible anatomical variations. Reconstruction of a post opposite the existing digit by the distraction-lengthening method maintains initial sensibility, and complications are infrequent.

▶ This unique type of monodigital hand is seen sporadically in large congenital hand services but seldom is discussed because the hook function is usually accepted, despite the plethora of techniques available to provide an opposition post. (One technique the authors did not mention is to mobilize a long radial flap, permitting skin and soft tissue lengthening, then to stabilize it with a bone graft.) I agree with the method they selected but wonder why they chose to lengthen so fast (over 2.5 cm/day) and why it was necessary to use two distraction episodes (perhaps a distal decubitus threatened during the first

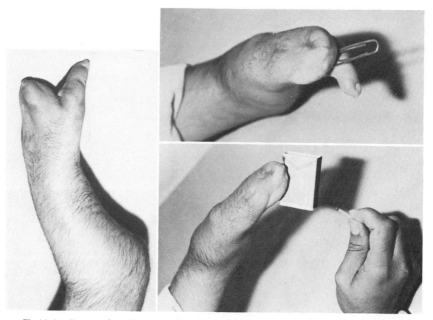

Fig 14–3.—Functional results 1 year after post construction. (Courtesy of Baruch, A.D., and Hecht, O.A.: J. Hand Surg. 8(Pt. 1):604–606, September 1983.)

lengthening, but might not have with a slower distraction). In any event, the results fully justify the reconstruction decision.—J.H.D.

Ulnar Dimelia

Peter T. Gropper (Univ. of British Columbia)
J. Hand Surg. 8:487–491, July 1983   14–3

Ulnar dimelia is a rare congenital anomaly of the upper extremity characterized by duplication of the ulna, absence of the radial ray, and polydactyly. An infant with 7 triphalangeal digits who underwent one-stage thumb reconstruction with the use of the pollicization method of Buck-Gramcko is described.

Infant boy, aged 2 months, had 7 triphalangeal digits in the left hand, 3 in a radial cluster and 4 in an ulnar group (Fig 14–4). Each digit was held in semiflexion and moved actively. The wrist was slightly radially deviated and hyperflexed to 110 degrees, with 60 degrees of passive extension. Rotation of the forearm was limited to 20 degrees in supination and pronation. A skin dimple was present on the ulnar side about 3 cm above the wrist. Films (Fig 14–5) showed polydactyly, absent radius, and two rather well-formed ulnas. Manipulation by the mother maintained elbow motion of 30 to 75 degrees during 22 months of observation, after which reconstruction was carried out by a modified pollicization technique.

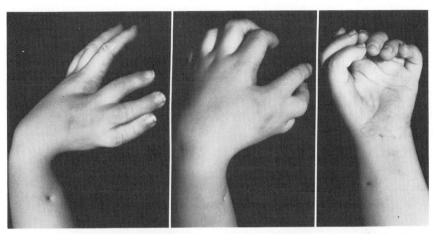

Fig 14–4.—Polydactyly of ulnar dimelia. Ulnar cluster of four triphalangeal digits and radial cluster of three triphalangeal digits. Skin dimple on ulnar aspect of forearm is typical. (Courtesy of Gropper, P.T.: J. Hand Surg. 8:487–491, July 1983.)

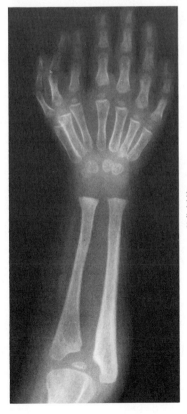

Fig 14–5.—Anterior film of forearm and hand. In forearm there is ulnar duplication with absence of radius. Duplication of carpal bones and seven triphalangeal digits are seen. (Courtesy of Gropper, P.T.: J. Hand Surg. 8:487–491, July 1983.)

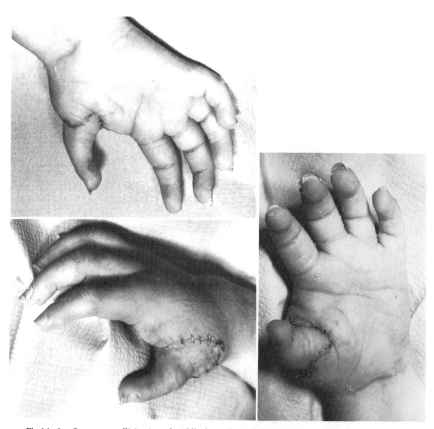

Fig 14–6.—One-stage pollicization of middle digit of radial cluster has been achieved. Tendon transfer in which supernumerary tendons were used provided intrinsic muscle stabilization. Shortening and skeletal reconstruction were achieved by diaphyseal excision of metacarpal and rotating epiphysis into hyperextension (as described by Buck-Gramcko). (Courtesy of Gropper, P.T.: J. Hand Surg. 8:487–491, July 1983.)

The middle of the 3 radial digits was isolated on its neurovascular pedicle. Adequate skin was available for reconstruction of the first web space after amputation of the most ulnar digit. The metacarpal was amputated at the proximal joint level and through the physis. The diaphysis was removed, and the epiphysis was hyperextended and sutured in place. The pollicized digit was fixed to the carpus with two sutures. The rudimentary flexor tendon to the most radial digit was transferred as the abductor pollicis brevis. The most radial extensor tendon was shortened and sutured to the base of the proximal phalanx as the abductor pollicis longus. The ulnar extensor tendon was shortened and sutured to the extensor hood of the pollicized digit to act as the extensor pollicis longus. The outcome is shown in Figure 14–6. Increasing functional use of the pollicized digit was apparent at 6 months, with active extension and intrinsic muscle strength.

This one-stage thumb reconstruction provided skeletal readjustment and satisfactory web space as well as muscle stabilization and intrinsic muscle control through appropriate tendon transfers.

▶ All that one can expect from a case report is achieved. Current provider preferred management for the usual reconstructive need is described and the sparse literature concerning other methods is summarized.—J.H.D.

Dysplasia Epiphysealis Hemimelica of Carpal Bones: Report of a Case and Review of the Literature
Alfred J. Lamesch (Children's Hosp. Med. Center, Luxembourg)
J. Bone Joint Surg. [Am.] 65-A:398–400, March 1983   14–4

Dysplasia epiphysealis hemimelica is a development disorder of the skeleton characterized by unilateral, asymmetric proliferation of cartilage associated with endochondral ossification in an epiphysis or tarsal bone, or, exceptionally, a carpal bone. The case report of a patient with disease involving the scaphoid bone and trapezium is presented.

Patient, aged 4½ years, had swelling over the radial aspect of the right wrist and valgus deformity of the hand. The scaphoid bone, trapezium, and distal radial epiphysis were enlarged and irregular, with multiple centers of ossification. Biopsy of the scaphoid showed a zone of hyperplastic cartilage, active normal endochondral ossification, and irregular ossification centers. There were no signs of inflammation. Splints were applied continuously at first and later at night only. Good

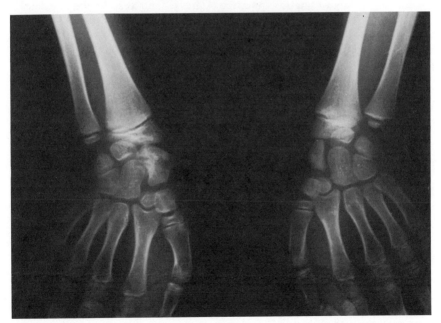

Fig 14–7.—X-ray film shows similar ulnar deviation in hand and in wrist. (Courtesy of Lamesch, A.J.: J. Bone Joint Surg. [Am.] 65-A:398–400, March 1983.)

progress was made. After 4 years the scaphoid bone was more normal in shape (Fig 14–7). Swelling and wrist pain resolved, and wrist motion became equal to that of the other wrist. The valgus deformity decreased gradually.

About 85 patients with dysplasia epiphysealis hemimelica have been described, most with lower extremity involvement. The cause of the disorder is unknown; no hereditary factor has been demonstrated. It is definitely a benign condition. The lesion should be excised if it produces deformity or interferes with function. Carpal lesions progress faster than do those at the talus and ankle, but the prognosis for functional recovery appears to be better with carpal lesions.

▶ Tumor manifestations in the wrist skeleton of a child are frightening. It is well to keep all the possibilities, benign and malignant, in mind. Deformity and restricted motion do occur following carpal involvement by this condition.—I.H.D.

Five-Fingered Hand Associated With Partial or Complete Tibial Absence and Preaxial Polydactyly: Kindred of 15 Affected Individuals in Five Generations

D. W. Lamb, Ruth Wynne-Davies, and J. Margaret Whitmore
J. Bone Joint Surg. [Br.] 65-B:60–63, January 1983   14–5

Data are presented on a kindred of 15 affected persons in 5 generations with autosomal dominantly inherited bilateral 5-fingered hand. The defect was clearly documented in 10 cases. All these subjects had two 5-fingered hands. A sixth digit having some resemblance to a thumb was present on the preaxial side in 5 cases. The tibia was partly or completely missing in at least 4 subjects, and probably 6, with marked overgrowth of the fibula in adults. Subjects frequently had 6 or 7 toes, with the additional digits being preaxial and either biphalangeal or triphalangeal. In 2 patients the middle 3 toes were fused, but no syndactyly of the fingers was observed.

Function of the upper extremity is enhanced by pollicization, which is best done at age 6 to 12 months. The techniques used have included digital transfer and rotation on an intact digital neurovascular pedicle, rearrangement of the interossei, and rotation of the metacarpal head. The triphalangeal thumb requires only shortening to normal proportions by removal of parts of the proximal and middle phalanges with joint fusion. Complete absence of the tibia is best managed by disarticulation at the knee and prosthetic replacement. With partial tibial absence and the preservation of the upper end, the fibula can be transferred into the tibial remnant.

The triphalangeal thumb should be distinguished from the 5-fingered hand. Bilateral 5-fingered hands sometimes are accompanied by preaxial polydactyly, with or without total or partial tibial absence with intact fibula. The disorder is inherited in an autosomal dominant manner, with variable expressivity. Function of both the upper and lower extremities can be improved surgically.

▶ Differentiating a hypoplastic thumb from a finger is not just an academic exercise but has practical relevance when thumb function is inadequate or missing. The authors clearly identify the classic criteria for differentiation, and this is usually sufficient. Unfortunately, there are occasional digits that cannot be typed so clearly.—J.H.D.

Symmetric Hyperphalangism of the Index Finger in Palatodigital Syndrome: A Case Report

Mark S. Klug, Lynn D. Ketchum, and James H. Lipsey
J. Hand Surg. 8:599–603, September 1983   14–6

The palatodigital syndrome is a rare disorder that includes absence of the hard palate, glossoptosis, micrognathia, an accessory rectangular bone at the base of the proximal phalanx of the index fingers, various cardiac anomalies, and skeletal growth retardation. The eighth case of this disorder to be reported is presented here.

Girl, 3, presented with marked radial deviation of the left index finger, which interfered with grasp. Micrognathia had caused no respiratory complications. Height and weight consistently had been below the third percentiles for age. Examination showed a bifid uvula, a high arching palate with no defect, and extreme radial deviation in both hands with mild supination of the index fingers and the metacarpophalangeal (MP) joints (Fig 14–8). Moderate overall joint laxity was noted. An accessory ossicle was palpable at the base of the index proximal phalanx on both hands. The index finger was passively deviated radially to about 70 degrees with the MP joint extended. Radiographic study showed brachymetacarpia and brachyphalangia in both index fingers.

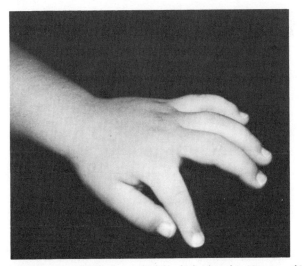

Fig 14–8.—Radial deviation of index finger of left hand of girl aged 3. (Courtesy of Klug, M.S., et al.: J. Hand Surg. 8:599–603, September 1983.)

The left accessory bone was rotated 90 degrees and pinned with Kirschner wires. The radial deviation was satisfactorily corrected when the pins were removed at 6 weeks. The correction was maintained at 1 year. There was 60 degrees of active motion at the MP joint. The right index ray was subsequently corrected by the same technique.

This form of hyperphalangism probably represents a variant of polydactylism. Holthusen et al. described a hand with typical features of this syndrome and a bifid first metacarpal head that articulated with the accessory ossicle. This supports the theory of a duplication mechanism in the etiology of the accessory bone in the palatodigital syndrome.

▶ Most instances of clinodactyly seem to be associated with accessory ossicles or accessory physes. When deformity is as extreme as that presented here, surgical correction is indicated either by the technique described by the authors, i.e., corrective osteotomy, or even removal and repositioning (deletion in some cases) of the ossicle. Because such operations are rare, one hopes that the authors have a better record of the surgical findings than is published.—J.H.D.

Duplication of the Thumb: A Retrospective Review of 237 Cases
Koichi Tada, Kazuo Yonenobu, Yuichi Tsuyuguchi, Hideo Kawai, and Tsuneichi Egawa (Osaka Univ.)
J. Bone Joint Surg. [Am.] 65-A:584–598, June 1983   14–7

The results of surgery were reviewed in a series of 237 patients (261 hands) seen in a 22-year period with duplication of the thumb. A total of

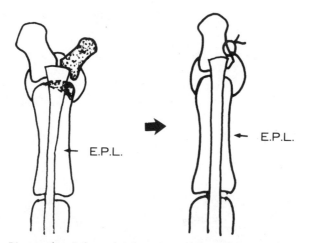

Fig 14–9.—Diagram of surgical procedure in treatment of type II duplication. Included are ablation of smaller portion of duplicated part of digit, shaving of articular cartilage of proximal phalanx, centralization of extrinsic tendons on distal phalanx, and reattachment and reefing of capsule of distal interphalangeal joint; *E.P.L.*, extensor pollicis longus. (Courtesy of Tada, K., et al.: J. Bone Joint Surg. [Am.] 65-A:584–598, June 1983.)

141 patients (group A) had not been operated on previously, whereas 96 (group B) had residual deformity after surgery. Surgery was performed on 125 hands in group A patients and on 68 in group B. Results were evaluable in 130 hands after an average of nearly 3 years.

The management of type II deformities, with a reduplicated distal pha-

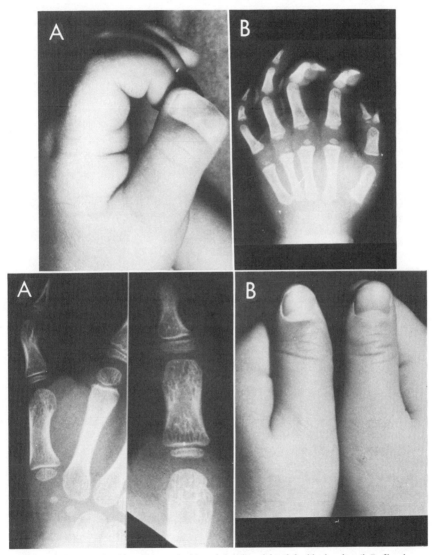

Fig 14–10 (top).—A, girl aged 1 year had broad thumb and fused double thumb nail. B, film shows duplication at interphalangeal joint.

Fig 14–11 (bottom).—Films (A) and photograph (B) 3½ years after surgery for type II duplication. Size and alignment of left thumb are satisfactory. Film shows good congruency and alignment of interphalangeal joint.

(Courtesy of Tada, K., et al.: J. Bone Joint Surg. [Am.] 65-A:584–598, June 1983.)

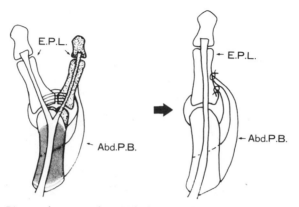

Fig 14–12.—Diagram of treatment of type IV duplication, including ablation of supernumerary thumb, arthroplasty of metacarpophalangeal joint and reattachment of abductor pollicis brevis *(Abd.P.B.)* capsule and collateral ligament. Accessory limb of extensor pollicis longus *(E.P.L.)* is bifurcated at same level as bone bifurcation and is resected. (Courtesy of Tada, K., et al.: J. Bone Joint Surg. [Am.] 65-A:584–598, June 1983.)

lanx, is illustrated in Figures 14–9 to 14–11, and that of type IV deformities, with reduplicated proximal and distal phalanges, is shown in Figures 14–12 to 14–14. Reconstruction of the zigzag deformity is illustrated in Figure 14–15.

Results of surgery in group A patients were rated good in 71 cases (75.5%), fair in 19 (20.2%), and poor in 4 (4.3%). All patients treated for bifurcation at the distal phalanx or carpometacarpal joint or for floating thumb had good results after simple resection or resection with tendon reinsertion or relocation. Thirteen group B patients were unimproved after further surgery, whereas 16 improved from fair to good and 7 from poor to fair. The results in 23 group B hands with angular deformity were disappointing. In hands with recurrent malalignment and residual joint instability, tendon reinsertion and arthroplasty were more effective than osteotomy in producing good alignment and stability of the thumb.

Duplication of the thumb is managed by reconstruction of the preserved thumb as well as excision of the supernumerary digit, preferably during the initial procedure. An attempt should be made to restore congruent interphalangeal and metacarpophalangeal joint surfaces and the balance of muscular forces about these joints. The present findings emphasize the importance of adequate initial surgery in cases of duplication of the thumb.

▶ That the principles of duplicate thumb treatment, outlined here, are generally accepted worldwide owes much to the extensive experience recorded in this article and to the prior publications (in Japanese) of the senior author, Doctor Egawa. Results are analyzed in so many different ways that they are difficult to follow, but they seem to reflect the current consensus that the appearance and function of all duplicate thumbs can be improved, none becomes completely normal, and inexperienced reconstruction can make them worse. Interestingly, the authors disregard the triphalangeal duplicates, which

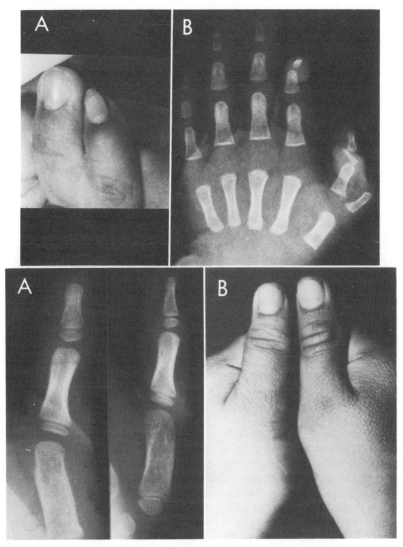

Fig 14–13 (top).—**A,** hand of boy aged 3 months when first seen. **B,** preoperative film of hand.

Fig 14–14 (bottom).—Films (**A**) and photograph (**B**) 8 years after surgery for type IV duplication. There is good alignment of left thumb, adequate congruency of metacarpophalangeal joint surfaces, and absence of any evidence of disturbed growth of affected thumb after arthroplasty of metacarpophalangeal joint.

(Courtesy of Tada, K., et al.: J. Bone Surg. [Am.] 65-A:584–598, June 1983.)

do occur. They properly advise caution regarding the use of the Bilhaut-Cloquet procedure, whose classic version of retaining symmetric portions of both bony and soft tissue augments bulk and strength at the expense of motion. They say nothing about those variations wherein asymmetric bonding of the duplicates (i.e., borrowing needed soft tissues but using one skeletal system) is

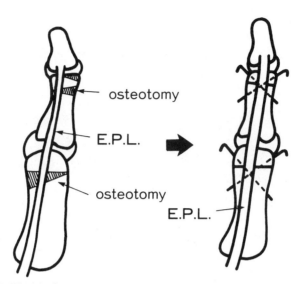

Fig 14–15.—Diagram of reconstruction of zigzag deformity in type III thumb in group B. Procedure includes shaving articular cartilage of head of proximal phalanx as well as wedge osteotomies of proximal phalanx and metacarpal to correct alignment; *E.P.L.*, extensor pollicis longus. (Courtesy of Tada, K., et al.: J. Bone Joint Surg. [Am.] 65-A:584–598, June 1983.)

carried out to obtain increased bulk and strength while retaining motion. These techniques are particularly intricate however, and the authors are probably wise in restricting their discussion to the standard complexities. It is good to have this extensive and excellent experience finally recorded in the English literature.—J.H.D.

Pathology of Involved Tendons in Patients With Familial Arthropathy and Congenital Camptodactyly
Takahiro Ochi, Rokuro Iwase, Norikazu Okabe, Chester W. Fink, and Keiro Ono
Arthritis Rheum. 26:896–900, July 1983   14–8

Two sisters with congenital camptodactyly and joint effusions who had tendon abnormalities were encountered. The abnormalities were restricted to the portion within synovial sheaths, implying a disorder of the tenosynovium rather than the tendon. The patients have been followed up for more than 3 years. Both patients had flexion deformity of both middle fingers at birth, and attempts to release the contractures failed. Painless swelling of the hands and knees developed in early childhood. The procedure showed some tendons in areas of chronic involvement that were replaced by fibrous tissue. Significant portions of the tendons in affected fingers were replaced by hard scar tissue. Synovial chondromas were present in synovial sheaths. Adhesions of synovial sheaths to tendons were very tight in regions of more advanced disease.

The cause of the pathology in this disease is unknown, but congenital camptodactyly found in association with familial arthropathy is probably the result of an intrauterine tenosynovitis rather than an isolated congenital anomaly. If the fibrosis and adhesions result from an existing persistent low-grade inflammation arising in the tenosynovium, tenosynovectomy and tenolysis might prevent tendon contractures and preserve finger motion. Synovectomy may be necessary if persistent hydrarthrosis is present.

▶ Both the article and its bibliography are surprisingly reticent regarding the more common forms of camptodactyly. Nevertheless, those workers called on to manage the more common camptodactyly should be aware of this alternate form, associated with a synovial disease whose cause is yet to be determined.—J.H.D.

Upper Limb Dysplasia, Form and Function
Douglas W. Lamb (Edinburgh)
J. R. Coll. Surg. Edinb. 28:203–213, July 1983   14–9

The author outlines the management of various forms of dysplastic upper limb deformity. The cause of transverse absence at the below-elbow level is unknown. Occasionally some vestigial terminal digits are present. A light nonfunctional prosthesis is fitted at age 4–6 months and a split hook is fitted at age 12–15 months. More than 40 children have been given a prosthesis originally designed for adult above-elbow amputees. It has a polycentric elbow mechanism and a new artificial hand design. The myoelectric controlled prosthesis has been used in 15 children aged 3–6 years. The appearance and quality of the hand and glove are not yet satisfactory, and repairs are frequently necessary.

Absence of the radius may be associated with anomalies elsewhere in the body. Occasionally only the distal two thirds of the bone is missing. Severe functional deficit can result from stiffness of the joints and limited muscles to move them. The wrist should be splinted in corrected position from an early age. An elbow that is stiff in extension should be mobilized by physiotherapy. The carpus is centralized over the lower ulna and the ulna is implanted to a depth equal to its transverse diameter. The periosteal flap raised from the carpus is closed to provide a new capsule. The intramedullary Kirschner wire used to maintain the position is left in place for up to a year.

An absent or nearly totally absent thumb is best managed by digital transfer on a neurovascular bundle or by free toe transfer. Indications for pollicization include the 5-fingered hand, the 4-fingered hand, and either a 4-fingered hand or "dangle thumb" associated with preaxial radial longitudinal deficiency. In the latter cases, pollicization should be preceded by correction of the wrist deformity. Transfer of the index finger on a neurovascular pedicle can provide good form and function. Free toe transfer may not provide the same quality of function and sensation, and some functional disability of the foot can result.

▶ There is nothing new in this published lecture, but the concise and authoritative summation of the topics discussed completely covers the current status of these subjects.—J.H.D.

Congenital Constriction Band Syndrome
Takayuki Miura (Nagoya Univ.)
J. Hand Surg. 9A:82–88, January 1984   14–10

The findings in and treatment of 55 patients seen since 1968 with congenital constriction band syndrome affecting the upper extremity were reviewed. Ninety-one hands were involved. A ring deformity only was present in 8 patients, 21 also had peripheral amputation, and 26 had fenestrated syndactyly with or without amputation. Forty-one patients had involvement of the foot as well, and 9 patients had associated anomalies, most frequently clubbed feet and cleft lip-palate. Graphs of the metacarpal pattern profile distinguished between constriction band syndrome and failure of formation (Figs 14–16 and 14–17). Bone formation and maturation proximal to the constriction rings were unimpaired.

Two thirds of patients required more than one operation. Half the circumference of the constriction ring was treated by Z-plasty, and the other half was treated by Z-plasty at a later stage. A few patients with severe lymphedema had a combination of Y-V-plasty and W-plasty. More extensive syndactyly necessitates division and skin grafting. Small sinus tracts usually are excised and grafted but occasionally can be incorporated into local flaps. Where short, webbed digits are present, the interdigital spaces are deepened with local flaps. The functional results have been satisfactory, but the cosmetic results are sometimes poor (Fig 14–18).

Six patients had improved function after the thumb web space was deepened by the sliding dorsal flap procedure. The digital transfer described by Soiland is useful for short thumbs. Occasionally the thumb can be lengthened by adding the shortened index ray to the thumb (Figs 14–19 and 14–20). Digital lengthening by osteotomy and distraction is likeliest to succeed in older children. Transplantation of the toe by microsurgery is rarely indicated, because most patients gain good function from local reconstructive procedures, and vascular anastomoses are technically difficult in the digits of small children.

▶ Professor Miura's resumé of an extensive experience with congenital constriction band syndrome presents one new idea to Western readers (the use of relative metacarpal lengths to aid in classification) and reiterates good standard treatment methods. Web depth should be set at the appropriate level (normal depth for normal-length fingers, deeper for short fingers) and at the initial operation if feasible (the fenestrations are never at an adequate depth).

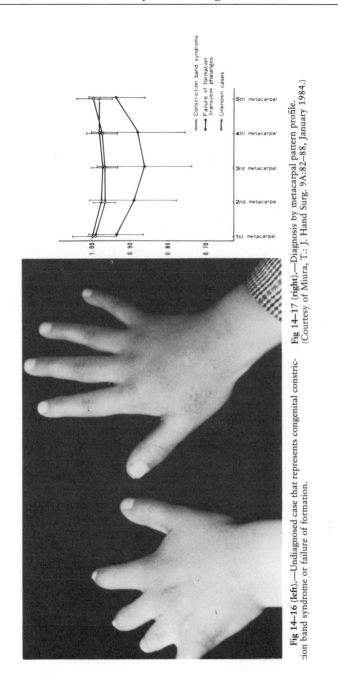

Fig 14–16 (left).—Undiagnosed case that represents congenital constriction band syndrome or failure of formation.

Fig 14–17 (right).—Diagnosis by metacarpal pattern profile. (Courtesy of Miura, T.: J. Hand Surg. 9A:82–88, January 1984.)

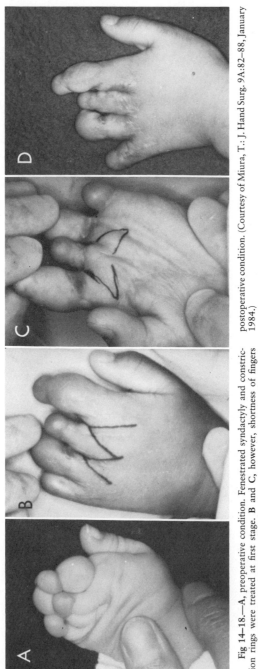

Fig 14–18.—A, preoperative condition. Fenestrated syndactyly and constriction rings were treated at first stage. B and C, however, shortness of fingers remained. Same procedure as syndactyly release was used to lengthen fingers. D, postoperative condition. (Courtesy of Miura, T.: J. Hand Surg. 9A:82–88, January 1984.)

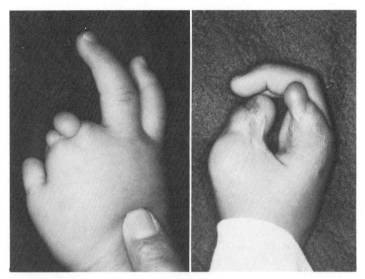

Fig 14–19 (left).—Preoperative condition.
Fig 14–20 (right).—"On top" thumb plasty by index finger transfer.
(Courtesy of Miura, T.: J. Hand Surg. 9A:82–88, January 1984.)

The on-top-plasty can be very useful, as indicated but it is unfair to deprecate lengthening after only one trial. Toe-to-hand transfer or even hand-to-hand transfer of digits rarely will be indicated but has been done; the long-term usefulness of these procedures is yet to be determined.—J.H.D.

Upper Extremity Gangrene of the Newborn Infant
William O. Shaffer, Pat L. Aulicino, and T. E. DuPuy (Portsmouth, Va.)
J. Hand Surg. 9A:88–90, January 1984   14–11

Twenty-two cases of neonatal upper extremity gangrene have been reported, 15 occurring at birth.

Male infant, aged 9 days, had had a cyanotic right upper extremity since birth to a borderline hypertensive woman with excessive weight gain during pregnancy. Labor had been prolonged, requiring mechanical rupture of the membranes 7 hours before delivery. The affected right arm presented posteriorly. Meconium staining was noted, and the 1-minute Apgar score was 5. The right arm below the elbow was intensely cyanotic. The cord blood hemoglobin was 20.1 gm/dl. At 8 hours there was no movement in the right upper arm, and a blue-black mottled appearance was noted distal to the elbow, with extensive epidermolysis on the dorsum of the forearm and hand and an eschar covering the ulnar border of the forearm. Doppler study failed to show pulsations distal to the axillary artery. Demarcation was present just below the elbow at age 9 days, with increasing cellulitis proximally. Cultures of the eschar yielded *Staphylococcus aureus,* and oxacillin was given intravenously. On day 11, the arm was amputated through the elbow (Fig 14–

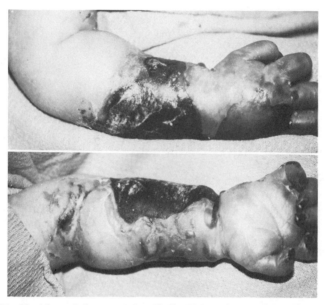

Fig 14–21.—The right arm before amputation. (Shaffer, W.O., et al.: J. Hand Surg. 9A:88–90, January 1984.)

21). All muscle distal to the elbow was necrotic, and organized thrombus was present in the radial and ulnar arteries. No vascular anomalies were found. The child did well after the amputation.

Many causes of neonatal gangrene exist. In the present case, the position of the extremity may have caused it to be compressed against the sacrum during a prolonged labor during which hypoxia occurred. Complete recovery has been described with conservative management in 2 cases of upper extremity gangrene and 1 of lower extremity neonatal gangrene. Supportive care, sterile dressings, prophylactic antibiotic therapy, and heparinization may be sufficient in cases of acral or incomplete ischemia. Early arteriography is indicated if complete ischemia is present; conservative treatment may be continued if collateral circulation is demonstrated. Early surgery with balloon catheter thrombectomy may be helpful in the severely or progressively ischemic limb that lacks muscle contractility.

▶ Upper extremity gangrene is rare, but is a crisis when encountered. A useful summary of one's options is given in this article.—J.H.D.

Isolated Radial Nerve Lesion in the Newborn

David Ross, H. Royden Jones, Jr., Julian Fisher, and Richard J. Konkol
Neurology (Cleve.) 33:1354–1356, October 1983   14–12

Two cases of neonatal radial nerve palsy are described. The neonates presented at ages 1 and 9 days, respectively, with isolated unilateral flaccid paralysis of the wrist and finger extensors. The lesion was documented electromyographically. The finding of fibrillation potentials in 1 patient at age 7 days suggested the possibility of an onset in utero. This infant had been born by cesarean section and was noted on the first day of life to have a wristdrop and an indurated area near the elbow. No treatment was given, and the findings at age 6 weeks were normal. The other infant had several bruises and a prominent hematoma above the elbow. The palsy was proximal to the triceps branch. No treatment was given, and the findings at age 4 months were normal.

A variety of peripheral nerve injuries of the upper extremities occur during the perinatal period. Twelve cases of radial nerve palsy in neonates have been reported. Seven cases involved prolonged or abnormal labor. In 9 cases, there was localized subcutaneous fat necrosis overlying the course of the radial nerve proximal to the radial epicondyle of the ipsilateral humerus. All patients but 1 recovered fully within 3 months. The fat necrosis may result from abnormal intrauterine positioning, amniotic bands, or other, unidentified trauma. Complicating infection in soft tissues or underlying bone should be ruled out. If infection is excluded or treated, the prognosis should be favorable. It is important to distinguish an isolated radial nerve lesion from the more serious medial brachial plexus lesion.

▶ Peripheral nerve palsy in the newborn is almost surely more common than is generally thought, as this review of radial palsies suggests. The excellent prognosis for most cases is not shared by those associated with congenital constriction band disorder (though even these vary). The case reported by Weeks et al (*Plast. Reconstr. Surg.* 69:333–336, 1982) was associated with peripheral nerve disruption, and I am aware of several similar unreported cases. The lack of quick recovery in the infant suggests a severe lesion requiring decompression or reconstruction.—J.H.D.

Wringer Washer Injuries in Children
Edmond B. Cabbabe and Stanley W. Korock (St. Louis Univ.)
Ann. Plast. Surg. 10:135–142, February 1983   14–13

Wringer washer injuries continue to occur despite the introduction of safer automatic washers. The injuries result from the forces exerted on an extremity between the rotating rollers and involve thermal, crushing, and avulsion types of injury. Data on 104 children (average age, 4.8 years) seen in 1970–1980 with wringer washer injuries were reviewed. The average hospital stay was 5.05 days. Admission for observation and treatment became much more frequent later in the review period. Most injuries involved the forearm and elbow regions. Thirteen patients received skin grafts or flaps for full-thickness losses. Thirteen had lacerations in the first web space, the thenar area, and the third and fourth web spaces. Four patients had fractures, and 4 had nerve injuries.

Most children with wringer injuries now are admitted to hospitals. Tetanus toxoid is given as indicated. Prophylactic antibiotics are not routinely used. Muscle compartments are decompressed promptly if intracompartmental pressure is elevated. Reasonably clean lacerations are repaired, and fractures are reduced and splinted as indicated. The patient can be discharged when edema has subsided and there are no sensory, motor, or soft tissue deficits. Tendon or nerve repair is done when necessary as a delayed primary or secondary procedure. Most closed nerve injuries are of the neuropraxia type and can be expected to resolve spontaneously. Patients with contraction may require later treatment.

All children with a history of wringer washer injury should be admitted and observed for 48 hours after injury. Current management emphasizes elevation rather than pressure dressing. The extremity must be observed closely. Physical therapy is mandatory. The patients in the present series who had permanent disability were the 2 who had amputations.

▶ This is an entity from the past that still occurs. The authors present a rational update on treatment.—R.L.L.

Computed Tomographic Localization of Wooden Foreign Bodies in Children's Extremities.
A. Robert Bauer, Jr., and Dennis Yutani (St. Mark's Hosp., Salt Lake City)
Arch. Surg. 118:1084–1086, September 1983   14–14

Wooden foreign bodies embedded in an extremity have been difficult to identify and locate with previous roentgenographic methods. The authors evaluated computed tomography (CT) for this purpose because of its ability to distinguish subtle differences in density. The usefulness of CT in a boy aged 12 who had intermittent purulent drainage from an old knee wound incurred when falling on a dead branch is shown in Figure 14–22. Routine roentgenograms were normal in this case, but the CT study defined a wooden foreign body and permitted its precise surgical removal. Another patient, a boy aged 5 who impaled his thigh on a branch and had recurrent drainage after initial removal of a section of wood, had wooden foreign bodies deep in the thigh muscles accurately localized by CT. These then were removed without difficulty. Both patients healed without evidence of damage to nerves or vessels.

Computed tomography permits the accurate localization of wooden foreign bodies, which have a density close to that of normal tissue, and aids a planned surgical approach. General anesthesia and heavy sedation usually are not necessary with use of a high-speed scanner. Fistulous tract injection and instrumentation can be avoided. The radiation dose from CT is less than that from many of the previously used methods. Noninvasive follow-up to confirm the complete resolution of inflammation is feasible using CT, on an outpatient basis. Considerable cost savings may result through the avoidance of complicated diagnostic measures and prolonged treatment.

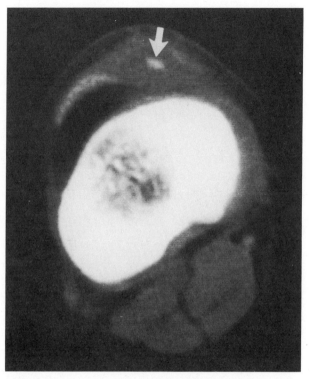

Fig 14–22.—Accurate computed tomographic (9.6 second; 5-mm collimator) demonstration of wooden foreign body *(arrow)* 1 cm × 3 mm in soft tissue of anterior aspect of right knee. (Courtesy of Bauer, A.R., and Yutani, D.: Arch. Surg. 118:1084–1086, September, 1983; copyright 1983, American Medical Association.)

▶ Computed tomography (CT) has proved extremely helpful in evaluating a variety of soft tissue problems. Localization of foreign bodies such as wood that do not show up well on routine radiography is another demonstration of the clinical utility of this diagnostic tool. In the cases presented in this article, CT helped confirm the presence of a foreign body, thus explaining the persisting symptoms. Because both patients had draining wounds, however, the necessity of performing the diagnostic study could be questioned. Exploration of the draining sinus clearly was indicated in both cases; in my experience in similar cases, the foreign body has been localized within a fairly well-defined abscess cavity. I would think that the usefulness of this procedure would be more in the acute setting when an inflammatory reaction has not yet developed around the foreign body.—P.C.A.

15 Microsurgery

Primary Microsurgical Repair of Ring Avulsion Amputation Injuries
Tsk-Min Tsai, Carl Manstein, Richard DuBou, Thomas W. Wolff, Joseph E.
Kutz, and Harold E. Kleinert (Univ. of Louisville)
J. Hand Surg. 9A:68–72, January 1984   15–1

The symbolic importance of the ring-bearing part of the hand has led to requests by patients with ring avulsion injuries of the fourth and fifth digits, particularly female patients for reconstruction rather than completion of the amputation. The authors report the results obtained in 4 left and 3 right ring finger avulsion injuries with total amputation, managed by primary microsurgical replantation. The 4 male and 3 female patients (average age, 30 years) had crushing avulsion of skin, tendon damage, loss of both neurovascular bundles, joint dislocation, and phalangeal fracture.

Six patients had a viable repair. One patient had bilateral digital nerve grafting 3 months after initial operation to correct segmental losses of the digital nerves. No primary nerve grafts were utilized. Four patients required multiple interpositional vein grafts for the arteries or veins, or both. Sensation was protective in all cases and good in 3, paralleling the severity of injury. Four patients had minor cold intolerance at follow-up. None had significantly limited motion of adjacent fingers. Average ranges of motion were 0/84 degrees at the metacarpophalangeal joint and 15/90 degrees at the proximal interphalangeal joint, with distal interphalangeal joint ankylosis at 0–15 degrees of flexion. All 4 patients questioned were satisfied with the outcome. Two laborers were able to return to work after 4 and 6 months, respectively.

Primary microsurgical repair is indicated in carefully selected patients with complex ring avulsion injuries, which tend to occur during the time of maximum patient productivity and responsibility. The average hospital stay is about a week. Early mobilization of fingers is recommended. Vascular complications are most likely due to intimal disruption that is not recognized and excised at the time of initial vascular repair.

▶ The outstanding results presented in this report should perhaps encourage reassessment of management considerations for complete ring degloving injuries.—M.B.W.

AV Anastomosis as Solution for Absent Venous Drainage in Replantation Surgery
Arlan R. Smith, G. Jan Sonneveld, and Jacques C. van der Meulen
Plast. Reconstr. Surg. 71:525–532, April 1983   15–2

The survival rate of "artery only" replantations of amputated digits is much less than that after procedures in which both arteries and veins are anastomosed. In an attempt to obtain adequate circulation in the replanted part to assure sufficient arterial perfusion, the authors used the contralateral artery in the replanted digit as a venous outflow pole, connected with or without a vein graft to a vein in the proximal stump of the digit.

Man, 23, underwent amputation of the thumb at the level of the interphalangeal (IP) joint (Fig 15–1, A) due to an electric saw injury. Ischemia time at admission was 2 hours, and surgery began within an hour. Extensive débridement was carried out, two Kirschner wires were passed through the IP joint, and the extensor and flexor tendons were repaired. Nerve repair was followed by arterial repair at the radial side of the thumb; the ischemia time was then 4½ hours. Excellent perfusion was obtained, but no suitable veins were found for drainage; therefore, the ulnar artery of the replanted thumb, which had excellent backflow, was connected to a vein at the dorsum of the proximal stump at the level of the metacarpophalangeal joint by using a vein graft from the lower forearm. The transcutaneous Po_2 was monitored for 5 days postoperatively. The patient received aspirin, Persantine, dextran, and antibiotics. Sensation was normal 6 months postoperatively, by which time the patient had returned to his previous work. An angiogram done at 4 months showed all anastomoses to be patent (Fig 15–1, B).

Early postoperative Po_2 measurements in the authors' 3 patients had the same curves as oxygen levels in replantations with normal inflow and outflow. The results can be attributed to the value of hypoxia as a stimulus to neovascularization, as in congenital arteriovenous malformations when the nutrient circulation is bypassed. The sudden high arterial pressure presumably leads mechanically to the opening of multiple communications that already exist with the associated vein. Blood flow continues as the nutrient circulation is essentially bypassed, resulting in hypoxia in the adjacent region. Surgical trauma accentuates hypoxia and ischemia, and

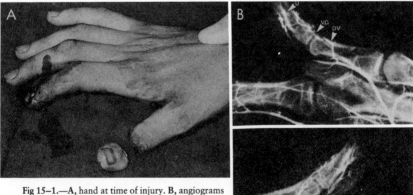

Fig 15–1.—A, hand at time of injury. B, angiograms 4 months postoperatively show results of replantation. R, radial digital artery; U, ulnar digital artery; VG, venous graft; and DV, dorsal vein. (Courtesy of Smith, A.R., et al.: Plast. Reconstr. Surg. 71:525–532, April 1983.)

also promotes angiogenesis. James W. May, Jr., agrees that this is a useful alternative when vein-to-vein reconstruction is not feasible.

▶ Replantation of digits amputated distal to the interphalangeal joint is controversial. While replantation is technically possible at this level, many authors report cold intolerance and incomplete sensibility, suggesting that most patients would be better off without the replanted fingertip. Others, such as the present authors, believe that there is considerable cosmetic as well as functional advantage in reimplanting these distal-level amputations. The authors, furthermore, have devised a technique of arteriovenous (AV) anastomosis when dorsal veins are lacking. Survival of digits without venous return is usually unsuccessful. In the few we have had survive, we have found a hypotrophic and unsensitive digit resulting.

The authors report 3 cases in which they successfully used AV anastomosis when there was absent venous drainage. They carefully selected their cases, limiting the technique to an amputation of the thumb, to the index finger in a professional pianist, and to a ring avulsion injury in a young man. In cases like the last, with an extreme avulsion injury, ray amputation might be preferable because satisfactory sensation without cold intolerance is difficult to obtain.

In the invited comments on this article, James May brings up a number of questions as to how the terminal portion of the digit would survive with an AV shunt. One would expect AV steal from the distal portion of the digit and—as a result—questionable viability and, at best, poor sensibility. The authors propose hypoxia as a stimulus to neovascularization. We would agree with May that studies to date suggest that this probably is not the correct explanation. Possibly the reversal of flow through the AV shunt into the venous system as well as perfusion of the nutrient capillary bed might occur. Our experience with an AV anastomosis in 2 patients has not been successful, and we would question the general advisability in such distal amputations.—W.P.C.

Low-Dose Fibrinolytic Therapy in Hand Ischemia

Jaime Tisnado, Dennie T. Bartol, Shao-Ru Cho, Frederick S. Vines, Michael C. Beachley, and William R. Fields (Virginia Commonwealth Univ., Richmond)
Radiology 150:375–382, February 1984   15–3

Low-dose streptokinase was administered intra-arterially to 5 patients with acute hand ischemia of 2–48 hours duration and 1 with ischemia of 3 months' duration. Excellent restoration of the patency of occluded hand arteries was obtained in the acute cases, but the patient with iatrogenic chronic occlusion required bypass surgery. No complications occurred during or after the procedure.

Man, 30, a drug abuser, presented with a painful, cold, ischemic left hand secondary to the self-administered intra-arterial injection of dissolved tablets of pentazocine hydrochloride and codeine phosphate 18 hours before. The radial pulse was markedly reduced, and the ulnar pulse was absent. A stellate ganglion block was not helpful, and a brachial angiogram showed occlusion of the radial and ulnar arteries at the wrist and no opacification of the palmar arches. No change followed intra-arterial vasodilator and local anesthetic administration. A dose of 100,000 units of streptokinase was infused in 30 minutes via a distal brachial artery catheter. The ulnar artery was recanalized, and the superficial palmar arch opacified. A streptokinase infusion of 5,000 units per hour was continued for 12 hours, with further opacification occurring on arteriography. The infusion rate was halved when the fibrinogen level fell to 110 mg/dl and rate was restored to 5,000 units per hour when the fibrinogen level rose to normal. The hand and fingers became pink and warm the next day, with good capillary refill and much improved sensation. Streptokinase was infused for a total of 96 hours, after which systemic heparinization was given for 3 days. The hand was normal when the patient was discharged.

Severe hand ischemia is an uncommon disorder carrying a serious prognosis. Good results have been obtained with low-dose streptokinase therapy in patients with acute hand ischemia. The successful treatment of chronic occlusions up to 12 months old also has been reported. Possibly, the catheter should be embedded in the clot. The current loading dose of streptokinase is 50,000 units in 30 minutes. Systemic heparin usually is given after low-dose fibrinolytic therapy. Fibrinolysis can be useful in cases of impending gangrene where reconstructive surgery is technically extremely difficult or impossible.

▶ The authors present additional evidence that intra-arterial streptokinase therapy is effective in the treatment of acute hand ischemia caused by thromboembolic disease. We have had experiences similar to the authors in lysing these acute vascular occlusions. We have found, however, that the situation is entirely different in replantation cases in which there is vascular ischemia, and in these cases the use of low- or even high-dose fibrinolytic therapy has been ineffective. The authors present some excellent case examples and emphasize the important fact that intra-arterial direct release of the fibrinolytic substance near the clot is essential for this to be therapeutically effective. I agree with the authors that fibrinolytic therapy with streptokinase offers effective treatment for patients with severe, acute hand ischemia with impending gangrene.—W.P.C.

Dynamic Radionuclide Imaging as a Means of Evaluating Vascular Perfusion of the Upper Extremity: Preliminary Report
L. Andrew Koman, James A. Nunley, Robert H. Wilkinson, Jr., James R. Urbaniak, and R. Edward Coleman (Duke Univ.)
J. Hand Surg. 8:424–434, July 1983   15–4

Vascular competence was evaluated in the upper extremities of 35 male and 9 female patients (mean age, 38 years), 22 symptomatic after documented arterial injury and 22 with symptoms suggesting vascular insufficiency of unknown origin. Flow was correlated with the contrast angiographic or operative findings in 50 extremities. Rapid-sequence dynamic radionuclide imaging (DRI) was accompanied by immediate postinjection "blood pool" imaging and delayed imaging at 3–4 hours. The DRI was done using 20–25 mCi of ^{99m}Tc-medronate and a wide-field-of-view scintillation camera. Nine sequential images were obtained in each hand at a rate of 5 seconds per image. Where possible, computer data were acquired and stored simultaneously.

The presence or absence of hemodynamically significant vascular changes in the forearm was appreciated correctly in all posttraumatic extremities. Anatomical detail in the wrist and hand was more difficult to visualize accurately. All 14 arteries that were thrombosed or not in continuity were identified correctly, as were a posttraumatic arteriovenous fistula and a radial artery aneurysm. Flow in 12 arterial reconstructions was confirmed. In the nontraumatic cases, all DRI studies correlated with the contrast angiographic and operative findings. A correct diagnosis was made by DRI in all but 4 extremities. Limited resolution precluded the precise definition of aneurysms in 3 extremities and of digital artery occlusion with adequate collateral circulation in 1 case.

The use of DRI of the upper extremity is a rapid means of providing the relatively inexperienced examiner with information equivalent to that obtainable clinically through classic digital and wrist Allen testing. It can be done as part of a bone scan study, and it avoids the morbidity and discomfort of arteriography. Bilateral information is obtained from DRI. Anatomical detail is relatively limited, however, and long sequencing intervals are necessary. Repeat testing is limited by radiation exposure.

▶ Dynamic radionuclide imaging represents a particularly useful method for anatomically assessing vascular perfusion, with the additional advantage of being at least a semiquantitative technique.—M.B.W.

▶ A similar technique can be used to evaluate patients preoperatively and postoperatively when microlymphaticovenous anastomosis is being considered. An excellent review of this subject can be found in *Clinics in Nuclear Medicine* (8:309–311, 1983).—P.C.A.

Functioning Free Muscle Transplantation
Ralph T. Manktelow, Ronald M. Zuker, and Nancy H. McKee (Univ. of Toronto)
J. Hand Surg. 9A:32–39, January 1984   15–5

Twelve patients were followed for a mean of 3 years after free muscle transplantation to the arm. The indication for functioning free muscle transplantation is a major loss of skeletal musculature leading to significant functional deficit. There usually has been major injury to the forearm with the loss of all the flexor musculature and some damage to the extensor muscles. The chief functional complaint is a lack of grip capacity. Good motivation is necessary to insure that the patient will comply with a prolonged postoperative program of resisted exercises. The gricilis, latissimus dorsi, or percoralis major muscle may be considered for transplant. Technically perfect vascular anastomoses are essential. The nerve repair should be done as close as possible to the neuromuscular junction. Tendon fixation is carried out at a tension that provides good muscle balance and optimal grip strength. Good flap coverage in the distal forearm is necessary for tendon gliding. Resisted exercises are begun when there is a full range of excursion, usually 6–12 months postoperatively.

Eleven of the 12 transplants survived completely and 1 partially. Eleven procedures were successful by supplying a useful range of motion and adequate grip strength under volitional control. Full muscle contraction was achieved within 6–9 months after surgery. Nine patients had full motion in the finger. Grip strength continued to increase for up to 3 years after operation. The patient with only partial muscle survival had occlusion of the anterior interosseous artery supplying a pectoralis major transfer for Volkmann's ischemic paralysis.

The gracilis muscle can be transplanted successfully to the forearm to provide finger flexion after muscle loss at this site. Full finger motion and considerable grip strength can be regained, but some time is needed to achieve maximum function. Heavy labor may not be possible until 2 years after free muscle transplantation.

▶ This is a good concept to provide some functional movement with a free muscle transfer when there are no available local muscles or tendons to serve this purpose. The authors present a good number of cases, outline valid criteria for success, and point out some helpful technical points.—G.B.I.

Reconstruction of the Hand With Free Microneurovascular Toe-to-Hand Transfer: Experience With 54 Toe Transfers
Graham D. Lister, Michael Kalisman, and Tsu-Min Tsai (Univ. of Louisville)
Plast. Reconstr. Surg. 71:372–384, March 1983   15–6

The results of 54 toe-to-hand transfers performed on 27 male and 7 female patients between 1974 and 1980 were reviewed. Forty operations were performed on 36 hands. The mean age of the patients was 29 years. The dominant hand was involved in 17 patients. Most absent digits had been amputated traumatically by industrial machinery or farm and yard implements. Thumb reconstruction was done in 24 instances; the great toe was used in 13 and the second toe in 11. Thirteen combined second and third toe-to-hand transfers were done in 12 patients with severely mutilating transmetacarpal amputations. A patient with congenital absence of all digits had two second toe transfers for finger reconstruction. All transfers were done as secondary elective procedures. A groin flap procedure was done first in 77% of cases. Nerve repairs, in contrast to tendon repairs, were done as far distally as possible. Osteosynthesis was by type A interosseous wiring. No anticoagulants, vasodilators, or antiaggregating agents were used.

Forty-nine of the transferred toes (91%) survived. Exploration for circulatory compromise was necessary after about one third of operations. Secondary operations were performed after about two thirds of the procedures; tendolyses were most frequent. Both power grip and pinch varied widely on follow-up an average of 21 months after operation. Nine of 12 patients evaluated more than 2 years after operation had static two-point discrimination of less than 10 mm. All patients were bothered by cold intolerance. Few significant foot problems were described.

A large majority of toe-to-hand transfers in this series survived. The choice of which toe to transfer to the thumb position is open, but the authors generally transfer second toes in children. Vascular considerations are critical in this surgery. Survival itself does not insure good function, and efforts to improve the functional outcome must continue. A method of osteosynthesis that permits early motion will help keep the joints supple and avoid tendon adhesions. Sensory return can be enhanced by using only nerve that is totally free from scarring and from as far distal in the hand as is possible. Early and sustained sensory reeducation is also important.

▶ This well-written article presents the comprehensive results of a large series of toe-to-hand transfers. It also presents helpful and factual information regarding general reconstructive options for thumb loss.—M.B.W.

▶ These techniques also can be used to salvage more proximal amputations, as in the case reported by Furnas and Achauer (*J. Hand Surg.* 8:453–457, 1983) in which a great toe was transferred to the radius to provide prehension in a patient with a proximal transmetacarpal amputation.

It is important, however, to remember that surgical ingenuity and dexterity are not proper substitutes for patient selection and good judgment when considering treatment options in the severely mutilated hand. Some of these patients may be better served by prosthetic devices.—P.C.A.

Immediate Reconstruction of the Wrist and Dorsum of the Hand With a Free Osteocutaneous Groin Flap
William M. Swartz (Univ. of Pittsburgh)
J. Hand Surg. 9A:18–21, January 1984   15–7

The author describes a patient with traumatic loss of the first and second metacarpals and the radial carpal bones who was managed by immediate soft tissue and bone reconstruction with a free osteocutaneous groin flap.

Man, 24, sustained a punch press injury to the dorsum of the dominant right hand that included extensive soft tissue loss over the dorsoradial aspect of the wrist and loss of the thumb and index metacarpals and the scaphoid, trapezium, and trapezoid bones (Fig 15–2). Regional tendons were crushed, but the thumb and index finger were both well vascularized. Primary wrist fusion and metacarpal stabilization were planned, with use of an osteocutaneous groin flap based on the deep circumflex iliac vessels (Fig 15–3). The skin island measured 8 × 18 cm and the bone graft, 15 × 4 cm. Kirschner wires were used for bony stabilization. A conventional iliac bone graft was used to replace the thumb metacarpal. A dorsal wrist vein was sutured to the deep circumflex iliac vein. Aspirin was the only anticoagulant used. The skin flap and split-thickness graft survived completely. Wrist fusion was solid at 12 weeks. A contour deformity of the dorsum of the

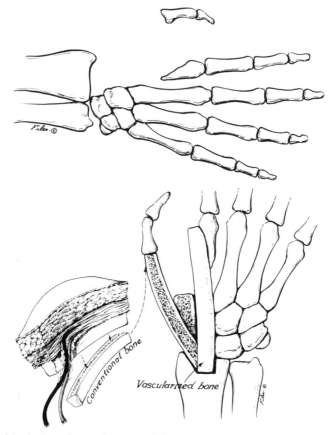

Fig 15–2 (top).—Bony elements that remained after punch press injury to dorsum of wrist that severely damaged thumb and index metacarpal bones and scaphoid, trapezoid, and trapezium.

Fig 15–3 (bottom).—Reconstruction of wrist and metacarpal bones with free vascularized groin flap. (Courtesy of Swartz, W.M.: J. Hand Surg. 9A:18–21, January 1984.)

wrist required secondary revision. Cast immobilization was continued for 6 weeks because of fracture of the thumb metacarpal bone graft. The patient was working as a laborer 19 months after initial operation. The thumb could be used for pulp-to-pulp pinch with the index and long fingers.

The osteocutaneous vascularized groin flap provided both soft tissue coverage and vascularized bone in a one-stage repair in this case. Composite free tissue transfers can be used in immediate or delayed primary reconstruction of traumatic defects where all nonviable tissue can be removed, contamination is minimal, and vascular access can be made reliably outside the zone of injury.

▶ This concept of one-stage repair of a multitissue traumatic wound of the hand with tissue loss is appealing. Although not the conventional approach, this method challenges one's judgment in case selection and technical ability in execution of the procedure, but the potential gain is quicker wound healing and resultant shorter hospitalization, lower cost, and a shorter period of disability.

I think there will be a trend in this direction in the future.—G.B.I.

The Use of the Free Parascapular Flap in Midpalmar Soft Tissue Defect
J. Fissette, Th. Lahaye, and G. Colot (Liège Univ., Liège, Belgium)
Ann. Plast. Surg. 10:235–238, March 1983   15–8

Distant flaps are needed to reconstruct extensive deep palmar and dorsal hand lesions, and thin, pliable, hairless skin from an inconspicuous donor site is desirable. Early mobilization of the groin flap is difficult when it is pedicled, and abdominal flaps often require defatting. The dorsalis pedis flap requires skin grafting of the donor site. The parascapular area can provide a safe flap 8 × 12 cm or larger in size. The flap pedicle is a posterior branch of the inferior scapular artery and is constant in location and easy to find. Emergence of the cutaneous artery is checked by the Doppler method; the upper flap border is 2 cm above the artery. A vascular pedicle more than 6 cm long and 2 mm in diameter can be obtained.

Free flaps are preferred to pedicled flaps, particularly in hand surgery. The parascapular flap can provide a safe, pliable, often hairless skin flap with minimal subcutaneous fat. Sequelae at the donor site are minimal. This flap is considered quite reliable, but it lacks sensory nerves. It therefore is recommended for use in the midpalm or, in some cases, the dorsum of the hand, where sensitivity is less important than in other areas of the hand.

▶ Reconstructive hand surgery welcomes any additions to the inventory of thin cutaneous free flaps with a donor site that may be primarily closed without a skin graft. The parascapular flap therefore may prove to be quite useful. We do not believe the absence of a sensory nerve to the flap is a major disadvantage.—M.B.W.

Upper-Extremity Free Skin Flap Transfer: Results and Utility as Compared With Conventional Distant Pedicle Skin Flaps
Michael B. Wood and George B. Irons (Mayo Clinic)
Ann. Plast. Surg. 11:523–526, December 1983   15–9

Free flap transfers in the upper extremity would appear to have many advantages over conventional distant pedicle flaps. A review was made of 12 cases of free flap transfer to the upper extremity, excluding other free tissue transfers, collected in a 25-month period in 1979–1981. Thirteen conventional distant pedicle flaps to the upper extremity done in the same period also were reviewed.

No failures of free skin flap transfer occurred. The most common flap donor sites were the tensor fascia lata and latissimus dorsi. Five procedures were done for exoskeletal fixation that prevented a conventional flap, and 4 were performed because of the need for a sensory flap. Two patients were reluctant to have a conventional flap procedure, and 1 patient was of advanced age. Massive defects exceeding 100 sq cm were present in 5 cases. Three patients required further procedures for complications, which included 1 case of deep sepsis. The complications increased hospital time and expense, but did not compromise the final outcome. All the distant pedicle flaps also succeeded. The donor site was the groin in all cases. Eleven patients had medium-sized defects, and 2 had small defects. Minor complications occurred in 2 cases.

Usual problems of major skin coverage of the hand or forearm can be managed effectively using a distant pedicle flap if direct closure, skin grafting, or local flap surgery is not feasible; however, free skin flap transfer is the best procedure in some situations. An innervated free skin flap transfer is indicated when sensibility of the flap will contribute substantially to the functional outcome and no local flap options exist. Free flap transfer offers the benefits of a single-stage procedure. A compound flap can be transferred. Also, "permanent" blood supply to the flap is maintained. The presence of exoskeletal fixation is another indication for free flap transfer in the upper extremity.

▶ The authors present socioeconomic data to support their conclusions that traditional distal pedicle flaps (e.g., groin flaps) are equal to—and, in most circumstances, superior to—free tissue transfers for soft tissue coverage in the upper extremity. When large defects exist or exoskeletal fixation is required, the increased risks of free tissue transfer are offset by the benefits of this procedure of rapid revascularization of the underlying tissues and versatility of application.—W.P.C.

Ring Finger Transfer in Reconstruction of Transmetacarpal Amputations

Wayne A. Morrison, Bernard McC. O'Brien, and Alan M. MacLeon (St. Vincent's Hosp., Melbourne)
J. Hand Surg. 9A:4–11, January 1984   15–10

Toe transfers for finger reconstruction after transmetacarpal amputation are limited by inadequate length for palmar-digital grip and the difficulty of reconstructing active intrinsic muscle power. The authors used the opposite ring finger for finger reconstruction in 4 cases of transmetacarpal mutilating injury. Thumb restoration was achieved by hallux transfer, second toe transfer, and a tube pedicle and free neurovascular first web foot flap, respectively, in the 3 cases where it was necessary.

Man, 27, a butcher, sustained a crushing transmetacarpal amputation of the left hand at the proximal metacarpal level. The thumb was amputated at the mid-metacarpal level. Considerable thenar musculature remained. The stump was initially covered with a groin flap. A one-stage procedure subsequently was done to transfer a hallux to reconstruct the thumb and to transfer the ring finger, including the metacarpal ray, from the opposite hand to the site of the third metacarpal.

Arterial and venous anastomoses were carried out for both transfers, with the finger joined to the palmar arch. Both finger flexors and the extensor tendon were repaired. A superficialis tendon extended by a palmaris longus graft was placed in the radial wing tendon expansion of the extensor mechanism 3 months later because of a tendency toward clawing of the ring finger. Metacarpophalangeal joint flexion and control of pinch were significantly improved, and the interphalangeal joints could extend more fully. Good functional sensibility was present in both transfers 5 years postoperatively. Function was adequate for the patient to work as a butcher. He could carry heavy objects by palmar-digital grip, and the hand had strong lateral and pulp pinch. He was able to manipulate objects without visual control. The secondary defects have not caused disability in the dominant hand or in the donor foot.

The ring finger has an excellent capacity for restoring palmar-digital grip. The sensory capacity of a finger is potentially greater than that of a toe. Grip span is much increased by ring-finger transfer, compared with lesser toe transfer, permitting larger objects to be manipulated. The defect in the donor hand has caused only minimal functional problems. If thumb function is compromised, the greater length and better function provided by the ring finger can significantly compensate for impaired thumb function.

▶ This article adds significantly to the topic of digit reconstruction by free tissue transfer, with convincingly demonstrated excellent results.—M.B.W.

16 Rehabilitation

Functional Comparison of Upper Extremity Amputees Using Myoelectric and Conventional Prostheses
R. B. Stein and M. Walley (Univ. of Alberta, Edmonton)
Arch. Phys. Med. Rehabil. 64:243–248, June 1983   16–1

A substantial number of myoelectric hands have been used by upper extremity amputees, but relatively few studies of their acceptance and use have been done. Twenty upper extremity amputees who used a myoelectric hand, and 16 who used a conventional cable-controlled hook prosthesis were evaluated by the authors with tests of functional range of motion, speed, strength and endurance. Subjects also answered a questionnaire relating to activities of daily living. Most subjects were below-elbow amputees.

Subjects who had used only a conventional prosthesis regularly used it for an average of 14 hours a day, compared to 9½ hours of use of the myoelectric hand. Some of the latter subjects continued using a conventional prosthesis for some jobs. Amputees with myoelectric prostheses had a greater functional range of motion than the others. The subjects took about 2.5 times as long to complete test tasks with a conventional prosthesis than with the normal hand, and about 5 times as long with a myoelectric prosthesis. Over half the below-elbow amputees, however, preferred the myoelectric hand to the conventional prosthesis previously fitted. Another one fourth of the subjects preferred using no prosthesis.

Most below-elbow amputees appear to prefer the myoelectric hand over a conventional prosthesis because of its function, range of motion, and appearance, despite its longer performance times. Above-elbow amputees are slower to accept either myoelectric or conventional prostheses, and a major effort is needed to improve this situation.

▶ Although great progress has been made in the design of upper extremity prostheses, we are still far away from a completely satisfactory prosthesis, as this report indicates. Hopefully, this and similar reports will stimulate additional research in this area.—A.H.S.

Electromyographic Biofeedback Applications to the Hemiplegic Patient: Changes in Upper Extremity Neuromuscular and Functional Status
Steven L. Wolf and Stuart A. Binder-MacLeod (Emory Univ.)
Phys. Ther. 63:1393–1403, September 1983   16–2

A lack of adequate restitution of hand function often impedes rehabilitation after a stroke. Meaningful upper extremity function is dependent on the restoration of finger and thumb movements. Brudny et al. have reported on the benefits of electromyogram (EMG) biofeedback in restoring upper extremity function in stroke patients. Wolf and Binder-MacLeod examined the effects of a specific EMG biofeedback treatment protocol on neuromuscular function in 22 chronic stroke patients, who were compared with 9 untreated patients. All patients had had a stroke at least a year previously and lacked evidence of receptive aphasia. Sixty biofeedback sessions were held over about 6 months, each lasting 45–60 minutes. Patients were trained to relax specific hyperactive muscles through both audio and visual feedback detected with surface electrodes. Attempts to recruit weakened antagonist muscles followed. Training proceeded in a proximal to distal direction. Patients progressed from isolated joint movements to manipulative efforts requiring voluntary stabilization of the proximal musculature.

The trained patients showed significant improvement in many neuromuscular measures, but not in function. The patients who gained the most functional benefit from biofeedback training had more active motion at major upper extremity joints initially and had less hyperactivity within typically "spastic" muscles. As antagonist muscles were recruited, patients sometimes received feedback from spastic muscles to reinforce previous training directed at their inhibition.

Electromyogram biofeedback can lead to substantial neuromuscular improvement in some chronic stroke patients and can be of considerable functional benefit to other patients. Better results might be obtained by using this method as an informational resource during other treatment approaches, rather than by itself as in the present study.

▶ This useful report points out both the benefits and the limitations of electromyographic biofeedback in the rehabilitation of stroke patients. Although patients with less severe involvement do show some improvement over control patients, the gains are small and the duration of treatment (6 months) is fairly long. For those interested in pursuing this avenue of therapy, the authors provide guidelines for patient selection based on pretreatment functional parameters that help select those patients most likely to receive practical benefit from biofeedback techniques.—A.H.S.

Exercise Therapies in Peripheral Neuropathies
Gerald J. Herbison, M. Mazher Jaweed, and John F. Ditunno, Jr. (Thomas Jefferson Univ.)
Arch. Phys. Med. Rehabil. 64:201–205, May 1983   16–3

Current stretching methods for use in treating contractures are based on the effects of heat on connective tissues. Psychologic support is needed in taking the joint beyond the point of pain to increase the range of motion. With respect to the management of weakness, overwork can apparently damage muscle tissue. Stretching does not increase strength. Electrical stimulation can retard the atrophy of totally denervated muscle, but it probably is not helpful in patients with total nerve injuries from crushing or complete transection and resuture. In addition, damage can result from electric stimulation with microelectrodes.

Use of an orthosis has been recommended to avoid chronic positioning of muscles in an elongated posture. Patients with motor unit disease sometimes report loss of strength when exposed to a cold environment. This may be a result of decreased synchrony of fiber depolarization because of slowing in the peripheral sprouts; inhibition of depolarization because of potassium accumulating in the transverse tubular system; increased viscosity of the juxta-articular skeletal muscle system; or a decreased spindle bias associated with decreased anterior horn cell activity. Strength can be improved by a brief isometric or progressive resistive exercise program performed 5–6 times a day. Surgery is another approach, but immobilization is a disadvantage. Retraining has been proposed for a patient who has had tendon transfer surgery.

Patients with peripheral nerve disease should be taught to maximize function through compensatory mechanisms and to minimize abnormal habit patterns. They should be encouraged to localize muscle contraction in order to prevent disuse and to build the strength of isolated muscles. Sensory training should be attempted where appropriate.

▶ I feel that this is an excellent summary article on the various treatment modalities, exercises, and therapies in peripheral neuropathies.—A.H.S.

Vibratory Sensory Testing in Acute Peripheral Nerve Compression
Robert M. Szabo, Richard H. Gelberman, Richard V. Williamson, A. Lee Dellon, Nicholas C. Yaru, and Mary P. Dimick
J. Hand Surg. 9A:104–109, January 1984   16–4

Vibratory stimulation offers a noninvasive means of diagnosing compartment syndromes, but several problems arise from the use of the tuning fork for this purpose. The authors used a calibrated vibrometer to quantitate vibratory thresholds and control stimulus amplitudes in studies on 12 healthy subjects aged 19–65 years. Intracarpal canal pressures were monitored with a wick catheter as compression was gradually applied to the wrist using an external device and sensory, motor, and electric tests were performed. A complete sensory block was produced for 10–20 minutes. Vibratory sensibility was tested with a 120-Hz, variable-amplitude vibrometer. Tuning fork and static and moving two-point discrimination tests also were done, and the von Frey cutaneous pressure threshold was determined using the Semmes-Weinstein pressure aesthesiometer.

All sensory abnormalities were immediately reversed on the release of compression. Compartment pressures of 50 mm Hg were produced. Five subjects had numbness and paresthesias simultaneously with a significant rise in vibratory threshold and 2 subjects, before the rise in threshold (Fig 16–1). Five subjects had a rise in threshold 5 minutes before the onset of paresthesias. The vibratory threshold always increased before two-point

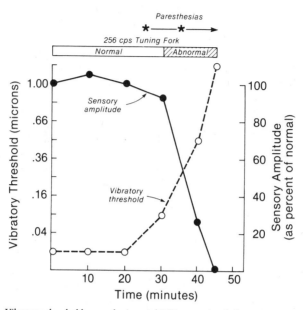

Fig 16–1.—Vibratory threshold, paresthesias, and 256 cps tuning fork perception and sensory amplitude versus time. Vibratory threshold is in microns of vibratory amplitude. Paresthesias are indicated by asterisk. Tuning fork perception is shown as normal or abnormal. Amplitude is in percentage of normal baseline value. (Courtesy of Szabo, R.M., et al.: J. Hand Surg. 9A:104–109, January 1984.)

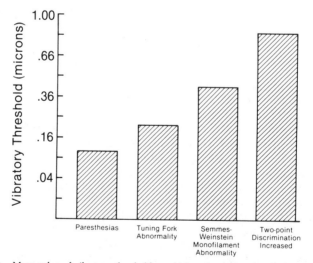

Fig 16–2.—Mean value of vibratory threshold at which each sensory abnormality was first noted. Vibratory threshold is in microns of amplitude. (Courtesy of Szabo, R.M., et al.: J. Hand Surg. 9A:104–109, January 1984.)

discrimination scores. The mean vibratory threshold at which two-point discrimination became abnormal was 0.89 μ (Fig 16–2). Both the vibrometer readings and the Semmes-Weinstein results closely paralleled the decreasing amplitude of the compound sensory action potential. An increasing vibratory threshold occurred simultaneously with an increase in sensory latency, and an increased threshold was present when the sensory amplitude was reduced by a mean of 12%.

The vibrometer holds potential as both a clinical and a research instrument in the assessment of nerve compression syndromes. Consistent specific values for normal vibratory sensation can be established using the vibrometer, and subsequent changes can be compared with the normal values.

▶ This excellent and practical article supports the use of vibratory testing in the evaluation of peripheral nerve compression syndromes. It would appear that the amplitude-variable 120-cycles-per-second vibrometer is most sensitive; probably even more sensitive than electric conduction studies. The 256-cycles-per-second tuning fork, however, is nearly as sensitive and appears to outperform not only two-point discrimination, but also the Semmes-Weinstein monofilaments.

Testing of vibration sensation is rightly becoming more commonly performed in hand centers around the United States and should become a part of the diagnostic armamentarium of all hand surgeons.—P.C.A.

The Vibrometer
A. Lee Dellon (Johns Hopkins Hosp., Baltimore)
Plast. Reconstr. Surg. 71:427–431, March 1983   16–5

Vibratory stimulation is useful in evaluating nerve regeneration and in diagnosing peripheral nerve injury and compression neuropathy, but use of the tuning fork is an uncontrolled method, and the results are expressed qualitatively. Daniel et al. found that a quantitative instrument, the vibrometer, is an inexpensive and convenient means of producing vibratory stimulation. Dellon therefore evaluated the vibrometer in 35 patients with 55 injured peripheral nerves and in 37 with 58 chronic nerve compression syndromes. The digital and median nerves were most often injured. The most common nerve compression syndromes involved the carpal tunnel and the cubital tunnel. The patients were aged 11–72 years. A portable vibrometer with a fixed frequency of 120 Hz and variable amplitude was used. The voltage readout is calibrated to convert to microns of displacement (Fig 16–3).

The vibrometer aided the diagnosis of difficult cases of nerve injury, including patients "missed" in the emergency room setting and those with a single digital nerve injury. Vibratory thresholds did not correlate with the results of the moving two-point discrimination tests. Thresholds were increased in 55% of patients with moderate and 85% of those with severe carpal tunnel syndrome. The test was not generally better than patient

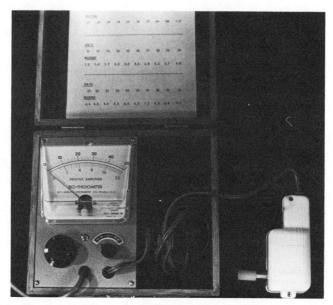

Fig 16–3.—The vibrometer. (Courtesy of Dellon, A.L.: Plast. Reconstr. Surg. 71:427–431, March 1983.)

perceptions of tuning fork stimuli in diagnosing either carpal tunnel syndrome or cubital tunnel syndrome. However, the vibrometer was clinically more useful than the tuning fork in 3 instances. It can be helpful in patients with bilateral nerve compression and where the patient cannot verbalize well or understand the test procedure.

The vibrometer is a rapid and simple means of producing vibratory stimulation, but it usually has not added new or better information compared with that obtained using a tuning fork and paper clip. The vibrometer findings are not of prognostic value after nerve repair. The instrument can provide useful quantitative sensory data in patients with bilateral peripheral nerve problems. It also can provide follow-up data to patients who may be unaware of improvement.

▶ This is a method of quantitatively gathering sensory data that is useful in evaluating patients with bilateral nerve problems. It allows longitudinal data on nerve function in a research setting. It is very important in evaluating nerve innervation density. This instrument, however, does not add new information nor improve information derived from evaluating sensitivity with a tuning fork or paper clip (tuning fork for vibrative stimulus and paper clip for innervation densities).—A.H.S.

17 Biomechanics

Form, Function, and Evolution of the Distal Phalanx
Marvin M. Shrewsbury and Richard K. Johnson (San Jose State Univ.)
J. Hand Surg. 8:475–479, July 1983   17–1

The human distal phalanx is characterized by a broad spadelike tuberosity with a proximal projecting spine and a wide diaphysis, which is concave palmarly to form an ungual fossa. These features are not found in any other primate (Fig 17–1). The distal ungual pulp provides for a more even distribution of direct forces to the surface of the digit. The papillary skin ridges over the distal pulp aid in resisting dorsal-palmar loads. The overlying nail plate absorbs some pinch pressure. All these elements contribute to stable tip-to-tip pinch with minimal pressure. The thick, mobile proximal pulp allows soft tissue to mold firmly about an object and hold it against the buttress of the distal pulp. The ability to hyperextend the distal phalanx passively, unique to the human being and the gibbon, facilitates proximal pinching between the finger pulp and thumb.

The definition of the proximal and distal pulp spaces, the strong bony elements of the distal phalanx, and passive hyperextension of this phalanx all set the hominid hand apart from that of other primates. There is substantial fossil evidence for progressive changes in the hominid distal phalanx. The early hominids living 2–3 million years ago had a robust bony

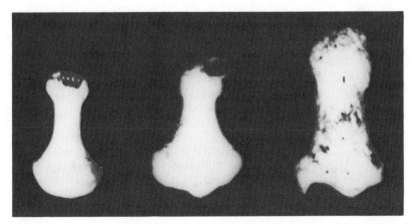

Fig 17–1.—Comparative morphology of the distal phalanges of the long finger of the monkey *(left)*, the gorilla *(center)*, and man *(right)*. (Courtesy of Shrewsbury, M.M., and Johnson, R.K.: J. Hand Surg. 8:475–479, July 1983.)

distal phalanx. Early man must have exploited this feature as he became a tool user.

▶ This is a brilliant glimpse into the past to understand the present. But again, did design permit function, or did function produce design?—R.L.L.

Determination of Forces in Extensor Pollicis Longus and Flexor Pollicis Longus of the Thumb
K. N. An, W. P. Cooney, E. Y. Chao, L. W. Askew, and J. R. Daube (Mayo Clinic and Found.)
J. Appl. Physiol. 54:714–719, March 1983   17–2

Force analysis of the thumb during function should provide a sound basis for devising thumb joint prostheses and for designing better reconstructive procedures. The authors developed a mathematical model for calculating internal forces in the thumb. Because the number of unknown forces exceeded the equations available in a static force analysis and the solution was indeterminate, muscle forces were assessed in conjunction with quantitative electromyography (EMG). Flexion-extension isometric force tests were carried out and pinch and grasp function evaluated in 3 normal male and 2 normal female subjects.

The relation between muscle force and the integrated EMG was obtained in terms of polynomial function. A multiple polynomial regression analysis of the measured force and integrated EMG data was used to determine correlation coefficients. The muscle forces calculated with the thumb performing tip, key, and pulp pinches and grasp were in the range of 3 to 120 newton for the flexor pollicis longus and 4 to 40 newton for the extensor pollicis longus.

Predicted muscle force data can be used to help design artificial prostheses for replacement of injured tendons and to calculate joint constraints in designing thumb joint prosthetic components and their fixation in bone.

▶ Precise force measurements are necessary to increasing our understanding of tendon biomechanics. Such research may lead to our ability to measure tendon forces actively in the clinical situation, with applications to both diagnosis and treatment.—R.L.L.
▶ This study is complimented well by a clinical report by Srinivasan (*J. Hand Surg.* 8:194–196, 1983), who evaluated postural changes in median, ulnar, and combined paralyses secondary to leprosy in a report that reminds us that careful observation is still our most important investigational tool. His clinical study demonstrates the role that each of the intrinsic muscles plays in maintaining normal thumb mechanics. Both these reports should be studied by all those who treat disorders of thumb function.—P.C.A.

Mechanical Strain in Forearm Bones

A. Opitz (Univ. of Vienna)
Wien. Klin. Wochenschr. [Suppl. 141] 95:1–27, 1983   17–3

Knowledge of the physiologic distribution of strain in bone is essential for a successful osteosynthesis by means of compression plate. If the side of tensile stresses varies within the bone, strain may not only occur on the side of the plate, but also on the opposite side of the cortex. In such cases the distribution of pressure in the fracture gap is of special importance.

In determining the distribution of strain on the radius, it is necessary to examine the forces caused by the flexor and extensor muscles of the wrist and fingers as well as of the elbow. The frame formed by the bow-shaped radius and the ulna is of further importance for the distribution of strain.

Anatomical studies on postmortem specimens showed how the direction of muscle action to wrist and fingers changed in relation to the position of a plate fixed to the proximal shaft of the radius. This relationship already demonstrates possible variations in the bending forces caused by forearm rotation (Fig 17–2).

An analysis of the distribution of strain in the forearm bones was performed on a biomechanical model using strain gauges. Six muscles and two muscle groups were simulated by means of wire pulls with calibrated strain gauges; these muscles and muscle groups act, because of the physiologic cross section and their position, as bending forces to the forearm bones in a dorsovolar plane. The tensile forces on radius and ulna were each controlled by three strain gauges in four sections. The characteristic quantities of these sections were determined by evaluation of the appropriate computed tomogram. With the aid of three strain gauges per section, it was possible to assess the strain at any one desired point. Distribution of strain was determined by pull to each "muscle" in the extreme position of forearm rotation and three different positions of flexion to the elbow. The tensile force was expressed on graphs as muscle tension of 2 kp/sq cm per cross section. All strains introduced to bone under different working conditions were summarized to determine the resulting distribution of strain. Where equal strains meet, the results are absolutely clear; where unequal strains occur, the relationship of acting muscles and muscle groups becomes of decisive importance.

There is no method capable of determining the contribution of one individual muscle from a group of synergists to the total force. The mechanical strains in the quadrants of the radial cortex had to be expressed partly as clear results and partly only as a trend. The strains measured on the radial shaft were compared with the tension force of a compression-plate osteosynthesis. Maximal tension forces occurring under physiologic conditions may lead to widening of the fracture gap.

Finally, the interosseous membrane caused positive strain on the ulnar side and negative strain on the radial side when the bow-shaped radial shaft was stretched in pronation, but there was no essential change to the distribution of strains to the extension and bending side of the radius. The surgical approach to the proximal radial shaft is possible from the volar side or from the dorsal side. As the dorsal approach could endanger the

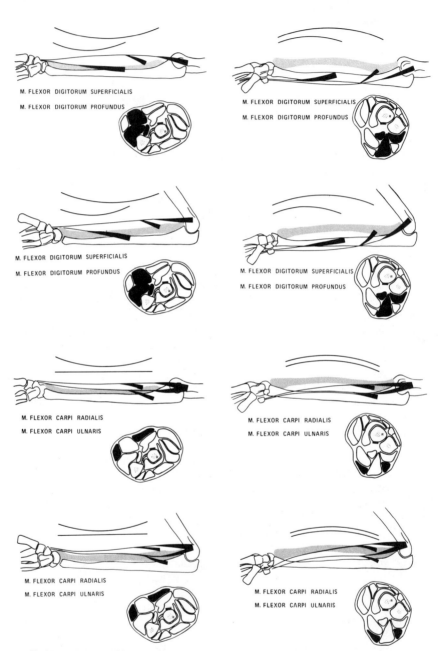

Fig 17–2.—Position of flexed wrist and finger in relation to compression plate fixed to proximal volar shaft of radius. Curved lines show expected flexion deformation of radius in flexed and extended position of elbow joint in pronation *(left)* and supination *(right)*. (Courtesy of Opitz, A.: Wien. Klin. Wochenschr. [Suppl. 141] 95:1–27, 1983.)

deep branch of the radial nerve, the volar access is recommended. Mechanically, the position of the plate is of secondary importance.

▶ This is a clever experiment that shows that stresses around the cortex of the forearm bones change according to position of the elbow and the degree of pronation and supination. This also has implications for study of the transfer of compressive stresses down the bone, for fracture studies, for the development of the arthritides, and for other problems associated with forearm rotation positioning.—R.L.L.

Pyrolite Carbon Implants in the Metacarpophalangeal Joint of Baboons
Stephen D. Cook (Tulane Univ.), Robert Beckenbaugh (Mayo Clinic), Allan M. Weinstein (Dublin, Calif.), and Jerome J. Klawitter (Austin, Texas)
Orthopedics 6:952–961, August 1983   17–4

Baboons were used to evaluate a nonconstrained, uncemented Pyrolite carbon prosthesis for replacement of the metacarpophalangeal (MCP) joint. A deep-cupped ball-and-socket implant with an offset stem was designed to provide for a proper center of rotation, and a cam effect at the MCP joint was incorporated to provide for stability of the collateral ligaments in flexion. Five Pyrolite carbon prostheses and 1 cemented Steffee design polyethylene-metal prosthesis were inserted into the long finger MCP joints of 4 baboons and were removed 9 months later.

The uncemented Pyrolite carbon implants were well tolerated. Evidence of direct appositional bone fixation along the medullary stem was noted in 1 specimen, and a combination of bone fixation with an interposed fibrous tissue membrane was noted in another. No bone resorption was seen around the implant stems, and functional fixation was obtained in all instances. There was no foreign body reaction in the soft tissues and no evidence of intracellular particles. Both a cemented Pyrolite carbon implant and the cemented polyethylene-metal implant showed evidence of bone resorption or gross implant loosening.

Pyrolite carbon-stemmed implants have the potential of biologic fixation when used for prosthetic replacement of the metacarpophalangeal joint. Adverse bone remodeling has not occurred with uncemented prostheses in baboons. Pyrolite carbon appears to be a superior material for use in prosthetic joint reconstruction.

▶ Early animal experience with pyrolytic carbon suggests that the material is well tolerated by both bone and soft tissue and can be designed to provide a press fit that offers long-term stability. The shallow ball-and-cup design probably only presents a first approximation to the contour of the metacarpophalangeal joint.—R.L.L.

The Importance of the Correct Resting Tension in Muscle Transplantation: Experimental and Clinical Aspects

Manfred Frey, Helmut Gruber, and Gerhard Freilinger (Univ. of Vienna)
Plast. Reconstr. Surg. 71:510–518, April 1983   17–5

When a muscle is being transplanted with microvascular anastomoses, the maintenance of optimal resting muscle tension seems to be essential so that optimal functional results can be obtained. Rabbit rectus femoris muscle was used by the authors to assess the effects of reduced resting tension 6 months after elongation of the patellar tendon. This was done by tensiometry, histologic and histochemical studies, and computer-assisted planimetry. The right rectus femoris was exposed. The patellar tendon was split longitudinally, cutting half the tendon from the patella and the other half from the tibial tuberosity. The rectus femoris with the patella and half the patellar tendon were freed from connections to vastus muscles. The retinacula patellae were cut, and the patellar tendon was elongated 5 mm before reconstructing the retinacula. The elongation represented 4.25% of the total muscle length. Studies were done 6 months after the operation.

The muscles with elongated tendons were somewhat smaller and had more fat and connective tissue than the normal control side. Muscle weights on the experimental side were 80% of those on the control side on the average. Optimal initial tensions were similar, but twitch tension on the experimental side reached only 73.5% of the control mean, and tetanic tension reached 78% of the control. The time for development of maximal tetanic tension was somewhat longer after tendon elongation. The mean values for force per gram showed almost no differences. An abnormal range of fiber diameters was found, and connective tissue appeared to be slightly increased in the operated muscles. Fat tissue was not augmented. Small, atrophic fibers were seen in the operated muscles.

Although these findings cannot be applied directly to human muscle transplantation, resting tension seems to be very important to the functional success of a muscle transplant with microneurovascular anastomosis. A simple measurement device has been made to insure that the transplanted muscle will have the same optimal resting tension it had in the donor position.

▶ The findings here seem to be quite important in understanding the changes associated with muscle transplantation. The authors have not used the findings of Brand in regard to the geometric determination of fiber length of muscle. This might make the resting length measurements and techniques of insertion somewhat more accurate.—R.L.L.

18 Research in Hand Surgery

The Role of Cutaneous Afferents in Position Sense, Kinesthesia, and Motor Function of the Hand
Erik Moberg (Univ. of Göteborg)
Brain 106:1–19, March 1983   18–1

Both joint and musculocutaneous receptors have been implicated as the primary source of propioceptive information, but little attention has been given to cutaneous factors. The preservation of very good kinesthesia in the absence of joint receptors militates against their importance, and a number of clinical observations suggest the importance of cutaneous afferents. Experience with patients having ulnar or median nerve block at the wrist, or both, and a block of the dorsal branches during operations suggests that muscle afferents alone cannot subserve an adequate sense of finger movement. A role for receptors in the skin or muscle or both is confirmed by observations in reconstructive surgery. It was hypothesized that information may come not only from the compression and stretching of skin over the finger joints during movements, but also from skin regions overlying contracting muscles and moving tendons remote from the joints.

Cutaneous and musculotendinous factors were assessed independently in the forearm and hand in test subjects by using an extensive nerve blocking technique and also in studies of the type developed by Gelfan and Carter. The results of thumb experiments are given in the table. No kinesthetic information reaching consciousness could be shown to arise from the musculocutaneous system, and cutaneous afferents appeared to provide the dominant input. Signals arising from skin displaced over contracting muscle bellies or moving tendons remote from activated parts of the extremity could be an important source of error in previous studies.

More precise knowledge of the role of cutaneous afferents in proprioception and motor function of the hand is important in reconstructive surgery and in rehabilitation. Information from distant cutaneous receptors apparently can be a significant source of error in studies of muscle sensation.

▶ Moberg's pioneering efforts in the understanding of sensibility of the hand and its role in hand function are well known. In this article, he presents a strong argument for the importance of cutaneous sensation in joint position sense. The table basically summarizes his concept, although it represents only one of the many clinical experiments carried out by Moberg and described in his article. Basically, as increasing cutaneous anesthesia is added by infiltration only subcutaneously around and proximal to the involved joint, the ability to

(Courtesy of Moberg, E.: Brain 106:1–19, March 1983.)

		No. of obs.	Maximum		Error	
Subject			Neg.	Pos.	Mean	SD
1	No anaesthesia	76	20	20	−2	8
2		67	10	10	0	6
3		68	10	10	1	5
1	Anaesthesia from wrist	27	90	0	37	26
2	level distally; volar	40	30	40	6	17
3	and dorsal aspects	40	30	40	1	16
1	Added anaesthesia of	26	60	60	−28	31
2	whole forearm	40	30	50	19	19
3	cutaneous sleeve	40	40	40	−11	19

ACTIVE THUMB POSITIONING WITH AND WITHOUT DIFFERENT LEVELS OF CUTANEOUS ANESTHESIA—LONG MUSCLES UNIMPAIRED

determine joint position is gradually decreased even though all feedback from the muscle and tendon remained intact.

The importance of this information to the hand surgeon is clear. Sensate skin is not only important because of the information it can impart regarding external objects with which it comes in contact, but, just as importantly, it provides critical information regarding the internal environment below it with regard to joint position.—P.C.A.

Effects of High-Peak Pulsed Electromagnetic Field on Degeneration and Regeneration of the Common Peroneal Nerve in Rats

A. R. M. Raji and R. E. M. Bowden
J. Bone Joint Surg. [Br.] 65-B:478–492, August 1983   18–2

The high-peak pulsed electromagnetic field (PEMF) has been reported to enhance axonal regeneration in the spinal cord of cats and accelerate the recovery of nerve conduction in rats. The authors used histologic, cytologic, and morphometric methods to assess the effects of PEMF on common peroneal nerve lesions in pairs of male rats matched for age, environmental conditions, and the level and type of lesion. The nerves were lesioned by crushing just above the knee or severing and immediately suturing it at the same level. Treated animals received PEMF produced by a Diapulse machine for 15 minutes a day for 3½ days to 8 weeks after sustaining the injury.

The use of PEMF appeared to accelerate the recovery of injured limbs and degeneration, regeneration, and maturation of myelinated axons. Epineural, perineural, and intraneural fibrosis was reduced compared with sham treatment, and the luminal cross-sectional area of the intraneural vessels was increased in the treated animals with both types of lesion. Comparison of fiber diameters indicated that significantly larger fibers were present at and below the level of crush injury in PEMF-treated animals.

The degree of maturation in the distal segment appeared to be greater in treated animals. Undamaged nerves exhibited no effects of PEMF treatment.

The recovery of injured peripheral nerves appears to be accelerated by PEMF. A controlled study of patients matched for age, level and type of lesion, and delay in repair would be needed before the routine use of this adjuvant therapy could be recommended. Thermal effects have not been noted in clinical work with PEMF, but possible effects on deep-tissue temperatures have not been assessed.

▶ The mode of action of pulsed electric magnetic fields in the regeneration of nerves and the healing of fractures is not specifically known. The authors have certainly pointed out, however, the potentials for improvement in the results of nerve repair with this technique utilizing very brief periods of time. Their work suggests the need for clinical controlled trials of this technique.—R.D.B.

Axonal Growth in Mesothelial Chambers: The Role of the Distal Nerve Segment
Nils Danielsen, Lars B. Dahlin, Yo Fon Lee, and Göran Lundborg
Scand. J. Plast. Reconstr. Surg. 17:119–125, 1983   18–3

The authors have investigated nerve regeneration in vivo in mesothelial chambers interposed between the segments of a transected rat sciatic nerve. A well-organized nerve structure is generated to bridge the gap, showing directional growth from the proximal to the distal segment. In the present study, an attempt was made to determine the critical gap length and to examine axonal growth in an "open" chamber where no distal nerve end is present. Silicone rods with an outer diameter of 2 mm were used. Chamber lengths ranged from 10 to 50 mm.

The new nerve structure generated in the mesothelial chamber was well developed when the gap length was 10 mm or less; axons from the left sciatic nerve reinnervated muscles in the right extremity via the right sciatic nerve. No such regeneration occurred with a 15-mm or larger gap. Where no distal nerve end was present, limited growth of only 5–6 mm into the chamber was observed. Without a mesothelial chamber, a neuroma was formed, extending over 6–8 mm from the original level of nerve resection.

There is increasing evidence that factors produced by the distal nerve segment itself may influence the growth and orientation of regenerating nerve fibers. In the present study using mesothelial chambers, the axons regenerate a certain distance when no distal nerve segment is present until no further outgrowth occurs. The observations may have clinical potential for preventing neuroma formation. The limited growth may reflect the lack of "trophic" or cellular support from a distal nerve segment.

▶ This report expands the body of knowledge developed by Lundborg and associates on regulators of nerve growth and regeneration. Here he discusses the effect of the presence or absence of the distal nerve segment and the size of the nerve gap on the quality of proximal nerve regeneration. He concludes with some interesting thoughts concerning the use of his mesothelial chambers in the prevention of neuroma formation. Lundborg's work in this area should be studied by all those who are interested or involved in operations on peripheral nerves.—P.C.A.

Peripheral Nerve Allograft: An Immunological Assessment of Pretreatment Methods
Susan E. Mackinnon, Alan R. Hudson, R. E. Falk, D. Kline, and D. Hunter
Neurosurgery 14:167–171, February 1984   18–4

Both experimental and clinical efforts in nerve allografting have focused on reducing the antigenicity of allografts. The authors used an in vivo immunologic assay to quantify nerve allograft responses in a rat model. Lewis rats received donor sciatic nerves from ACI rats. Allografts were placed beside the intact recipient sciatic nerve without suturing. Groups of allografts were irradiated; predegenerated for 1 to 10 weeks; frozen; lyophilized; and predegenerated, frozen, and irradiated. The in vivo ^{51}Cr cytotoxicity assay was performed as a measure of sensitization 16 days after exposure to the donor nerve. Labeled ACI splenocytes were used.

The index of recognition did not vary significantly from that of autografts after a high dose of radiation or lyophilization. Indices of recognition were significantly lower in all other groups than in the control group and did not differ from that of fresh, untreated allografts. Marked cellular infiltration of the epineurium and the nerve itself was noted in these cases. Infiltrating cells were very infrequent in the lyophilized and high-dose radiation groups. The cells were identified ultrastructurally as being activated lymphocytes. The degree of nerve fiber degeneration in each group did not vary significantly from that in the fresh allografts.

Lyophilization and high-dose irradiation can modify nerve allografts so that they are less immunogenic to host rats. Allografts treated by predegeneration, freezing, or low-dose irradiation are no less antigenic than fresh untreated allografts. Lyophilization and high-dose irradiation may hold promise for use in clinical nerve grafting.

▶ Nerve grafting is a useful procedure, but there are current limitations relating to the amount of graft nerve available for some extended segmental defects for multiple nerve injuries and also related to the disability of donor sites. These problems could be overcome if some nonautogenous material or device could be used to channel the axons successfully from the proximal nerve end to the distal end across a significant gap. One such possibility is the allograft. Clearly, there are tremendous obstacles to be overcome with regard to rejection and subsequent fibrosis that would interfere with the axonal migration. This report introduces some preliminary work in this area.—P.C.A.

Axoplasmic Transport Block Reduces Ectopic Impulse Generation in Injured Peripheral Nerves

Marshall Devor and Ruth Govrin-Lippmann (Hebrew Univ. of Jerusalem)
Pain 16:73–85, May 1983   18–5

Afferent discharges generated in regions of nerve injury are blamed for many of the chronic pains and paresthesias associated with amputation and other injury involving peripheral nerves. Sensory axons ending in chronic nerve-end neuromas are sensitive to adrenergic agonists and to the stimulation of sympathetic efferent fibers. The authors attempted to determine whether a partial block of rapid axoplasmic transport at a point central to the cut would alter the development of discharges from ectopic neuroma or even reverse it. Studies were done on the sciatic nerves of adult male rats. Afferent fibers ending in nerve-end neuromas in rats generate a substantial ectopic discharge and are sensitive to light pressure and to circulating adrenaline. Electrophysiologic studies were carried out with exposure of the nerves to colchicine and vinblastine.

Both colchicine and vinblastine produced marked concentration-dependent reductions in the incidence of spontaneous discharge generated in neuromas (Fig 18–1) and that of discharges evoked by intravenous adrenaline. The rate and pattern of ectopic discharge in fibers that remained active after treatment with colchicine and vinblastine were similar to those in untreated neuromas. The drugs also affected the activity of neuromas that already had begun to produce spontaneous discharges.

Colchicine and vinblastine reduce the rate of both spontaneous and adrenaline-induced discharges arising in distal neuromas when applied to the perineurium at midnerve. The effects do not appear to reflect fiber degeneration. The effects could result from prevention of the required number of sodium or calcium channels, or both, from being incorporated into the sprout membrane through partial blockade of rapid axoplasmic transport, or from a change in gating properties as a result of disruption of the axonal cytoskeleton in the region of the neuroma. It also is possible

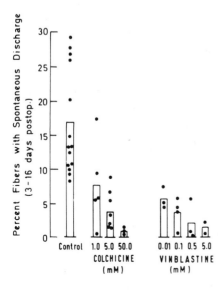

Fig 18–1.—Colchicine and vinblastine applied to the sciatic nerve reduce the incidence of spontaneous discharge in nerve-end neuromas. Bars show mean values, and filled circles are values for individual rats. (Courtesy of Devor, M., and Govrin-Lippmann, R.: Pain 16:73–85, May 1983.)

that the drugs act on the local cytoskeleton of the neuroma, directly on the local membrane, or on the cell body. Clinical use of the drugs would require an understanding of their effects on neighboring uninjured nerve fibers and on nerve regenerative processes.

▶ The better understanding of neurophysiology may soon improve the reliability of treatment for the vexing problem of painful neuromas. The study reported here, however, must be considered only the first step, because neither the toxicity nor the maximum duration of beneficial effect from the drugs used were evaluated in this study.—P.C.A.

Sensibility Testing in Peripheral Nerve Compression Syndromes: An Experimental Study in Humans
Richard H. Gelberman, Robert M. Szabo, Richard V. Williamson, and Mary P. Dimick (Univ. Hosp. Med. Center, San Diego, Calif.)
J. Bone Joint Surg. [Am.] 65-A:632–638, June 1983   18–6

Controversy continues regarding the reliability of sensory testing in the assessment of peripheral nerve compression. The authors evaluated four standard tests of sensibility in 12 healthy subjects aged 19–41 years who submitted to controlled external compression of the median nerve at the carpal tunnel at pressures ranging from 40 to 70 mm Hg. A wick catheter was placed, with the use of local anesthesia, for intracarpal canal pressure monitoring. Subjects were monitored for up to 4 hours with the two-point discrimination, moving two-point discrimination, Semmes-Weinstein pressure monofilament, and vibration tests. Abductor pollicis brevis strength also was assessed.

Arterial inflow and venous return were not significantly altered by the local pressure. All subjects had symptoms of median nerve compression, starting when the median sensory amplitude was 87% of baseline (Fig 18–2). The threshold tests consistently reflected gradual reductions in nerve function as reflected by both subjective reports and electric testing (Fig 18–3), while the two-point discrimination measures remained normal until sensory conduction had practically ceased. Muscle strength did not decline until all of the sensory tests were abnormal. Both sensory and motor fiber recordings rapidly returned to normal when compression was released.

The vibration and Semmes-Weinstein monofilament tests correlated well with both subjective and electrodiagnostic measures of median nerve compression in normal subjects in this study. The Semmes-Weinstein pressure test was the most accurate quantitative measure of early nerve compression. Vibratory sensation may be as effective a parameter, but there is a problem in quantifying responses. A calibrated vibration system is under study. Threshold tests may prove useful in evaluating patients for a variety of peripheral nerve compression syndromes.

▶ This is an excellent study that correlates some of the common clinical sensibility testing modalities with nerve conduction studies in an experimental

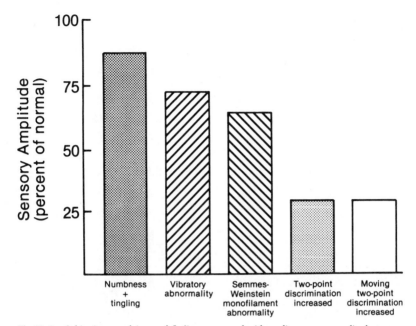

Fig 18–2.—Subjective complaints and findings compared with median sensory amplitude as percent of normal baseline amplitude (summary of data from 12 subjects). (Courtesy of Gelberman, R.H., et al.: J. Bone Joint Surg. [Am.] 65-A:632–638, June 1983.)

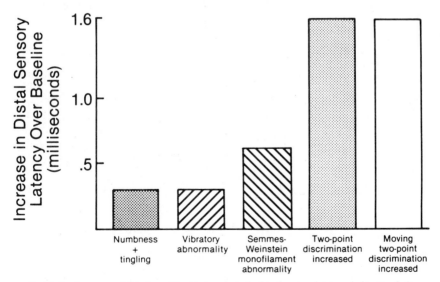

Fig 18–3.—Summary of data from 12 subjects: onset of subjective complaints and objective findings compared with increase in distal sensory latency. (Courtesy of Gelberman, R.H., et al.: J. Bone Joint Surg. [Am.] 65-A:632–638, June 1983.)

acute carpal tunnel syndrome. Several important observations have been made. Sensory amplitude is the most sensitive of the parameters studied, followed by subjective change in perception of vibration and threshold sensation to pressure using the Semmes-Weinstein monofilaments. The more traditional two-point discrimination actually lagged far behind as an indicator of median nerve compression. By applying multiple sensibility evaluations to patients with peripheral nerve compression syndromes, fixed sensibility deficits can be detected more accurately and treatment decision making should be facilitated.—P.C.A.

Combined Morphological and Electrophysiologic Study of Conduction Block in Peripheral Nerve
L. Sedal, M. N. Ghabriel, Fensheng He, G. Allt, Pamela M. Le Quesne, and M. J. G. Harrison
J. Neurol. Sci. 60:293–306, August 1983   18–7

Local demyelination is seen at sites of peripheral nerve damage in man, and its presence often is inferred from the electrophysiologic demonstration of conduction block or slowed conduction velocity. The authors produced local demyelination in the rat tibial nerve by intraneural microinjection of 1% lysophosphatidylcholine (LPC) to determine the reliability of electrophysiologic criteria in documenting conduction block in a mixed motor and sensory nerve. Rats received single intraneural injections of 4.5 μl of LPC or saline, or two separate injections of 3 μl of 1% LPC 8 mm apart.

The single injections of LPC produced lesions of variable severity. Double injections more consistently produced severe lesions with marked conduction block. Occasional nerves exhibiting severe demyelination had slight axonal damage. The postinjection ratio of amplitudes of muscle action potentials evoked by stimulation proximal and distal to the injection site was more than 2 SD below the control mean in 86% of nerves showing signs of demyelination. No such findings were obtained in nerves given saline injections. The degree of electrophysiologic abnormality was not, however, a reliable indicator of the histologic findings. Electrophysiologic recovery was observed even after double injections of LPC.

The findings suggest that caution be used in interpreting the presence or absence of signs of conduction block in clinical work. The absence of conduction block, defined as a reduced amplitude of muscle response after proximal stimulation, appears not to exclude the presence of local demyelination. The extent of an electrophysiologic block does not reflect the histologic severity of a peripheral nerve lesion accurately.

▶ This very interesting article reports on an experimental model for focal demyelination of a peripheral nerve. The study correlates the drop in conduction velocity over the demyelinated segment with the histologic evidence of demyelination.

The study shows that the conduction block is specific in that it does not occur in nerves that were treated by control injections. The extent of slowing was generally proportional to the amount of demyelination present, but there is a considerable degree of overlap so that direct correlation between the amount of observable demyelination and the amount of nerve slowing cannot be made.

In summary, this study is useful in that it confirms in an experimental model that nerve conduction slowing is rarely, if ever, a false positive finding. On the other hand, absence of slowing may be a false negative finding in that histologic damage may be present in nerves that conduct in an apparently normal way. Clinically, this information is useful, particularly in the evaluation of patients suspected of compression neuropathy. An abnormal nerve conduction study can be accepted as fairly conclusive evidence that there is indeed some degree of nerve compression, probably sufficient to cause histologic changes in the nerve. A normal study, however, does not rule out disease and should not be taken as a contraindication to surgical intervention if clinical signs indicate a focal compression, and nonsurgical treatment is unsuccessful.

Hopefully, the authors will continue to pursue their studies and identify a more sensitive electrophysiologic parameter to reduce the number of false negative nerve conduction studies.—P.C.A.

Effect of Acute Compartmental Pressure Change on Response to Vibratory Stimuli in Primates
A. L. Dellon, R. J. Schneider, and R. Burke
Plast. Reconstr. Surg. 72:208–216, August 1983   18–8

The group A beta fibers mediate vibration sensation, and vibratory perception has been found to be compromised in acute and chronic compartment syndromes. The authors examined the effects of increased compartment pressures on sensory conduction and vibratory perception in adult *Macaca mulatta* monkeys. Acute carpal tunnel syndromes were produced by placing an angiocatheter into the carpal tunnel and infusing sterile Ringer's lactate solution. Anterior compartment syndrome was produced by infusing fluid beneath the muscle fascia midway between the head of the fibula and the lateral malleolus. Somatosensory evoked potentials were recorded and psychophysical studies carried out.

The time needed for the height of the A beta wave to decline lessened with the height of pressure in monkeys with induced carpal tunnel syndrome. The height of the A beta wave regularly recovered, and the time needed for recovery was related to the time required to produce a complete conduction block, not to the compartment pressure itself. In the study of an awake monkey trained to discriminate differences in amplitude of a 10-Hz vibratory stimulus to the hairs on the dorsum of the foot, an anterior compartment pressure of 37 mm Hg for 90 minutes significantly reduced the ability to discriminate between the two amplitudes. Further impairment was evident at an anterior compartment pressure of 50 mm Hg.

This model provides a means of assessing the effects of relatively low compartment pressures on the peripheral nerves of subhuman primates. Noninvasive vibratory stimuli, like those produced by a tuning fork, can be used to investigate acute compartment syndromes. The increased sensory amplitude observed at a low level of increased compartment pressure could represent a perceived increase in vibratory stimulation in early nerve compression. It also might represent the physiologic basis of the "double-crush syndrome," in which a proximal nerve injury increases susceptibility of the nerve to further compression.

► This appears to be an important article that brings to our attention a useful diagnostic tool for compressive neuropathies. Moreover, it adds to our understanding of the pathophysiology of chronic nerve compression and recovery following decompression.—M.B.W.

Separation of Sutured Tendon Ends When Different Suture Techniques and Different Suture Materials Are Used: Experimental Study in Rabbits
Bengt Nyström and Dan Holmlund (Univ. of Umeå)
Scand. J. Plast. Reconstr. Surg. 17:19–23, 1983   18–9

Many different suture materials and various techniques have been used for anastomosing tendons. The authors investigated whether the suture techniques should be varied according to the suture materials used for tendon anastomosis. Calcaneal tendons of rabbits were divided 15 mm from their insertion and were repaired with 3–0 Prolene, Ethiflex, or stainless steel wire sutures. Bunnell's classic crisscross technique was compared with placement of a single small loop "near" suture, with or without ligatures of Dexon applied about the tendon ends inside the suture loop. Immobilization was for 16 or 35 days.

Separation of the tendon ends was biphasic in all instances (Fig 18–4). The duration of immobilization did not influence the time course of late separation, but early removal was followed by considerable late separation when Dexon rings were used, and late removal was followed by marked separation when a simple near suture was used without Dexon rings. With Bunnell suturing, Ethiflex resulted in significantly more initial separation than Prolene. Initial separation was least when steel sutures were used. Dexon rings did not reduce early separation when near sutures were utilized.

New suture materials should not replace current types without their different physical properties being taken into account. Steel wire sutures are appropriately used with the Bunnell suturing method. Neither Dexon rings nor complicated suturing techniques are necessary. A single loop can be used successfully for suturing a tendon.

► This interesting study reviews the effect of different suture materials on gap formation after tendon suture. The lack of rigidity of suture like Ethiflex and Prolene was shown to affect gap formation adversely when a multiple crisscross suture of the Bunnell type was used. The stiffer steel wire apparently did not allow a similar degree of accordion effect and was associated with much less gap formation. When a simple suture was performed, there was no difference in the three suture materials.

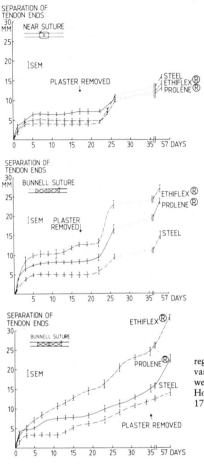

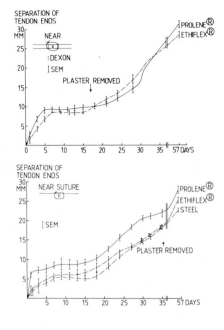

Fig 18–4.—Curves representing continuous registration of tendon end separation when various suture materials and suture techniques were used. (Courtesy of Nyström, B., and Holmlund, D.: Scand. J. Plast. Reconstr. Surg. 17:19–23, 1983.)

This information should be of interest to all hand surgeons. The modified Kessler suture used widely today is a form of loop suture, and any of these suture materials would appear appropriate for that sort of repair. If a multiple crisscross suture is to be used, however, it would appear that the wire suture initially recommended by Bunnell would remain the suture material of choice.—P.C.A.

The Pseudosynovial Sheath: Its Characteristics in a Primate Model
James M. Hunter, Scott H. Jaeger, Takeshi Matsui, and Naotsune Miyaji (Hand Rehabilitation Center, Philadelphia)
J. Hand Surg. 8:461–470, July 1983   18–10

The pseudosynovial sheath concept has been increasingly used in clinical work with satisfactory results. Most often a silicone, Dacron-reinforced implant is utilized. The authors examined the long-term outcome of the pseudosynovial sheath formed in response to a gliding tendon implant in mature stumptail monkeys. Number 3 Hunter passive gliding tendon implants were placed in 32 digits of 8 monkeys, half of which had had tendon lacerations repaired primarily and had contractures, adhesions, and scarred beds. Long implants were used to insure uniform gliding, and all annular pulleys were preserved or reconstructed. Syndactylism was created to the adjacent active digits to allow passive digital motion. The extremity was immobilized for 2 weeks.

The average implant excursion on radiography was 2.5 cm. The inner surface of the pseudosynovial sheath appeared smooth and glistening at the time of biopsy. Intimal, medial, and adventitial sheath layers were distinguished. The sheath was mature and stable at 8 weeks, when the intima cells contained a glycosaminoglycan and exhibited secretory capacity. The media cells had large amounts of collagen. The adventitia was a highly vascular structure containing clefts that may represent gliding planes. Sheaths from the area of the A-2 pulley were consistently thicker than those from the palm or forearm.

The pseudosynovial sheath in this primate model, which closely simulates the clinical situation, is a useful structure not susceptible to contracture. It appears to have the characteristics needed to provide a good bed for a tendon graft. The gliding implant can transform an injured, scarred flexor system into a coherent framework that can support a tendon graft for a prolonged period. Adverse mechanical elements must be avoided, and stage II tendon graft juncture should be done in the forearm, well away from scarred or contracted tissue planes.

▶ This article characterizes the histologic appearance of the sheath formed by a gliding silicone implant. Although the two-staged tendon reconstruction procedure has certainly improved the results of tendon grafting in the presence of severe scarring of the tendon bed, further studies are indicated to characterize better the secretory products of the pseudosynovial sheath and, more particularly, the durability of the sheath and its secretions in the presence of a living tendon graft as opposed to an inert tendon implant.—P.C.A.

The Healing of Superficial Skin Wounds Is Stimulated by External Electric Current
Oscar M. Alvarez, Patricia M. Mertz, Richard V. Smerbeck, and William H. Eaglstein (Univ. of Pittsburgh)
J. Invest. Dermatol. 81:144–148, August 1983   18–11

Electrically stimulated bone healing and regeneration have been described by many investigators. Alvarez et al. found that direct electric current promotes epidermal resurfacing and dermal collagen biosynthesis in partial-thickness wounds in Yorkshire pigs. Keratome-induced wounds 0.3 mm deep were made on the skin of young pigs, and direct current (DC) of 50–300 μA was delivered by an energized silver-coated electrode. An unenergized electrode was used as a placebo treatment. Wounds were excised after 1 to 7 days. The separated epidermis was evaluated for reepithelialization, and the dermis was assayed for collagen biosynthetic capacity using ^{14}C-proline.

The rate of wound epithelialization was significantly accelerated in DC-treated wounds. Collagen synthetic capacity increased substantially on days 5–7 after wounding in DC-treated wounds, but no significant effect was apparent when collagen production was corrected for DNA content. The amount and type of microflora did not differ significantly in the DC-treated and control wounds. Treatment with DC did not influence the amount of silver present in the serum or feces.

External DC enhances both epidermal wound repair and dermal collagen production in superficial wounds in domestic pigs. The effects appear unrelated to any antimicrobial action of silver that is liberated during the treatment. The findings suggest that the proliferative or migratory capacity of the epithelial and connective tissue cells involved in wound repair and regeneration can be influenced by an electric field.

▶ While these authors focus on other tissue than discussed by other investigators in demonstrating the beneficial effects of electric stimulation and has many clinical implications, it is obvious that further work and clinical trials are necessary before considering this a viable addition to standard care of patients. There seems little question, however, from the experimental data arising on both direct and pulsed electric field treatments that enhanced healing of tissues, including bone, vessel, nerve, and now skin, does occur. These conditions produce a biologic effect that appears to be a positive one in the experimental model.—R.D.B.

Vascularized Limb Transplantation in the Rat
Robert A. Lipson, Hisashi Kawano, Philip F. Halloran, Nancy H. McKee, Kenneth P. H. Pritzker, Fred Langer, and Rita Kandel (Mount Sinai Hosp., Toronto)
Transplantation 35:293–304, April 1983   18–12

I. Results with syngeneic grafts.—Interest has increased in using massive vascularized skeletal tissue allografts to reconstruct large skeletal defects resulting from congenital deformity, trauma, or tumor resection. The authors devised a microsurgical model for examining the characteristics of vascularized skeletal tissue transplants in inbred rats. Joint function and bone viability and growth have been followed for up to a year after orthotopic transplantation of the distal part of the femur, knee, intact tibia, and associated musculature in Fischer F344 rats. The femoral vessels were anastomosed microsurgically, and coverage was provided by recipient skin. Controls included syngeneic grafts without anastomoses, avascular free knee grafts, and distal femoral osteotomy.

A total of 79 vascularized limb transplantations were carried out, and 63 were followed for an average of 22 weeks. The bone and joint tissues survived and grew, and the joints functioned and appeared normal histologically. Bone growth in the grafts was readily apparent in adolescent rats. All the tissues were essentially normal histologically for up to 7 months, except for muscle, which exhibited denervation atrophy. The hypertrophic zone of epiphyseal cartilage survived the operation in a healthy, viable state. Bone scans showed a slight increase in uptake in the early postoperative period only. The nonvascularized control grafts rapidly became necrotic and inflamed. The nonvascularized knee grafts developed progressive degenerative changes.

This model is expected to be useful in determining the feasibility and potential clinical uses of large vascularized grafts of skeletal tissue. The possibility of using vascularized allografts to repair large skeletal defects that otherwise would require amputation warrants efforts to overcome any barriers to the clinical use of this approach.

II. Results with allogeneic grafts.—Assessment was made of 55 allogeneic grafts performed in rats, in which a model of vascularized orthotopic limb transplantation was used. Composite musculo-osseous grafts of the type that were shown to do well syngeneically were taken from brown-Norway rats aged 6 to 8 weeks and placed in Fischer 344 rats. Ten avascular knee allografts were made as controls for the effects of vascularization. All 10 rats given avascular allogeneic hindlimb grafts died of sepsis within 3 weeks of operation.

The initial anastomotic patency of the allografts was comparable with that of syngeneic grafts, but eventually the large vessels became occluded and fibrosed. Venous patency was compromised sooner than arterial patency. Bone healing was retarded, compared with syngeneic transplants, and the allogeneic grafts did not grow. A rapid decline in bone scan activity often was seen despite patent anastomoses. Histologic study of the allogeneic grafts showed changes of severe rejection leading to death of the epiphyseal cells, osteocytes and, later, articular chondrocytes. Alloantibody responses to the vascularized and nonvascularized allografts did not differ markedly.

Allogeneic vascularized limb grafts in rats undergo severe rejection, with cessation of new bone formation and eventual death of osteocytes, but bone healing and joint function are better than in avascular control grafts. This model may be useful in elucidating adverse immunologic effects on a variety of skeletal tissue components in their intact state, as may occur in the collagen diseases and other disorders.

▶ This two-part article presents an accurate account of the timing and mode of limb homotransplant rejection in the allogeneic rat and the success of the transplant in the syngeneic rat. It is certainly possible that immunology advances will permit syngeneic tolerance of allografts in the near future.— M.B.W.

▶ One of the problems with using small animals for microsurgical studies has been the necessity for surgical exposure of the anastomosis in order to assess patency. Recently, van Bemmelen, Hoynck, van Papendrecht, and Nieuborg (*Br. J. Plast. Surg.* 36:463–465, 1983) presented a technique that may avoid that necessity. Satisfactory angiograms have been obtained in their hands by the injection of contrast material within the medullary cavity of bone in the region of the surgical repair, which then is picked up by the intramedullary blood supply.

Dynamic radionuclide scanning (*Clin. Nucl. Med.* 8:309–311, 1983) is another possibility.—M.B.W.

Histologic Comparison of Experimental Microarterial End-in-End (Sleeve) and End-to-End Anastomoses
Jan B. Wieslander and Alf Rausing (Univ. of Lund)
Plast. Reconstr. Surg. 73:279–287, February 1984   18–13

As few histologic studies of the healing of end-in-end (EIE), or sleeve, anastomoses have been reported, the authors compared the healing of conventional end-to-end (ETE) and EIE anastomoses of vessels about 1 mm in diameter in rabbits. Twenty-five EIE and 21 ETE anastomoses were made on central arteries of the ear; Dermalon 10–0 sutures were used in all cases. After the adventitia was removed, the EIE anastomosis was made by placing two sutures 120 degrees apart, taking a full-thickness bite through the distal vessel end and a partial bite through the proximal stump 2 mm from the end, and telescoping the proximal vessel end into the distal lumen. The ETE anastomoses were made by placing three stay sutures 120 degrees apart and three to five interrupted sutures among them. Samples were taken for examination at intervals up to 90 days after anastomosis.

Two anastomoses of each type were occluded by thrombi. Two partial occlusions followed the ETE technique, and 4 occurred with the EIE technique. Considerable narrowing was present immediately after EIE anastomosis (Fig 18–5). A gradual increase in luminal diameter ensued. Platelets accumulated after both types of anastomosis, particularly after ETE anastomosis. Reendothelialization appeared to occur on top of organized aggregates of platelets. Both repairs were characterized by neointimal hyperplasia inside the internal elastic membrane and heavy fibrosis external to this at 90 days (Fig 18–6).

Reendothelialization occurs in a comparable manner after ETE and EIE anastomosis of small arterial vessels in the rabbit. There appears to be an increased risk of late anastomotic failure after use of the sleeve technique, which should be reserved for larger vessels or used in small vessels only if there is a favorable discrepancy between the diameters of the vessel ends.

▶ The authors clearly illustrate the histologic hazards and potential utility of the end-in-end anastomosis technique. This technique may have particular application for the rapid anastomosis of supranummary vessels when a significant vessel size discrepancy exists.—M.B.W.

▶ Cuffing techniques in microarterial surgery have been evaluated recently by Merrell, Zook, and Russell (*J. Hand Surg.* 9A:76–82, 1984). They report that cuffs of artery, vein, or polyglycolic acid tubing can reduce the average repair time by as much as 50% without compromising patency rates. Again, these techniques may have particular usefulness when multiple vessel repairs are indicated, as, for example, in the replantation of multiple digits.—P.C.A.

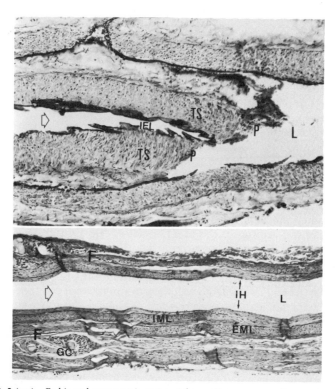

Fig 18–5 (top).—End-in-end anastomosis at 1 to 2 hours. Note pronounced narrowing of lumen. Platelets (P) adhere to raw vessel end of telescoped segment (TS). Internal elastic lamina (IEL) is folded, and distal part of sleeved segment shows signs of thickening. L, lumen. Open arrow indicates direction of blood flow. Weigert-van Gieson; original magnification ×200.

Fig 18–6 (bottom).—End-in-end anastomosis at day 90. Double vascular walls are clearly visible. Internal surface consists of thick, hyperplastic neointima (IH), making discontinuity between the two vessels smooth. Fibrous tissue (F) replaces most of atrophic external vascular walls. EML, external medial layer; IML, internal medial layer; and L, lumen. Open arrow indicates direction of blood flow. Weigert-van Gieson; original magnification ×130.

(Courtesy of Wieslander, J.B., and Rausing, A.: Plast. Reconstr. Surg. 73:279–287, February 1984.)

Vascular Knee Allograft Transplantation in a Rabbit Model

Michael J. Yaremchuk, Tamela Sedacca, Alan L. Schiller, and James W. May, Jr.

Plast. Reconstr. Surg. 71:461–471, April 1983   18–14

The problems encountered with nonviability of bone and joint allografts theoretically can be overcome by transplanting them as organs, with immediate vascularization through anastomosis of the donor and the host vessels. The authors examined the survival of vascularized knee allografts in a rabbit model and the effect of immunosuppression on allograft survival. Donor and host vessels were anastomosed microsurgically and, in some animals, immunosuppression with azathioprine and methylprednisolone was used. Outbred New Zealand white rabbits were employed in the study. Skin graft exchanges also were carried out.

The mean graft survival in nonimmunosuppressed rabbits was 9 days, and immunosuppression did not significantly increase graft survival. The longest allograft survival was 81 days. The survival of second-set control skin grafts did not differ significantly from that of skin grafted onto vascularized allografts and nonvascularized allografts. Vascularized allografts, with or without immunosuppression, resembled nonvascularized allografts histologically. There was no cellular evidence of graft rejection. Early studies showed changes of acute vascular rejection in the vascularized grafts. Vascularized autografts, in contrast, contained viable-appearing bone and cartilage and had an active circulation with patent vessels. Degenerative changes in articular cartilage were less than in the allografts.

Joint allografts appear to be immunogenic, but they do not undergo the same destructive rejection changes as soft-tissue grafts. The donor vessels do exhibit classic rejection changes that appear to lead to thrombosis and graft loss. The findings argue against the immediate clinical use of vascularized joint allografts. Immediate vascularization of bone and joint allografts seemingly benefits the grafts only if they can be supplied indefinitely by surgically anastomosed vessels or at least for longer than 6 months.

▶ This report is further documentation of the inadequacy of conventional means of immunosuppression to prevent rejection of vascularized allograft tissue. It is likely, however, that more effective methods of immunosuppression will permit such procedures in the future.—M.B.W.

Subject Index

Index to Authors